Heart Failure

Editor

HOWARD J. EISEN

CARDIOLOGY CLINICS

www.cardiology.theclinics.com

Consulting Editors
ROSARIO FREEMAN
JORDAN M. PRUTKIN
DAVID M. SHAVELLE
AUDREY H. WU

February 2014 • Volume 32 • Number 1

ELSEVIER

1600 John F. Kennedy Boulevard ● Suite 1800 ● Philadelphia, Pennsylvania, 19103-2899

http://www.theclinics.com

CARDIOLOGY CLINICS Volume 32, Number 1

February 2014 ISSN 0733-8651, ISBN-13: 978-0-323-27782-2

Editor: Barbara Cohen-Kligerman

Cardiology Clinics (ISSN 0733-8651) is published quarterly by Elsevier Inc., 360 Park Avenue South, New York, NY 10010-1710. Months of issue are February, May, August, and November. Business and Editorial Offices: 1600 John F. Kennedy Blvd., Ste. 1800, Philadelphia, PA 19103-2899. Customer Service Office: 3251 Riverport Lane, Maryland Heights, MO 63043. Periodicals post-age paid at New York, NY and additional mailing offices. Subscription prices are $320.00 per year for US individuals, $530.00 per year for US institutions, $155.00 per year for US students and residents, $390.00 per year for Canadian individuals, $665.00 per year for Canadian institutions, $455.00 per year for international individuals, $665.00 per year for international institutions and $220.00 per year for Canadian and international students/residents. To receive student/resident rate, orders must be accompanied by name of affiliated institution, data of term, and the *signature* of program/residency coordinator on institution letterhead. Orders will be billed at individual rate until proof of status is received. Foreign air speed delivery is included in all *Clinics* subscription prices. All prices are subject to change without notice. **POSTMASTER:** Send address changes to *Cardiology Clinics*, Elsevier Health Sciences Division, Subscription Customer Service, 3251 Riverport Lane, Maryland Heights, MO 63043. **Customer Service: 1-800-654-2452 (U.S. and Canada); 314-447-8871 (outside U.S. and Canada). Fax: 314-447-8029. E-mail: journalscustomerservice-usa@ elsevier.com (for print support); journalsonlinesupport-usa@elsevier.com (for online support).**

Reprints. For copies of 100 or more, of articles in this publication, please contact the Commercial Reprints Department, Elsevier Inc., 360 Park Avenue South, New York, NY 10010-1710. Tel.: 212-633-3874; Fax: 212-633-3820; E-mail: reprints@elsevier.com.

Cardiology Clinics is also published in Spanish by McGraw-Hill Interamericana Editores S. A., P.O. Box 5-237, 06500, Mexico D. F., Mexico; in Portuguese by Reichmann and Alfonso Editores Rio de Janeiro, Brazil; and in Greek by Dimitrios P. Lagos, 8 Pondon Street, GR115-28 Ilissia, Greece.

Cardiology Clinics is covered in *MEDLINE/PubMed (Index Medicus), Excerpta Medica, The Cumulative Index to Nursing and Allied Health Literature* (CINAHL).

Printed and bound by CPI Group (UK) Ltd, Croydon, CR0 4YY

Transferred to digital print 2012

Contributors

EDITORIAL BOARD

ROSARIO FREEMAN, MD, MS, FACC
Associate Professor of Medicine;
Director, Coronary Care Unit; Director,
Echocardiography Laboratory, University of
Washington Medical Center, Seattle,
Washington

JORDAN M. PRUTKIN, MD, MHS, FHRS
Assistant Professor of Medicine, Division of
Cardiology/Electrophysiology, University of
Washington Medical Center, Seattle,
Washington

DAVID M. SHAVELLE, MD, FACC, FSCAI
Associate Professor of Clinical Medicine,
Division of Cardiovascular Medicine, Keck
School of Medicine at USC; Director, Los
Angeles County/USC Cardiac Catheterization
Laboratory; Director, Interventional Cardiology
Fellowship, Los Angeles County/USC Medical
Center, Los Angeles, California

AUDREY H. WU, MD
Assistant Professor, Internal Medicine,
University of Michigan, Ann Arbor, Michigan

EDITOR

HOWARD J. EISEN, MD, FACC, FAHA, FACP
Thomas J. Vischer Professor of Medicine;
Chief, Division of Cardiology, Hahnemann
University Hospital, Drexel University College
of Medicine, Philadelphia, Pennsylvania

AUTHORS

SASIKANTH ADIGOPULA, MD
Mechanical Circulatory Support and Heart
Transplantation Program, Ahmanson-UCLA
Cardiomyopathy Center, David Geffen School
of Medicine, University of California,
Los Angeles, Los Angeles, California

ALLEN S. ANDERSON, MD, FACC, FAHA
Professor of Medicine, Feinberg School
of Medicine, Northwestern University;
Medical Director, Center for Heart Failure,
Bluhm Cardiovascular Institute,
Chicago, Illinois

DAVID A. BARAN, MD, FACC
Director, Heart Failure and Transplant
Research, Newark Beth Israel Medical Center;
Clinical Associate Professor of Medicine,
Rutgers New Jersey Medical School, Newark,
New Jersey

GEETHA BHAT, PhD, MD
Medical Director, Center for Heart Transplant
and Assist Devices, Advocate Christ Medical
Center, Oak Lawn, Illinois; Clinical Professor of
Medicine, University of Illinois at Chicago
College of Medicine, Chicago, Illinois

PATRICIA P. CHANG, MD, MHS
Director, Heart Failure and Transplant
Program; Associate Professor, Division of
Cardiology, Department of Medicine,
University of North Carolina at Chapel Hill,
Chapel Hill, North Carolina

MONICA COLVIN-ADAMS, MD, MS, FAHA
Assistant Professor of Medicine, Section on
Advanced Heart Failure, Transplant and
Mechanical Circulatory Support, Cardiovascular
Division, University of Minnesota Medical
Center, Lillehei Heart Institute, University of
Minnesota, Minneapolis, Minnesota

MARIO C. DENG, MD, FACC, FESC
Mechanical Circulatory Support and Heart
Transplantation Program, Ahmanson-UCLA
Cardiomyopathy Center, David Geffen School
of Medicine, University of California,
Los Angeles, Los Angeles, California

EUGENE C. DEPASQUALE, MD
Mechanical Circulatory Support and Heart
Transplantation Program, Ahmanson-UCLA
Cardiomyopathy Center, David Geffen School
of Medicine, University of California,
Los Angeles, Los Angeles, California

HOWARD J. EISEN, MD, FACC, FAHA, FACP
Thomas J. Vischer Professor of Medicine;
Chief, Division of Cardiology, Hahnemann
University Hospital, Drexel University College
of Medicine, Philadelphia, Pennsylvania

SCOTT FEITELL, DO
Division of Cardiology, Drexel University
College of Medicine, Philadelphia,
Pennsylvania

ASHWANI GUPTA, MBBS
Fellow, Division of Cardiology, Drexel
University College of Medicine, Philadelphia,
Pennsylvania

SHELLEY R. HANKINS, MD
Medical Director, Cardiac Transplant and
Mechanical Circulatory Support Programs;
Assistant Professor of Medicine, Division of
Cardiology, Drexel University College of
Medicine, Philadelphia, Pennsylvania

HENRY HSIA, MD
Division of Cardiology, San Francisco
Veterans Affairs Medical Center, University of
California San Francisco, San Francisco,
California

ABHISHEK JAISWAL, MD
Fellow, Advanced Heart Failure and Transplant
Medicine, Newark Beth Israel Medical Center,
Newark, New Jersey

FRANCES L. JOHNSON, MD
Associate Professor of Medicine, Division of
Cardiovascular Medicine, Carver College of
Medicine, University of Iowa, Iowa City, Iowa

MICHELLE M. KITTLESON, MD, PhD
Director, Post-Graduate Medical Education in
Heart Failure and Transplantation; Director,
Heart Failure Research, Division of Cardiology,
Cedars-Sinai Heart Institute, Los Angeles,
California

LIVIU KLEIN, MD, MS
Division of Cardiology, University of California
San Francisco, San Francisco, California

JON A. KOBASHIGAWA, MD
DSL/Thomas D. Gordon Chair, Heart
Transplantation Medicine; Director,
Advanced Heart Disease Section; Director,
Heart Transplant Program, Cedars-Sinai
Medical Center; Associate Director, Division of
Cardiology, Cedars-Sinai Heart Institute, Los
Angeles, California

LONGJIAN LIU, MD, PhD, MSc, FAHA
Department of Epidemiology and Biostatistics,
School of Public Health, Drexel University,
Philadelphia, Pennsylvania

ALI NSAIR, MD
Mechanical Circulatory Support and Heart
Transplantation Program, Ahmanson-UCLA
Cardiomyopathy Center, David Geffen
School of Medicine, University of California,
Los Angeles, Los Angeles, California

MARIA PATARROYO-APONTE, MD
Cardiology Fellow, Division of Cardiovascular
Medicine, University of Minnesota Medical
Center, Lillehei Heart Institute, University of
Minnesota, Minneapolis, Minnesota

DANIEL F. PAULY, MD, PhD
Section of Cardiology, Department of
Medicine, Truman Medical Centers, School of
Medicine, University of Missouri Kansas City,
Kansas City, Missouri

JOHN J. ROMMEL, MD
Cardiovascular Disease Fellow, Division of
Cardiology, Department of Medicine,
University of North Carolina at Chapel Hill,
Chapel Hill, North Carolina

LISA J. ROSE-JONES, MD
Clinical Instructor, Division of Cardiology,
Department of Medicine, University of North
Carolina at Chapel Hill, Chapel Hill, North
Carolina

HEATH E. SALTZMAN, MD, FACC
Division of Cardiology, Cardiac
Electrophysiology, and Pacing, Drexel
University College of Medicine, Philadelphia,
Pennsylvania

GABRIEL SAYER, MD
Advanced Heart Failure Transplant
Cardiologist, Center for Heart Transplant
and Assist Devices, Advocate Christ Medical
Center, Oak Lawn, Illinois; Clinical Assistant
Professor of Medicine, University of Illinois
at Chicago College of Medicine, Chicago,
Illinois

FAIZ SUBZPOSH, MD
Fellow, Division of Cardiology, Drexel
University College of Medicine, Philadelphia,
Pennsylvania

REY P. VIVO, MD
Mechanical Circulatory Support and Heart
Transplantation Program, Ahmanson-UCLA
Cardiomyopathy Center, David Geffen
School of Medicine, University of California,
Los Angeles, Los Angeles, California

DAVID Y. ZHANG, MD, PhD
Section of Cardiology, Department of Medicine,
University of Chicago, Chicago, Illinois

Contents

Heart failure is one of the most prevalent cardiovascular diseases in the United States, and is associated with significant morbidity, mortality, and costs. Prompt diagnosis may help decrease mortality, hospital stay, and costs related to treatment. A complete heart failure evaluation comprises a comprehensive history and physical examination, echocardiogram, and diagnostic tools that provide information regarding the etiology of heart failure, related complications, and prognosis in order to prescribe appropriate therapy, monitor response to therapy, and transition expeditiously to advanced therapies when needed. Emerging technologies and biomarkers may provide better risk stratification and more accurate determination of cause and progression.

Heart failure remains a major health problem in the United States, affecting 5.8 million Americans. Its prevalence continues to rise due to the improved survival of patients. Despite advances in treatment, morbidity and mortality remain very high, with a median survival of about 5 years after the first clinical symptoms. This article describes the causes, classification, and management goals of heart failure in Stages A and B.

ACC Stage C heart failure includes those patients with prior or current symptoms of heart failure in the context of an underlying structural heart problem who are primarily managed with medical therapy. Although there is guideline-based medical therapy for those with heart failure with reduced ejection fraction (HFrEF), therapies in heart failure with preserved ejection fraction (HFpEF) have thus far proven elusive. Emerging therapies such as serelaxin are currently under investigation and may prove beneficial. The role of advanced surgical therapies, such as mechanical circulatory support, in this population is not well defined. Further investigation is warranted for these therapies in patients with Stage C heart failure.

Over the last 4 decades, cardiac transplantation has become the preferred therapy for select patients with end-stage heart disease. Heart transplantation is indicated in patients with heart failure despite optimal medical and device therapy, manifesting as intractable angina, refractory heart failure, or intractable ventricular arrhythmias. This article provides an overview of heart transplantation in the current era, focusing on the evaluation process for heart transplantation, the physiology of the transplanted heart, immunosuppressive regimens, and early and long-term complications.

From humble beginnings in 1963 with a single desperately ill patient, mechanical circulatory support has expanded exponentially to where it is a viable alternative for advanced heart failure patients. Some of these patients are awaiting transplant but others will have a mechanical heart pump as their ultimate treatment. The history of MCS devices is reviewed, along with the 4 trials that define the modern era of circulatory support. The practical aspects of life with an MCS device are reviewed and common problems encountered with MCS devices. Future trends including miniaturization and development of completely contained MCS systems are reviewed.

Arrhythmias and Heart Failure

Heath E. Saltzman

Atrial fibrillation and ventricular tachyarrhythmias are frequently seen in patients with heart failure, and complicate the management of such patients. Both types of arrhythmia lead to increased morbidity and mortality, and often prove to be challenging issues to manage. The many randomized studies that have been performed in patients with these conditions and concomitant heart failure have helped in designing optimal treatment strategies.

Sudden Cardiac Death in Heart Failure

Liviu Klein and Henry Hsia

Sudden cardiac deaths account for 350,000 to 380,000 deaths in the United States annually. Implantable cardioverter-defibrillators have improved sudden death outcomes in patients with heart failure, but only a minority of patients with defibrillators receives appropriate therapy for ventricular arrhythmias. The risk prediction for sudden death and selection of patients for defibrillators is based largely on left ventricular ejection fraction and heart failure symptoms because there are no other risk stratification tools that can determine the individual patients who will derive the greatest benefit. There are several other pharmacologic strategies designed to prevent sudden death in patients with heart failure.

Managing Acute Decompensated Heart Failure

Daniel F. Pauly

Acute decompensated heart failure may occur de novo, but it most often occurs as an exacerbation of underlying chronic heart failure. Hospitalization for heart failure is usually a harbinger of a chronic disease that will require long-term, ongoing medical management. Leaders in the field generally agree that repeated inpatient admissions for treatment reflect a failure of the health care delivery system to manage the disease optimally. Newer management strategies focus on ameliorating symptoms by optimizing the hemodynamics, restoring neurohormonal balance, and making frequent outpatient adjustments when needed.

Heart Failure with Preserved Ejection Fraction: An Ongoing Enigma

Lisa J. Rose-Jones, John J. Rommel, and Patricia P. Chang

Heart failure with preserved ejection fraction (HFpEF) is a complex clinical syndrome based on traditional heart failure symptoms with documentation of increased left ventricular filling pressures and preserved left ventricular ejection fraction. The exact mechanisms that induce HFpEF are not known. End-diastolic ventricular stiffness does not seem to be acting alone. Substantial mortality exists compared with healthy age-matched controls, as well as significant health care expenditures on hospitalizations and readmissions. This article reviews the epidemiology, pathophysiology, and treatment of heart failure with preserved ejection fraction (HFpEF). Current practice guidelines focus on remedying volume overload, aggressively controlling hypertension, and treatment of comorbid conditions that contribute to decompensation.

Heart failure is a costly and difficult disease to treat. However, new metrics make it an imperative to keep these patients out of the hospital. Implementing and maintaining patients on successful treatment plans is difficult. A multitude of factors make transitioning care to the outpatient setting difficult. A careful and well-orchestrated team of cardiologists, general practitioners, nurses, and ancillary support staff can make an important difference to patient care. A strong body of literature supports the use of pharmacologic therapy, and evidence-based therapies can improve mortality and quality of life, and reduce hospital admissions. Adjunctive therapies can be equally important.

CARDIOLOGY CLINICS

NOW AVAILABLE FOR YOUR iPhone and iPad

Preface

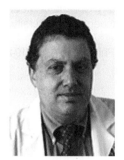

Howard J. Eisen, MD, FACC, FAHA, FACP
Editor

Heart failure has become one of the leading causes of morbidity and mortality in the United States and the developed world. The management of heart failure consumes considerable amounts of health care resources, and efforts to improve outcomes such as the CMS core measures and 30-day readmission and mortality rates have become important measures of hospital quality. Yet, heart failure is a complex group of diseases with a variety of causes and both established and evolving therapies.

The development of effective medical therapies became possible only when the role of neurohormonal activation and derangement in the development and progression of heart failure was understood. This provided insight into the structural, cellular, and molecular basis of the adverse remodeling seen as part of the progression of heart failure. The introduction of β-blockers to inhibit sympathetic nervous system activation and inhibitors of the renin-angiotensin-aldosterone system at a variety of steps has resulted in an improvement in patient symptoms, a reduction in mortality, and the halting or even reversal of the cardiac remodeling that occurs in these patients. Clinical trials of these agents have shown that their benefits extended beyond those with the worst stages of heart failure and could benefit those with asymptomatic left ventricular dysfunction in preventing progression to symptomatic heart failure. In addition, from an understanding of the epidemiology and causes of heart failure, it became clear that many of the same medications used for symptomatic heart failure could be used to treat the risk factors of heart failure, such as hypertension and ischemic heart

disease, before left ventricular dysfunction occurred. The result was the ACCF/AHA Staging System for heart failure, which includes stage A, representing patients with normal left ventricular function but with risk factors for heart failure such as hypertension, diabetes, ischemic heart disease, and others; stage B, which includes patients with asymptomatic left ventricular dysfunction; stage C, for patients with left ventricular dysfunction and symptomatic heart failure; and stage D for patients who have exhausted all other therapeutic options.

This issue of *Cardiology Clinics* begins by reviewing the epidemiology and enormous scope of the problem of heart failure. This is followed by a review of the pathophysiology and causes of heart failure and then the evaluation of heart failure to determine both the etiology and the severity of heart failure in individual patients and to develop diagnostic and therapeutic strategies. The cornerstones of heart failure pathophysiology and progression, the renin-angiotensin-aldosterone and sympathetic nervous systems, are discussed with particular attention paid to their role in the progression of heart failure. The management of the four ACCF/ AHA stages of heart failure is reviewed to provide insight into the management of each of these. Given the complexity of the management of stage D patients, the options of cardiac transplantation and mechanical circulatory support are given considerable emphasis. As arrhythmias, sudden cardiac death, and acute decompensated heart failure are critical issues of clinical importance, these are also reviewed in depth. The troubling and difficult-to-manage heart failure with preserved ejection fraction is reviewed in detail. This issue

Cardiol Clin 32 (2014) xiii–xiv
http://dx.doi.org/10.1016/j.ccl.2013.10.001
0733-8651/14/$ – see front matter © 2014 Published by Elsevier Inc.

cardiology.theclinics.com

ends with a discussion of adjunctive therapy and the management of transition of care, which has become and important measure of quality.

I am grateful to the contributing authors, whose hard work, diligence, and expertise is reflected in the articles in this issue. I would also like to thank my editor, Barbara Cohen-Kligerman, whose patience and attention to detail kept me in line and on a tight schedule.

Howard J. Eisen, MD, FACC, FAHA, FACP
Division of Cardiology
Drexel University College of Medicine and
Hahnemann University Hospital
245 North 15th Street
Philadelphia, PA 19102, USA

E-mail address:
heisen@drexelmed.edu

Epidemiology of Heart Failure and Scope of the Problem

Longjian Liu, MD, PhD, MSc, FAHA[a],*,
Howard J. Eisen, MD, FACC, FAHA, FACP[b]

KEYWORDS

- Heart failure • Epidemiology • Multiple comorbidity • Clinical correlation

KEY POINTS

- Of the major forms of cardiovascular disease, heart failure (HF) is the only disease that is increasing in incidence and prevalence in most developed countries.
- Elderly individuals are at particularly high risk of developing HF.
- Multiple comorbidity is one of the key characteristics in patients with HF.

INTRODUCTION

Heart failure (HF) is typically a chronic disease, with progressive deterioration occurring over a period of years or even decades. HF poses an especially large public health burden. It represents a new epidemic of cardiovascular disease, affecting nearly 5.8 million people in the United States, and more than 23 million people worldwide. Every year in the United States, more than 550,000 individuals are diagnosed with HF for the first time, and 1 in 5 have a lifetime risk of developing this syndrome.[1,2] In contrast to other major forms of cardiovascular diseases (ie, coronary heart disease and stroke), the prevalence, incidence, and mortality from HF are increasing, and prognosis remains poor.[1,3,4] HF results in high hospitalization rates and mortality; up to 40% of patients die within 1 year of first hospitalization, making the survival rate bleaker than that for nearly all cancers. In addition to the cost in human suffering, care for patients with HF places a large economic strain on the health care system, including the Medicare program. HF has caused very significant health and financial burdens on patients, their families, and society as a whole. In

2008, it was estimated that HF accounted for more than $35 billion in health care costs in the Unites States.[1] In the present article, the epidemiology of HF and challenges facing in HF prevention and treatment are described.

According to the American Heart Association (AHA) reports, HF was the underlying cause in 283,000 deaths in 2008, and mortality from HF with primary diagnosis or being diagnosed as a comorbidity was 281,437 (124,598 men and 156,839 women). In 2008, HF accounted for more than $35 billion in health care costs in the United States.[1]

DISEASE DESCRIPTION

HF is a multisystem disorder that is characterized by abnormalities of cardiac function, skeletal muscle, and renal function, as well as activation of the rennin-angiotensin-aldosterone and sympathetic nervous systems: a complex pattern of neurohormonal change that impairs the ability of either or both ventricles to fill or eject. HF syndromes are frequently fatal illnesses in which the heart loses its ability to pump effectively in response to the body's needs. Patients with HF may become incapable of performing even the

The authors have nothing to disclose.
a Department of Epidemiology and Biostatistics, School of Public Health, Drexel University, 1505 Race Street, Philadelphia, PA 19102, USA; b Division of Cardiology, College of Medicine, Drexel University, 245 N. 15th Street, Philadelphia, PA 19102, USA
* Corresponding author.
E-mail address: Longjian.Liu@Drexel.edu

Cardiol Clin 32 (2014) 1–8
http://dx.doi.org/10.1016/j.ccl.2013.09.009
0733-8651/14/$ – see front matter © 2014 Elsevier Inc. All rights reserved.

simplest activities of daily living and are at very high risk of medical complications and death. Three clinical pathophysiological models (hypotheses) for HF have been suggested: (1) HF is viewed as a problem of excessive salt and water retention that is caused by abnormalities of renal blood flow (eg, the "cardiorenal model"). (2) HF is thought to arise largely as a result of abnormalities in the pumping capacity of the heart and excessive peripheral vasoconstriction (eg, cardiocirculatory model or hemodynamic model). (3) The neurohormonal model, in which HF progresses as a result of the overexpression of biologically active molecules that are capable of exerting toxic effects on the heart and circulation.[5] According to the New York Heart Association (NYHA) Functional Classification, HF is classified into 4 classes that range from patients with asymptomatic left ventricular dysfunction (NYHA I) to those with severe symptoms at rest or with minimal exertion (NYHA IV). This classification helps clinicians assess the severity of a patient's symptoms, guides the choice of therapy, and helps with subjective documentation of response or lack of response to therapy.[6] However, this classification has a potential limitation. For example, an NYHA III class patient may improve to class II on initiation of treatment, indicating that the NYHA classification is essentially a functional/symptomatic score, not taking into account the underlying cardiac disorder that will almost inevitably progress. In 2001, the American College of Cardiology and American Heart Association proposed a new conceptual framework to help health professionals understand the continuum of disease progression in HF.[4] Rather than replacing the NYHA classification, the framework defines disease progression in 4 stages: A, B, C, and D, beginning with patients who have risk factors for developing HF all the way to patients with end-stage disease.[4,7,8] Of these, stage A is diagnosed in those who are at high risk for HF but without structural heart disease or symptoms of HF, such as patients with hypertension, atherosclerosis disease, or diabetes mellitus. Stage B is for those who have structural heart disease but without signs or symptoms of HF, such as patients with myocardial infarction (MI), left ventricular remodeling. These patients in fact have never had an episode of symptomatic HF. Stage C is for those who have structural heart disease with prior or current symptoms of HF, such as patients with known structural heart disease and shortness of breath and fatigue. Stage D is for those who have refractory HF requiring specified interventions; these patients have marked symptoms at rest despite maximal medical therapy.

RISK FACTORS

Hypertension is a common risk factor for HF, followed closely by antecedent MI, heart rhythm disorders (arrhythmias), diabetes, congenital heart disease, and heart muscle disease (cardiomyopathy). Other risk factors that are associated with these diseases in general also contribute to HF, including high cholesterol, inflammation, hyperglycemia, cigarette smoking, alcohol abuse, micronutrient deficiency, a family history of HF or other cardiovascular diseases, and poorer socioeconomic position over the life course are all identified as risk factors for HF. For example, in the Health Aging, Body, and Composition study, among 2934 participants, the incidence of HF was 13.6 per 1000 person-years. Men and African American participants of both genders were more likely to develop HF. Coronary heart disease (population attributable risk 23.9% for white participants, 29.5% for African American participants) and uncontrolled blood pressure (population attributable risk 21.3% for white participants, 30.1% for African American participants) had the highest population attributable risks in both races/ethnicities. There was a higher overall proportion of HF attributable to modifiable risk factors in African American participants than white participants (67.8% vs 48.9%). Hospitalizations were higher among African American participants. Inflammatory markers (interleukin-6 and tumor necrosis factor-α) and serum albumin levels were also associated with HF risk.[7,9–13] Data from the first National Health and Nutrition Examination Survey Epidemiologic Fellow-up study, from 5545 men and 8098 women participants during average follow-up of 19 years, suggested that more than 60% of HF that occurs in the US general population might be attributable to coronary heart disease, followed by cigarette smoking (17.1%), hypertension (10.1%), low physical activity (9.2%), male sex (8.9%), less than a high school education (8.9%), overweight (8.0%), diabetes (3.1%), and valvular heart disease (2.2%).[14] Micronutrients, such as vitamin D deficiency, and metabolic risk factors have been also suggested in relation to risk of HF, although further longitudinal studies are needed.[15–19]

INCIDENCE IN THE UNITED STATES AND WORLDWIDE

Data from the US National Heart, Lung, and Blood Institute (NHLBI)-sponsored Framingham Heart Study indicate that HF incidence approaches 10 per 1000 population after 65 years of age. Seventy-five percent of HF cases have antecedent hypertension.[20] In NHLBI-sponsored

Cardiovascular Health Study, the annual rates per 1000 population of new HF events for white men are 15.2 for those 65 to 74 years of age, 31.7 for those 75 to 84 years of age, and 65.2 for those ≥85 years of age. For white women in the same age groups, the rates are 8.2, 19.8, and 45.6, respectively. For African American men, the rates are 16.9, 25.5, and 50.6, and for African American women, the estimated rates are 14.2, 25.5, and 44.0, respectively.[1] In NHLBI-sponsored Multi-Ethnic Study of Atherosclerosis, African American participants had the highest risk of developing HF, followed by Hispanic, white, and Chinese Americans (4.6, 3.5, 2.4, and 1.0 per 1000 person-years, respectively). This higher risk reflected differences in the prevalence of hypertension, diabetes mellitus, and socioeconomic status. African Americans seemed to have the highest proportion of incident HF not preceded by clinical MI (75%).[1,21] Data from the US National Health and Nutrition Examination Surveys 2007 to 2010 indicate that in men, non-Hispanic (NH) blacks had about a 10-year younger age at diagnosis of HF than NH whites (48.16 vs 59.68 year older, P<.001) and women (51.87 vs 61.39 years older, P<.001, **Fig. 1**).[22]

At this moment, direct comparable data from different countries on the incidence of HF are not available because there has been much variation in the diagnostic criteria used in HF studies by different countries. However, testing for trends within a country and/or region that apply the same criteria is possible using, for example, data from the Rotterdam (The Netherlands) and Hillingdon (UK) HF studies.[23,24] Both studies are population based and used an expert panel to establish the presence or absence of HF. In the Hillingdon study (n = 101,855), the incidence of HF increased from 0.02/1000 person-years in those aged 25 to 34, to 0.2/1000 person-years in those aged 45 to 55 years, and to 12.4/1000 person-years in those aged ≥85 years. In Rotterdam (n = 7129), the incidence increased from 2.5/1000 person-years (age

55–64 years) to 44/1000 person-years (85 years or older), and HF occurs more frequently in men than in women (15 and 12 per 1000 person-years, respectively).[25,26]

PREVALENCE OF HF IN THE UNITED STATES AND WORLDWIDE

Data from National Health and Nutrition Examination Surveys 2007 to 2010 suggest that non-Hispanic blacks had the highest prevalence of HF, followed by NH whites and Mexican Americans (MA) (**Fig. 2**). Prevalence of HF significantly increased in those aged 65 and older (**Fig. 3**).[1,22]

It is estimated that by 2030, an additional 3 million people will have HF, a 25.0% increase in prevalence from 2010 in the United States.[27]

Data from the US National Hospital Discharge Surveys suggested that of 3 major forms of cardiovascular disease, age-adjusted hospitalization rates in patients aged 65 and older with primary diagnosis of coronary heart disease significantly decreased from early 1990s, and age-adjusted hospitalization rates in patients aged 65 and older with primary diagnosis of cerebrovascular disease significantly decreased from mid 1980s in both men and women. However, HF hospitalization rates have significantly increased, with an estimated annual rate increase of 1.20% in men, and 1.55% in women between 1980 and 2006 (**Fig. 4**).[3] Of 6 selected comorbidities, about 50% in men and 40% in women with HF had a coexisting disease of coronary heart disease, followed by chronic obstructive pulmonary disease, diabetes mellitus, renal failure, and pneumonia.[3]

The worldwide prevalence of HF seems to have been increasing over the past decades. This trajectory may reflect growing awareness and diagnosis of HF, an aging population, increasing incidence of HF, improvement in the treatment and management of cardiovascular disease, or a combination of some or all of these potential explanations. Extrapolating from available evidence,

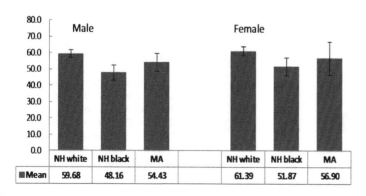

	Male				Female		
	NH white	NH black	MA		NH white	NH black	MA
▪Mean	59.68	48.16	54.43		61.39	51.87	56.90

Fig. 1. Mean age at diagnosis of HF by race/ethnicity. NH, non-Hispanic; MA, Mexican Americans. (*Data from* Centers for Disease Control and Prevention (CDC), National Center for Health Statistics (NCHS). National Health and Nutrition Examination Survey Data. Hyattsville (MD): US Department of Health and Human Services, Centers for Disease Control and Prevention; 2007–2010. Available at: http://www.cdc.gov/nchs/nhanes.htm. Accessed August 16, 2013.)

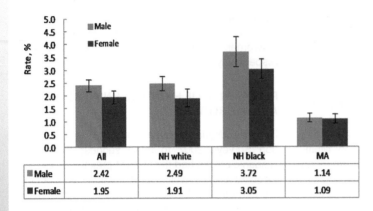

Fig. 2. Prevalence (%) of HF in US adults aged 20 and older by race/ethnicity. (*Data from* Centers for Disease Control and Prevention (CDC), National Center for Health Statistics (NCHS). National Health and Nutrition Examination Survey Data. Hyattsville (MD): US Department of Health and Human Services, Centers for Disease Control and Prevention; 2007–2010. Available at: http://www.cdc.gov/nchs/nhanes.htm. Accessed August 16, 2013.)

McMurray and colleagues[28] estimate a worldwide prevalence of 23 million individuals living with HF. However, incidence and prevalence data for HF are scarce in most countries, and current epidemiologic data from developing countries are inadequate for making an accurate assessment.[2,23]

MORTALITY OF HF IN THE UNITED STATES AND WORLDWIDE

Despite advances in therapy and management, HF remains a deadly clinical syndrome. In 2008, HF any-mention mortality was 281,437 (124,598 men and 156,839 women). HF was the underlying cause in 56,830 of those deaths in 2008. The 2008 overall any-mention death rate (per 100,000 population) for HF was 84.60. Any-mention death rates were 98.9 for white men, 102.7 for black men, 75.9 for white women, and 78.8 for black women. One in 9 deaths has HF mentioned on the death certificate. The number of any-mention deaths from HF was approximately as high in 1995 (287,000) as it was in 2008 (283,000). Survival after HF diagnosis has improved over time, as shown by data from the Framingham Heart Study and the Olmsted County Study.[29,30] However, the death rate remains high: almost 50% of people diagnosed with HF will die within 5 years.[30,31] In

the elderly, data from Kaiser Permanente indicate that survival after the onset of HF has also improved.[32]

Studies of prevalent cases in Europe have slightly more favorable estimates, with 1-year and 5-year mortality at 11% and 41%, respectively, from the Rotterdam study,[33] possibly owing to differences in patient selection and definitions of HF leading to inclusion of milder cases. Stewart and colleagues[34] suggested that HF was more "malignant" than cancer in a study of greater than 30,000 patients hospitalized for HF, MI, or 4 common cancers in Scotland; with the exception of lung cancer, HF was associated with the worst 5-year adjusted mortality.

CLINICAL CORRELATION
The Complex of Multiple-Comorbidity

As the prevalence of patients with HF continues to climb in the United States and worldwide, the clinical characteristics and management of these individuals have become increasingly complex. This complexity is attributed, in part, to the changing profile of the patients with HF, who are likely to be older adults, taking more medications, and to have multiple comorbid conditions. In the study using data from the US National Hospital

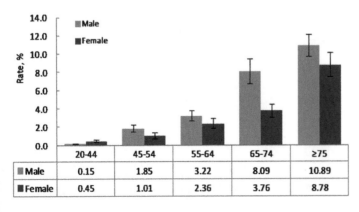

Fig. 3. Prevalence (%) of HF in US adults aged 20 and older by age and sex. (*Data from* Centers for Disease Control and Prevention (CDC), National Center for Health Statistics (NCHS). National Health and Nutrition Examination Survey Data. Hyattsville (MD): US Department of Health and Human Services, Centers for Disease Control and Prevention; 2007–2010. Available at: http://www.cdc.gov/nchs/nhanes.htm. Accessed August 16, 2013.)

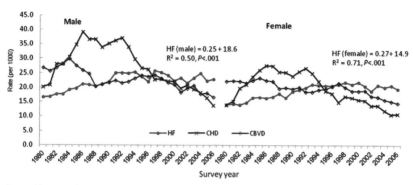

Fig. 4. Age-adjusted hospitalization rates (per 1000) in patients aged 65 and older with primary diagnosis of coronary heart disease (CHD), cerebrovascular disease (CBVD) and HF. (*Data from* Liu L. Changes in cardiovascular hospitalization and comorbidity of heart failure in the United States: findings from the national hospital discharge surveys 1980–2006. Int J Cardiol 2011;149(1):41.)

Discharge Surveys 1980 to 2006, HF patients had 2.4 times higher odds of having comorbid coronary heart disease, and renal failure, and 2 times higher odds of having chronic obstructive pulmonary disease, about 1.8 times higher odds of having diabetes and pneumonia.[3] A recent report by Wong and colleagues[35] using data from the National Health and Nutrition Examination Surveys 1988 to 2008 suggested that the proportion of patients with HF who were aged 80 years and older increased from 13.3% in 1988–1994 to 22.4% in 2003–2008 ($P<.01$). The proportion of patients with HF who had 5 or more comorbid chronic conditions increased from 42.1% to 58.0% ($P<.01$), and the main conditions driving this increase included hypercholesterolemia (41% to 54%), diabetes (25% to 38%), obesity (33% to 47%), kidney disease (35% to 46%), thyroid disease (10% to 23%), and osteoporosis (5% to 16%). The mean number of prescription medications increased from 4.1 to 6.4 prescriptions ($P<.01$). Although these comorbidities may share certain common risk factors and treatment approaches, each comorbid condition comes with a unique set of causes, symptoms, and clinical management requirements. Another example is studies related to cardiorenal syndrome and interaction of renal dysfunction and diabetes on HF, which have further demonstrated the complex nature of patient's self-care and clinical management.[3,4,36,37] There is no doubt that despite clinical guidelines for HF management, the heterogeneity of patient's trajectories in HF adds to the complexity of this problem for patients and clinicians alike.

DIAGNOSTIC CRITERIA

HF is defined, clinically, as a syndrome in which patients have typical symptoms (eg, breathlessness, ankle swelling, and fatigue) and signs (eg, elevated jugular venous pressure, pulmonary crackles, and displaced apex beat) resulting from an abnormality of cardiac structure or function.[4,38] Although HF is a common clinical syndrome, especially in the older adults, its diagnosis is often missed. A detailed clinical history is crucial and should address not only current signs and symptoms of HF but also signs and symptoms that point to a specific cause of the syndrome, such as hypertension or coronary heart disease. In North America, the commonly used criteria for the diagnosis of HF are the Framingham criteria, Duke criteria, and the Boston criteria.[39–41] The physical examination includes assessment of jugular venous distention, the presence of adventitious cardiac sounds such as the S3 and S4 and cardiac murmurs, the location and intensity of the left ventricular apical impulse, and the presence of a right ventricular heave. An electrocardiograph, chest radiography, and/or echocardiography of the heart helps differentiate systolic from diastolic dysfunction.[39] Coronary angiography provides information regarding concomitant coronary artery disease, whereas hemodynamic assessments, including pulmonary arterial pressure, pulmonary capillary wedge pressures, cardiac output, and cardiac index can provide valuable information about volume status and forward flow. In Europe, the criteria developed by the European Society of Cardiology are applied.[38] In general, the diagnosis of HF can be difficult because many of the symptoms of HF are nondiscriminating. At the international level, a formal standardization criterion for the definition of HF has been not established.

INTERVENTION AND TREATMENT

The current clinical guidelines have suggested the goals and clinical management by each stage of HF. In stage A, the goals are treatment for hypertension, encourage smoking cessation, treat lipid disorders, encourage regular exercise, and discourage alcohol intake, discourage illicit drug use, and control metabolic syndrome, and use of angiotensin converting enzyme inhibitor (ACEI) or angiotensin receptor blocker (ARB) in appropriate patients for vascular disease or diabetes. In stage B, the goals are treatment for all measures under stage A, and use of ACEI or ARB or β-blocker in appropriate patients, or use of implantable defibrillations in selected patients. In stage C, the goals are treatment for all measures under stages A and B, dietary salt restriction, and uses of diuretics for fluid retention, ACEI or/and β-blockers for routine care, and uses of aldosterone antagonist, ARBs, digitalis, and/or hydralazine/nitrates in selected patients, and use of devices in selected patients (biventricular pacing or implantable defibrillators). In stage D, specialized intervention and treatment are required for HF patients in this stage, including appropriate measures under stages A, B, and C. Options of compassionate end-of-life care/hospice, extraordinary measures, heart transplant, chronic inotropes, permanent mechanical support, experimental surgery or drugs should be considered appropriately.[4,42]

SUMMARY

HF has become the leading cause of morbidity, hospitalization, and death in the developed world. The prevalence and incidence of HF increase with age and are expected to constitute a considerable burden of health care and public health. There are no comparable data that could be used to have a direct international comparison because of the lack of standardized or internationally applied criteria of HF definition. In the United States and several other countries, the absolute number of patients with HF has increased. The association of multiple comorbidity in patients with HF makes disease treatment and prevention more complex. The heterogeneity of the disease causes, including the degrees and types of multiple comorbid disease among different racial/ethnic populations, raises further questions to be studied and addressed in disease control and research.

REFERENCES

1. Roger VL, Go AS, Lloyd-Jones DM, et al, American Heart Association Statistics Committee, Stroke Statistics Subcommittee. Executive summary: heart disease and stroke statistics–2012 update: a report from the American Heart Association. Circulation 2012;125:188–97.

2. Bui AL, Horwich TB, Fonarow GC. Epidemiology and risk profile of heart failure. Nat Rev Cardiol 2011;8: 30–41.

3. Liu L. Changes in cardiovascular hospitalization and comorbidity of heart failure in the United States: findings from the National Hospital Discharge Surveys 1980–2006. Int J Cardiol 2011;149:39–45.

4. Hunt SA, Abraham WT, Chin MH, et al. 2009 Focused update incorporated into the ACC/AHA 2005 guidelines for the diagnosis and management of heart failure in adults: a report of the American College of Cardiology Foundation/American Heart Association task force on practice guidelines: developed in collaboration with the International Society for Heart and Lung Transplantation. Circulation 2009;119:e391–479.

5. Batlle M, Perez-Villa F, Garcia-Pras E, et al. Downregulation of matrix metalloproteinase-9 (MMP-9) expression in the myocardium of congestive heart failure patients. Transplant Proc 2007;39:2344–6.

6. Caboral M, Mitchell J. New guidelines for heart failure focus on prevention. Nurse Pract 2003;28:13, 16, 22–3; [quiz: 24–5].

7. Newschaffer CJ, Liu LL, Sim A. Cardiovascular disease. In: Remington PL, Brownson RC, Wegner MV, editors. Chronic disease epidemiology and control. Washington, DC: American Public Health Association; 2010. p. 383–428.

8. Rasmusson KD, Hall JA, Renlund DG. The intricacies of heart failure. Nurs Manage 2007;38:33–40 [quiz 40–1].

9. Gopal DM, Kalogeropoulos AP, Georgiopoulou VV, et al, Health ABC study. Serum albumin concentration and heart failure risk the health, aging, and body composition study. Am Heart J 2010;160: 279–85.

10. Kalogeropoulos A, Georgiopoulou V, Kritchevsky SB, et al. Epidemiology of incident heart failure in a contemporary elderly cohort: the health, aging, and body composition study. Arch Intern Med 2009;169: 708–15.

11. Kalogeropoulos A, Georgiopoulou V, Psaty BM, et al, Health ABC study investigators. Inflammatory markers and incident heart failure risk in older adults: the health ABC (health, aging, and body composition) study. J Am Coll Cardiol 2010;55: 2129–37.

12. Liu L, Chen M, Hankins SR, et al, Drexel cardiovascular health collaborative education, research, and evaluation group. Serum 25-hydroxyvitamin D concentration and mortality from heart failure and cardiovascular disease, and premature mortality from all-cause in United States adults. Am J Cardiol 2012;110:834–9.

13. Liu L, Newschaffer CJ. Impact of social connections on risk of heart disease, cancer, and all-cause mortality among elderly Americans: findings from the

second longitudinal study of aging (LSOA II). Arch Gerontol Geriatr 2011;53:168–73.

14. He J, Ogden LG, Bazzano LA, et al. Risk factors for congestive heart failure in US men and women: NHANES I epidemiologic follow-up study. Arch Intern Med 2001;161:996–1002.

15. Liu L, Yin X, Ikeda K, et al. Micronutrients, inflammation, and congestive heart failure among the elderly; nutritional perspectives on primary prevention and clinical treatment. Clin Exp Pharmacol Physiol 2007;34:S14–6.

16. Liu L, Eisen HJ. Serum vitamin D concentration and congestive heart failure in the elderly [abstract 291]. J Card Fail 2006;12:S90.

17. Liu L, Nettleton JA, Bertoni AG, et al. Dietary pattern, the metabolic syndrome, and left ventricular mass and systolic function: the multi-ethnic study of atherosclerosis. Am J Clin Nutr 2009;90:362–8.

18. Sandek A, Doehner W, Anker SD, et al. Nutrition in heart failure: an update. Curr Opin Clin Nutr Metab Care 2009;12:384–91.

19. Zittermann A, Koerfer R. Vitamin D in the prevention and treatment of coronary heart disease. Curr Opin Clin Nutr Metab Care 2008;11:752–7.

20. Lloyd-Jones DM, Larson MG, Leip EP, et al, Framingham Heart Study. Lifetime risk for developing congestive heart failure: the Framingham Heart Study. Circulation 2002;106:3068–72.

21. Bahrami H, Kronmal R, Bluemke DA, et al. Differences in the incidence of congestive heart failure by ethnicity: the multi-ethnic study of atherosclerosis. Arch Intern Med 2008;168:2138–45.

22. CDC-NCHS. National health and nutrition examination survey data. Hyattsville (MD): U.S. Department of Health and Human Services, Centers for disease control and prevention, Available at: http://www.cdc.gov/nchs/surveys.htm. Accessed August 16, 2013.

23. Mosterd A, Hoes AW. Clinical epidemiology of heart failure. Heart 2007;93:1137–46.

24. Reitsma JB, Mosterd A, de Craen AJ, et al. Increase in hospital admission rates for heart failure in the Netherlands, 1980–1993. Heart 1996;76:388–92.

25. Cowie MR, Wood DA, Coats AJ, et al. Incidence and aetiology of heart failure; a population-based study. Eur Heart J 1999;20:421–8.

26. Mendez GF, Cowie MR. The epidemiological features of heart failure in developing countries: a review of the literature. Int J Cardiol 2001;80:213–9.

27. Heidenreich PA, Trogdon JG, Khavjou OA, et al, American Heart Association Advocacy Coordinating Committee, Stroke Council, Council on Cardiovascular Radiology and Intervention, Council on Clinical Cardiology, Council on Epidemiology and Prevention, Council on Arteriosclerosis, Thrombosis and Vascular Biology, Council on Cardiopulmonary, Critical Care, Perioperative and Resuscitation, Council on Cardiovascular Nursing, Council on the Kidney in Cardiovascular Disease, Council on Cardiovascular Surgery and Anesthesia, Interdisciplinary Council on Quality of Care and Outcomes Research. Forecasting the future of cardiovascular disease in the United States: a policy statement from the American Heart Association. Circulation 2011;123:933–44.

28. McMurray JJ, Petrie MC, Murdoch DR, et al. Clinical epidemiology of heart failure: public and private health burden. Eur Heart J 1998;19(Suppl P):P9–16.

29. Roger VL, Weston SA, Redfield MM, et al. Trends in heart failure incidence and survival in a community-based population. JAMA 2004;292:344–50.

30. Matsushita K, Blecker S, Pazin-Filho A, et al. The association of hemoglobin a1c with incident heart failure among people without diabetes: the atherosclerosis risk in communities study. Diabetes 2010; 59:2020–6.

31. Levy D, Kenchaiah S, Larson MG, et al. Long-term trends in the incidence of and survival with heart failure. N Engl J Med 2002;347:1397–402.

32. Barker WH, Mullooly JP, Getchell W. Changing incidence and survival for heart failure in a well-defined older population, 1970–1974 and 1990–1994. Circulation 2006;113:799–805.

33. Bleumink GS, Knetsch AM, Sturkenboom MC, et al. Quantifying the heart failure epidemic: prevalence, incidence rate, lifetime risk and prognosis of heart failure the Rotterdam study. Eur Heart J 2004;25: 1614–9.

34. Stewart S, MacIntyre K, Hole DJ, et al. More 'malignant' than cancer? Five-year survival following a first admission for heart failure. Eur J Heart Fail 2001;3: 315–22.

35. Wong CY, Chaudhry SI, Desai MM, et al. Trends in comorbidity, disability, and polypharmacy in heart failure. Am J Med 2011;124:136–43.

36. Dickson VV, Buck H, Riegel B. Multiple comorbid conditions challenge heart failure self-care by decreasing self-efficacy. Nurs Res 2013;62:2–9.

37. Liu L. Prevalence, comorbidity, and outcomes in hospitalized patients with heart failure for White and Africans: implications and benchmarks [abstract]. Circulation 2008;117:e273.

38. McMurray JJ, Adamopoulos S, Anker SD, et al, Task Force For The Diagnosis And Treatment Of Acute And Chronic Heart Failure 2012 Of The European Society Of Cardiology, ESC Committee for Practice Guidelines. ESC guidelines for the diagnosis and treatment of acute and chronic heart failure 2012: the Task Force for the Diagnosis and Treatment of Acute and Chronic Heart Failure 2012 of the European Society of Cardiology. Developed in collaboration with the Heart Failure Association (HFA) of the ESC. Eur J Heart Fail 2012;14:803–69.

39. Shamsham F, Mitchell J. Essentials of the diagnosis of heart failure. Am Fam Physician 2000;61: 1319–28.

40. McKee PA, Castelli WP, McNamara PM, et al. The natural history of congestive heart failure: the Framingham Study. N Engl J Med 1971;285:1441–6.

41. Harlan WR, oberman A, Grimm R, et al. Chronic congestive heart failure in coronary artery disease: clinical criteria. Ann Intern Med 1977;86:133–8.

42. Schocken DD, Benjamin EJ, Fonarow GC, et al, American Heart Association Council on Epidemiology and Prevention, American Heart Association Council on Clinical Cardiology, American Heart Association Council on Cardiovascular Nursing, American Heart Association Council on High Blood Pressure Research, Quality of Care and Outcomes Research Interdisciplinary Working Group, Functional Genomics and Translational Biology Interdisciplinary Working Group. Prevention of heart failure: a scientific statement from the American Heart Association Councils on Epidemiology and prevention, clinical Cardiology, cardiovascular Nursing, and high blood pressure research; Quality of care and Outcomes research Interdisciplinary Working group; and functional Genomics and Translational Biology Interdisciplinary Working group. Circulation 2008;117:2544–65.

Pathophysiology and Etiology of Heart Failure

Frances L. Johnson, MD

KEYWORDS

- Heart failure • Pathophysiology • Etiology • Diagnosis

KEY POINTS

- Diagnosis and treatment of heart failure require careful evaluation of each patient.
- Diagnostic testing is highly influenced by the quality of the initial evaluation and the identification of comorbid conditions.
- Categorizing a patient's cardiomyopathy will help guide therapy and lend prognostic value as standard and new treatments are applied.

INTRODUCTION

Examining the etiology and underlying pathophysiology of heart failure (HF) is an often neglected but important aspect of treating the condition. Identifying an underlying cause, whenever possible, will allow for optimal care of each patient and guide rational treatment. Treatment requires more than rote application of evidence-based pharmacotherapy. An example is the challenge of HF with preserved ejection fraction. Although therapy for systolic HF is well grounded in data from randomized clinical trials, the large ADHERE Registry showed that nearly half of all patients in the United States with acutely decompensated HF have preserved ejection fraction (>50%).[1] This equally morbid condition is one for which there are few randomized treatment trials.[2] Clinicians must still use knowledge and skills grounded in their understanding of pathophysiology.

This article reviews common mechanisms in the pathophysiology of HF, and categorizes some common cardiomyopathies. Testing that is informative about underlying pathophysiology is discussed within the context of mechanisms, while tests used to diagnose specific cardiomyopathy types are mentioned in the compendium of etiology.

COMMON PATHOPHYSIOLOGIC MECHANISMS IN HEART FAILURE

Our understanding of cardiac pathophysiology is well developed. Whole organ physiology has been informed over the past 30 years by discoveries of humoral and cellular mechanisms that were elucidated by techniques of molecular biology. Today, genetic and proteomic discoveries further deepen our understanding of old paradigms and identify new ones. Pathophysiologic mechanisms of HF coexist and evolve over the course of the condition.

Structural Heart Disease and Mechanical Stress: Pressure/Volume Overload

Hemodynamic principles are centered on knowledge of the heart as a pump. It has properties that allow for increased blood flow commensurate with bodily needs such as exercise under normal conditions by increasing heart rate, stroke volume,

The author has the following financial relationships: Intellectual property licensed with royalties: Comentis, Inc. Intellectual property with stock options: XDx, Inc. Paid consulting: Sorbent Therapeutics Executive Committee. Sponsored Clinical Trials: Biocontrol Medical (USA), Celladon, Inc, CardioMEMs, Inc, Corthera, Inc, NIH, Syncardia Systems, Inc.

Division of Cardiovascular Medicine, Carver College of Medicine, University of Iowa, 200 Hawkins Drive, 318-2 GH, Iowa City, IA 52242, USA

E-mail address: frances-johnson@uiowa.edu

Cardiol Clin 32 (2014) 9–19

http://dx.doi.org/10.1016/j.ccl.2013.09.015

or both. Increased ventricular preload augments contractility, but excessive pressure and volume causes a plateau, then reduction in contraction force. Frank and Starling illustrated this with landmark hemodynamic studies in the early twentieth century, and the term "Starling's Law of the Heart" was coined to describe it.[3] Subsequent study of chronic HF confirmed the validity of Starling's Law, but more importantly defined a spectrum of anatomic and hemodynamic profiles associated with chronic pressure and/or volume overload.[4]

The hemodynamic model of HF is one of ventricular remodeling. Abnormal hemodynamics leads to remodeling, which leads to further abnormalities in hemodynamics. Primary and compensatory changes in geometry and performance vary by the type of HF. Classic examples include pressure-overload conditions such as hypertension and stenotic valves, which result in hypertrophy of the affected ventricle, increased myocardial stiffness, and restricted stroke volume in relation to left ventricular mass. Volume-overload conditions such as valvular regurgitation usually lead to ventricular dilation, elevated end-diastolic pressure, and, ultimately, reduced systolic function. Conditions that affect contractility, such as myocardial infarction or primary myopathy, produce both pressure and volume overload. Reduced systolic function increases ventricular end-diastolic pressure, and causes both ventricular dilation and increased mass (**Fig. 1**). The ultimate result of all pathologic remodeling is a reduction in cardiac output over a range of loading conditions, and dyspnea or edema associated with chronically elevated filling pressures.

All patients with HF should have the extent of structural heart disease defined. Transthoracic echocardiography (TTE) remains the initial test of choice for the assessment of structural heart disease and hemodynamics. It can accurately delineate ventricular size, systolic and diastolic function, and valvular morphology in most patients. Doppler waveform velocities can accurately estimate key intracardiac and extracardiac pressures and valve areas when image quality is good. TTE is readily available in most practice settings, is noninvasive, and takes little time to perform. Its principal limitation is poor image quality in the obese, those with obstructive lung disease, and those with chest-wall deformities or implanted material that limits sonographic image quality. The right ventricle can be difficult to visualize with sufficient detail to accurately assess systolic function.[5,6]

In patients for whom TTE is not adequate, cardiac magnetic resonance imaging (CMR) or cardiac computed tomography (CT) can be performed. CMR has several advantages. Measurements of volume, mass, and ejection fraction of both ventricles are very accurate and reproducible. Abnormalities involving the great vessels, valvular lesions, shunts, and the extent of ischemic myocardial fibrosis can be well defined. It is particularly useful for early-stage disease, regurgitant valves, congenital heart disease, and specific cardiomyopathies.[7] A CMR scan performed for HF should include gadolinium perfusion when possible, which allows for quantitation of ischemic fibrosis and inflammation (**Fig. 2**). Patients with metal in situ are usually excluded from scans, and those with a glomerular filtration rate of less than 30 mL/min should not receive gadolinium because of the risk of cutaneous sclerosis.[8–15]

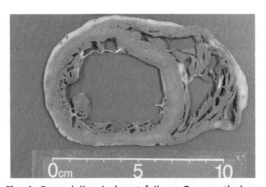

Fig. 1. Remodeling in heart failure. Gross pathology shows marked biventricular dilation with normal thickness in a patient with chronic systolic heart failure. Overall ventricular mass is increased. (*Courtesy of* Dennis Firchau, MD, Department of Pathology, University of Iowa Carver College of Medicine, Iowa City, IA.)

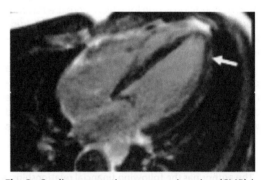

Fig. 2. Cardiac magnetic resonance imaging (CMR) in heart failure. Gadolinium-enhanced CMR in a patient with new-onset heart failure. Bright areas (*arrow*) delineate active inflammation. Myocarditis was confirmed by endomyocardial biopsy. (*Courtesy of* Robert Weiss, MD, Cardiovascular Medicine Division, University of Iowa Carver College of Medicine, Iowa City, IA.)

Hemodynamic measurements (pressure, volume, and flow) can often be deduced by knowledge of the HF etiology and structural lesions. Alternatively, they can be estimated using echocardiography. Understanding a patient's hemodynamics informs the use of medications, especially when side effects limit evidence-based therapies. The gold standard remains invasive right heart catheterization with a pulmonary artery catheter. Invasive hemodynamic monitoring has not been shown to improve mortality in the routine treatment of decompensated HF.[16] Nonetheless, it can still be valuable in some circumstances, the first of which is during diagnostic heart catheterization for new or worsening HF. Hemodynamic monitoring is the most accurate way to diagnose whether elevated pulmonary vascular resistance or intracardiac shunt is impeding circulatory performance, especially if concomitant coronary angiography and left ventricular end-diastolic pressure do not adequately explain symptoms. Another is when assessing acute response to potent pulmonary or peripheral vasodilators. A final indication is critical illness that is not responding to treatment. When performed, invasive hemodynamic measurements should be complete and performed with high fidelity, so that all pertinent calculations of cardiac output, intracardiac shunt, ventricular stroke work, and pulmonary and peripheral vascular resistance can be performed.[5,16]

Neurohormonal Dysregulation

The neurohormonal model of HF is largely responsible for improved treatment outcomes in chronic systolic HF. Acutely reduced cardiac output or vascular underfilling leads to baroreceptor-mediated sympathetic nervous activity with consequent elevation of heart rate, blood pressure, and vasoconstriction. Although this adaptation mitigates an acute drop in cardiac output, it is ultimately maladaptive and leads to myocardial β-receptor downregulation and uncoupling of contractility from normal stimuli. In chronic HF, increased adrenergic tone is accompanied by pathologic activation of the renin-angiotensin-aldosterone system (RAAS). Overproduction of angiotensin II stimulates the adrenal glands to release more catecholamines, which in turn stimulate the juxtaglomerular apparatus in the kidney to release renin. Renin increases vascular tone and pressure overload on a heart susceptible to hemodynamic injury. Angiotensin II also stimulates the adrenal secretion of aldosterone. Nonosmotic release of vasopressin and elevated aldosterone levels reduce renal excretion of water and sodium, leading to excessive preload, edema, and dyspnea. It is now appreciated that neurohormonal imbalances have direct tissue effects as well.[17]

The neurohormonal model of HF was a paradigm shift from the hemodynamic model. HF became a systemic disease amenable to pharmacologic blockade of hormonal pathways. This model has been highly effective and remains the foundation of chronic systolic HF therapy. Other neurohormone levels are altered in HF, including the natriuretic peptides atrial natriuretic peptide and brain natriuretic peptide (BNP), and endothelin-1, but they have not been proven as targets for effective therapy.[18]

Assessment and monitoring of neurohormonal activation is largely done on clinical grounds, such as heart rate, blood pressure, and volume status. The basic metabolic panel is informative if hyponatremia is present. Biomarkers such as BNP and its precursor N-terminal proBNP have been used to diagnose HF in patients with dyspnea of unclear etiology.[19] It is less clear whether it can be used to effectively guide medication titration. A study funded by the National Institutes of Health, GUIDE-IT (Guiding Evidence Based Therapy Using Biomarker Intensified Treatment), will test this hypothesis.

Ischemic Injury: Replacement Fibrosis and Hibernating Myocardium

Ischemic heart disease is thought to be the most common cause of HF in developed countries. Structural changes after myocardial infarction are due to permanent injury and remodeling. Ischemic replacement fibrosis leads to elevated intracardiac pressure and myocardial strain. The hemodynamic model of HF explains the consequences of myocardial infarction well.[20]

By contrast, hibernating myocardium is a potentially reversible condition. The term is used to describe poorly contracting myocardium resulting from constant hypoperfusion without acute injury. The subendocardium is most vulnerable to this type of injury. Canine models show that adequate subendocardial myocardial blood flow (SE-MBF) is requisite for normal systolic function. SE-MBF is disproportionately affected by a ratio of 2:1 to reductions in transmyocardial blood flow (TM-MBF), meaning that even small reductions in the transmyocardial pressure gradient will cause large changes in systolic function. For example, in dogs a 20% reduction in SE-MBF results in severe regional systolic dysfunction.[21] It is important to appreciate that conditions associated with HF, such as systemic hypotension and elevated ventricular end-diastolic pressures, further reduce TM-MBF and worsen systolic dysfunction independent of coronary disease.

Discrimination of hibernating myocardium from ischemic fibrosis has prognostic value. Revascularization procedures in persons with viable myocardium by imaging result in improved left ventricular systolic function, exercise capacity, and survival in comparison with medical therapy alone.[22,23] Diagnostic tests capitalize on 2 characteristics of hibernating myocardium: (1) resting metabolism that is more like normal myocardium than fibrotic scar, and (2) the presence of contractile reserve when stimulated with inotropic agents. Metabolic activity is typically assessed using ^{18}F-fluorodeoxyglucose positron emission tomography (FDG PET). Combination perfusion and metabolic imaging on a CT/PET scanner allows rest and stress [82]Rb perfusion images to be overlaid with FDG-uptake images. In half a day one can accurately identify areas of hibernating myocardium relative to areas of inducible ischemia and replacement fibrosis. Alternatively, CMR can be used to quantify ischemic fibrosis using late gadolinium enhancement, and contractile reserve can be evaluated with the low-dose dobutamine stress.[8,24]

Survival benefit appears to be present even when restoration of perfusion does not lead to improved systolic function.[25,26] It should be noted that published outcomes may censor patients with perioperative mortality. Preoperative risk assessment for revascularization procedures such as coronary artery bypass grafting and open transmyocardial laser should include the use of the Society of Thoracic Surgeons (STS) risk-assessment tool for calculating perioperative mortality. The STS Risk Calculator can be found online at http://riskcalc.sts.org/.

Ultrastructural Abnormalities: Hypertrophy, Fibrosis, and Apoptosis

Cardiac remodeling depends on changes in cell structure, the relative number and activity of cells present, and changes in the extracellular matrix (ECM). Increased ventricular mass and varying degrees of myocyte hypertrophy, fibrosis, and myocyte drop-out are consistent histopathologic findings in cardiomyopathy (**Fig. 3**). In pathologic hypertrophy, myocyte size, volume, and sarcomere number all increase while the rate of apoptosis increases. Pressure and volume overload combine with neurohormonal and cytokine signaling to create a complex pro-hypertrophic milieu. The tissue mediators of hypertrophy are numerous. Key pathways involve catecholamine stimulation of G-protein–coupled β-adrenergic receptors, myocyte and fibroblast stretch activation of integrins, G-protein–mediated intracellular

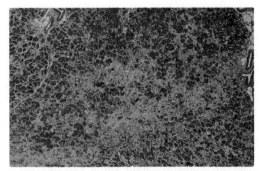

Fig. 3. Ultrastructural changes in heart failure. Microscopic pathology using trichrome staining to highlight excess collagen deposition (*blue*) and myocyte hypertrophy with cell drop-out (*red*). (hematoxylin-eosin, original magnification 4×). (*Courtesy of* Dennis Firchau, MD, Department of Pathology, University of Iowa Carver College of Medicine, Iowa City, IA.)

signaling by way of numerous protein kinases, and the regulatory-action microRNAs. At the gene expression level, these histologic changes are associated with changes toward a fetal pattern.[27–29]

The ECM provides essential scaffolding for the heart, and is an important factor in determining its mechanical properties and function. The ECM is a complex and biologically active mixture of cross-linked collagen fibers, proteoglycans, and signaling molecules. In HF, cardiac fibroblasts and smooth muscle cells proliferate and produce abundant ECM that is rich in fibrillar collagen. The abnormal ECM quantity and composition is not merely the result of changes in production. There is also dysregulation of matrix metalloproteinases (MMPs), which degrade ECM and tissue inhibitors of matrix metalloproteinases (TIMPs). There is experimental evidence that transcriptional regulation of MMPs and TIMPs play a key role the different patterns of hypertrophy and fibrosis seen in cardiomyopathy phenotypes.[30–32]

Another cardinal feature of cardiomyopathy is an increased rate of myocyte apoptosis, or programmed cell death. Increased apoptosis may begin with an initiating ischemic, inflammatory, or toxic injury, but is perpetuated by continual oxidative stress and elevation of death, promoting inflammatory cytokines such as tumor necrosis factor α, norepinephrine, and angiotensin II. Increased apoptosis, which is important when differentially regulated in fetal heart development, may be part of a comparatively unregulated fetal gene program induced by HF. The result over time is a gradual depletion of myocytes and loss of contractile function.[33–35]

Abnormal Intracellular Calcium Handling

Cytoplasmic calcium flux is central to the function of the myocyte contractile apparatus. Thick (myosin) and thin (actin) myofilaments couple and decouple via calcium-dependent events. Intracellular calcium rises by entry of Ca^{2+} from outside the cell via L-type Ca^{2+} channels in the transverse tubules, and by release of calcium from stores in the sarcoplasmic reticulum (SR) through calcium channels known as ryanodine receptors (RyR2). Release of calcium from the SR is the primary activator of contraction, while active reuptake of calcium into the SR concludes contraction and promotes relaxation. Calcium is sequestered in the SR by the action of the adenosine triphosphate–driven Ca^{2+} pump (SERCA2a). In HF, cytosolic calcium levels are elevated. The 2 primary mechanisms by which this occurs are reduced SERCA2a activity and depletion of SR stores from excessive efflux from RyR2 receptors.[36] Both of these mechanisms are potential new targets of therapy. A phase II gene therapy trial to test whether increasing SERC2a gene expression will improve HF outcomes, CUPID 2b, is ongoing. Another active area of research is whether modulation of enzymes that regulate the phosphorylation of the RyR2 receptor, such as Ca^{2+}/calmodulin-dependent kinase II or phosphokinase A, may improve SR reuptake and reduce RyR2 receptor "leak."[37,38]

Genetic Mutations

Once considered rare, it is now clear that many genetic mutations cause cardiomyopathy, either singly or in the context of a specific genetic background. From an etiologic perspective, genetic abnormalities can be classified as structural disease caused by errant development (complex congenital heart disease), mutations of structural and contractile proteins, muscular dystrophies, and mutations of ion channels. From a phenotypic viewpoint, the World Health Organization (WHO) recognizes 4 phenotypes of cardiomyopathy: hypertrophic (HCM), dilated (DCM), restrictive (RCM), and arrhythmogenic right ventricular cardiomyopathy (ARVC). It is now appreciated that ARVC can also affect the left ventricle, and the term arrhythmogenic cardiomyopathy (ACM) is also used. Left ventricular noncompaction (LVNC) is an additional phenotype that is now widely recognized (**Fig. 4**).[39]

Guidelines exist for genetic testing in all the HF phenotypes, and gene test panels are available for the most common mutations. Genetic testing is strongly recommended for individuals with HCM, and is recommended for those with familial cardiomyopathy of other phenotypes. Familial cardiomyopathy is defined as a cardiomyopathy of unknown cause in 2 or more close family members. Testing is recommended for the most affected individual in the family, followed by "cascade

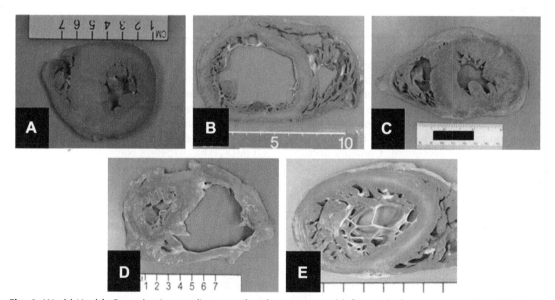

Fig. 4. World Health Organization cardiomyopathy phenotypes and left ventricular noncompaction. (*A*) Hypertrophic cardiomyopathy. (*B*) Dilated cardiomyopathy. (*C*) Restrictive cardiomyopathy. (*D*) Arrhythmogenic right ventricular cardiomyopathy. (*E*) Left ventricular noncompaction. (*Courtesy of* Dennis Firchau, MD, Department of Pathology, University of Iowa Carver College of Medicine, Iowa City, IA.)

screening" of asymptomatic first-degree relatives if a causative gene is identified.[40,41] Despite published guidelines, rates of genetic testing remain low, perhaps reflecting a lack of physician awareness combined with economic and social barriers.[42] If genetic testing is not performed or is negative for a known mutation, clinical screening of first-degree relatives is recommended at intervals that vary by phenotype, but typically range from 1 to 5 years.[43]

HEART FAILURE BY ETIOLOGY

Although the WHO recognizes 4 classes of primary cardiomyopathy, there are many specific types that can be categorized either by phenotype or underlying etiology. Common types are detailed here.

Ischemic Cardiomyopathy

Occlusive coronary artery disease (CAD) is widely acknowledged as the most common reason for symptomatic HF in United States adults, but prevalence data are sparse. Ischemic cardiomyopathy is typified by regional hypokinesis, ventricular enlargement, and thinning of the ventricles in areas of full-thickness injury. One or both ventricles often become more spherical and exhibit atrioventricular valve incompetence, owing to annular dilatation over time. The result is combined systolic and diastolic HF, with systolic dysfunction predominating in the majority of patients.

Because of its prevalence, it is imperative that occlusive coronary disease be excluded in adult patients presenting with new-onset HF. In children and young adults, ischemia from coronary anomalies and other congenital malformations should also be excluded; this can be done either invasively or noninvasively. The American Heart Association/American College of Cardiology (AHA/ACC) guidelines for CAD diagnostic testing are primarily driven by the presence or absence of typical angina and the patient's suitability for undergoing a revascularization procedure. Coronary angiography remains the gold standard for accuracy, but carries an average procedural complication rate of 7.4 in 1000 and a mortality rate of 0.7 in 1000.[44] Noninvasive testing is therefore recommended for patients with a low ejection fraction who are free of angina or evidence of active ischemia (**Table 1**).[5,45]

Noninvasive imaging studies, although less sensitive and less specific than invasive coronary angiography, all carry less procedural risk. Risk is generally confined to the potential toxicity of perfusion agents and radiation exposure. Pharmacologic or exercise stress testing combined with

Table 1
AHA/ACC recommendations for diagnostic testing for occlusive CAD

Patient Characteristics	Coronary Angiography	Noninvasive Imaging
Typical angina or demonstrated ischemia	Class I LOE B	—
CP of uncertain etiology, no prior CAD screening, revascularization eligible	Class IIA LOE C	—
No CP, known or suspected CAD, revascularization eligible	Class IIA LOE C	Class IIA LOE B
No CP, no prior CAD screening, reduced LVEF, revascularization eligible	—	Class IIB LOE C

Abbreviations: ACC, American College of Cardiology; AHA, American Heart Association; CAD, coronary artery disease; Class I, should be performed; Class III, not beneficial/harmful; Class IIA, reasonable to perform; Class IIB, may be considered; CP, chest pain; LOE, level of evidence; LOE A, multiple randomized clinical trials; LOE B, single or nonrandomized trials, registries; LOE C, expert opinion; LVEF, left ventricular ejection fraction.

Data from Yancy CW, Jessup M, Bozkurt B, et al. 2013 ACCF/AHA guideline for the management of heart failure: a report of the American College of Cardiology Foundation/American Heart Association Task Force on Practice Guidelines. Circulation 2013. [Epub ahead of print]; and Jessup M, Abraham WT, Casey DE, et al. 2009 Focused Update: ACCF/AHA Guidelines for the Diagnosis and Management of Heart Failure in Adults. Circ 2009;119:1977–2016.

single-photon emission CT or PET imaging remain the primary screening methods for CAD in patients with HF, because of the accuracy and wide availability of the equipment. 64-Slice multidetector CT (MDCT) has excellent coronary imaging resolution and CMR has acceptable resolution; both are reasonable alternatives.[15,46] The primary limitation of both MDCT and CMR is the need for long breath holds, a regular heart rhythm, and a low enough heart rate to accurately gate the imaging sequences in patients.[47] Echocardiography alone is inadequate for CAD detection, even when regional wall-motion abnormalities exist. Dobutamine stress echo can be used if the baseline ejection fraction is preserved, but should be interpreted with caution when the baseline left ventricular ejection fraction is depressed, as differences in contractility with stress may be subtle. Testing should be tailored to minimize risk and optimize diagnostic accuracy in a given individual.[48–50]

Idiopathic Dilated Cardiomyopathy

Idiopathic dilated cardiomyopathy describes a DCM for which no clear etiology has been identified. It is second in prevalence, and the most common reason for heart transplantation recorded in the International Society of Heart and Lung Transplant registry. DCM is a heterogeneous group. This diagnosis of exclusion reflects how difficult it is to diagnose early inciting events and uncommon genetic mutations. The natural history of myocarditis suggests that many of these cases can be attributed to remodeling after acute inflammation, and an additional 20% to 35% of cases are estimated to be hereditary in nature.[40] Typical features are biventricular enlargement and global hypokinesis. Mitral and tricuspid valve annular dilatation and central valve regurgitation are common. The echocardiographic appearance of the myocardium is normal. Wall thickness is normal to thin, and CMR usually shows faint midmyocardial late gadolinium enhancement. Histology is bland, with diffuse myocyte hypertrophy, fibrosis, and reduced capillary density.

Specific cardiomyopathies should be excluded, with AHA/ACC strongly recommending diagnostics including a 3-generation family history, complete physical examination, and the following screening tests: complete blood count, comprehensive metabolic panel, fasting lipids, thyroid-stimulating hormone, BNP level, chest radiograph, 12-lead electrocardiogram (ECG), and 2-dimensional echocardiogram with Doppler. Further diagnostics are recommended when there is suspicion for a specific disease; these include stress and myocardial viability testing for CAD, and screening tests for autoimmune diseases, amyloidosis, hemochromatosis, human immunodeficiency virus, and secondary forms of hypertension. Endomyocardial biopsy is not recommended for the routine diagnosis of HF.[5]

Hypertensive Heart Disease

The strongest risk factor for the development of HF remains hypertension, and it is a common comorbidity in persons with ischemic heart disease.[51] As the population ages and HF with preserved ejection fraction (HFpEF) increases in prevalence, the terms hypertensive heart disease and HFpEF may become almost synonymous. The cardinal features include left ventricular hypertrophy and abnormal diastolic function ascertained by echo Doppler or cardiac catheterization in a patient with a history of systemic hypertension. If left ventricular hypertrophy and diastolic dysfunction are present without a history of hypertension, an infiltrative etiology should be strongly suspected.

Valvular Cardiomyopathy

Valvular cardiomyopathy can be either inherited or acquired. Excluding complex congenital and syndromic heart disease, the most common congenital valvular lesions are bicuspid aortic valve, with a prevalence of approximately 1%, and myxomatous mitral valve, with a prevalence of 2% to 3% in adults.[52,53] Acquired lesions are typically calcific degeneration or are caused by postinflammatory changes from infective endocarditis, rheumatic fever, rheumatologic disorders, carcinoid, or fenfluramine/phentermine exposure. Among acquired lesions, calcific aortic stenosis is the most common, and primarily affects the elderly. The HF phenotype in valvular cardiomyopathy is determined by the hemodynamic profile caused by the lesion, and compensatory changes in the heart and pulmonary vascular bed. Transthoracic and transesophageal echocardiography are excellent diagnostic tests for defining valvular pathology, and have largely replaced invasive cardiac catheterization. The advent of transcatheter aortic valve replacement is a significant advance for HF patients with calcific aortic stenosis who are poor surgical candidates.[54]

Familial Cardiomyopathy

In contrast to idiopathic cardiomyopathy, familial cardiomyopathy is defined by a clear family history of HF or sudden cardiac death in at least 2 close family members, or positive genetic testing for a specific mutation. Most familial cardiomyopathies are autosomal dominant in inheritance and are described by WHO phenotypes. One must be aware that phenotypic overlap can exist in families and that our understanding of the genotype-phenotype connection remains incomplete.

Familial HCM is the most common form of familial cardiomyopathy, with an estimated frequency of 1 in 500 adults.[42] There are several well-defined mutations in sarcomeric proteins for HCM. The genetic mutations for DCM and their prevalence are less well defined, but include mutations in structural proteins, ion channels, and membrane transporter proteins. Several gene mutations have also been identified for ARVC and LVNC.[55,56] Duchenne and Becker muscular dystrophies, which may also lead to DCM, are remarkable for X-linked rather than an autosomal dominant inheritance pattern.

Diagnosis of familial cardiomyopathy depends on a combination of family history and imaging that defines the phenotype. CMR is especially helpful in establishing whether structural criteria for HCM, ARVC, or LVNC are met. Confirmatory gene testing for known mutations is beneficial for prognosis in some cases, but is primarily helpful in family screening. Genetic counseling resources should be made available to all those who undergo genetic testing.

Inflammatory Cardiomyopathy

This heterogeneous group of secondary cardiomyopathies is caused by inflammatory injury to the myocardium, pericardium, and/or valvular structures. The archetype is acute lymphocytic myocarditis attributed to viral infection. There is strong experimental evidence that postviral autoimmune reactions lead to DCM after the acute phase, and some evidence in humans that viral persistence and the formation autoantibodies to heart proteins are poor prognostic signs.[57,58] To date, human studies have not shown that routine application of immunosuppression prevents progression to DCM or improves clinical outcomes.[59–61] Giant-cell myocarditis is worth special mention because of its fulminant course and association with life-threatening ventricular arrhythmias. This diagnosis can only be made with endomyocardial biopsy. Cardiac manifestations of autoimmune disease or hypersensitivity are often overlooked, but should be considered in the differential diagnosis. Peripartum cardiomyopathy is probably also autoimmune mediated in most cases.

Expert panel recommendations on the diagnosis and management of acute myocarditis and inflammatory cardiomyopathy encourage greater use of viral polymerase chain reaction tests, CMR to identify focal inflammation, and immunohistochemistry when endomyocardial biopsies are obtained.[59] Screening for collagen-vascular diseases and hypereosinophilia should be done in suspected cases. At present, endomyocardial biopsy is strongly recommended only when symptoms are short in duration, hemodynamic compromise is present, and/or if the patient is not responding to conservative treatment.[5,62]

Infiltrative Cardiomyopathy

Though uncommon, the infiltrative cardiomyopathies are important to distinguish from hypertensive heart disease and HCM. Amyloidosis, sarcoidosis, glycogen and liposomal storage diseases, and hemochromatosis can all be considered in this category. Left ventricular hypertrophy is typically present without a history of high blood pressure or elevated voltage on 12-lead ECG.

CMR is especially helpful in detecting abnormal myocardial tissue characteristics that discriminate these entities from "benign" left ventricular hypertrophy. Appropriate treatment of infiltrative cardiomyopathies requires confirmatory biochemical or genetic testing, and sometimes tissue sampling.

Toxic Cardiomyopathy

The most common toxic injuries to the heart include excessive alcohol ingestion, allergens that cause allergic myocarditis, radiation exposure from radiation therapy for cancer, and exposure to chemotherapeutic agents. Newer chemotherapeutic agents are of particular interest, and clinicians should be aware of the potentially reversible nature of HF caused by these agents. Traditional cytostatic agents such as anthracyclines, cyclophosphamide, and cisplatins cause irreversible damage through myofibrillar changes and cell death. By contrast, newer agents target cellular signaling pathways and blood vessels. Examples include monoclonal antibodies against growth factor receptors (including HER2 and epidermal growth factor), tyrosine kinase inhibitors, and antiangiogenic drugs. After cessation of the causative agent and medical management of HF, chemotherapy can often be resumed.[63]

SUMMARY

The diagnosis and treatment of HF require careful evaluation of each patient. Diagnostic testing is highly influenced by the quality of the initial evaluation and the identification of comorbid conditions. Categorizing a patient's cardiomyopathy will help guide therapy and lend prognostic value as standard and new treatments are applied.

REFERENCES

1. Owan TE, Hodge DO, Herges RM, et al. Trends in prevalence and outcome of heart failure with preserved ejection fraction. N Engl J Med 2006; 355(3):251–9.
2. Alagiakrishnan K, Banach M, Jones LG, et al. Update on diastolic heart failure or heart failure with preserved ejection fraction in the older adults. Ann Med 2013;45:37–50.
3. Sarnoff SJ, Berglund E. Ventricular function: I. Starling's law of the heart studied by means of simultaneous right and left ventricular function curves in the dog. Circulation 1954;9(5):706–18.
4. Holubarsch C, Ruf T, Goldstein DJ, et al. Existence of the Frank-Starling mechanism in the failing human heart: investigations on the organ, tissue, and sarcomere levels. Circulation 1996;94(4):683–9.

5. Yancy CW, Jessup M, Bozkurt B, et al. 2013 ACCF/AHA guideline for the management of heart failure: a report of the American College of Cardiology Foundation/American Heart Association Task Force on Practice Guidelines. Circulation. Int J Cardiol 2013;62(6):e147–239.

6. van der Zwaan HB, Geleijnse ML, McGhie JS, et al. Right ventricular quantification in clinical practice: two-dimensional vs. three-dimensional echocardiography compared with cardiac magnetic resonance imaging. Eur J Echocardiogr 2011;12(9): 656–64.

7. Pennell DJ. Cardiovascular magnetic resonance. Circulation 2010;121(5):692–705.

8. Kim RJ, Wu EE, Rafael AA, et al. The use of contrast-enhanced magnetic resonance imaging to identify reversible myocardial dysfunction. N Engl J Med 2000;343(20):1445–53.

9. McCrohon JA, Moon JC, Prasad SK, et al. Differentiation of heart failure related to dilated cardiomyopathy and coronary artery disease using gadolinium-enhanced cardiovascular magnetic resonance. Circulation 2003;108(1):54–9.

10. Rajappan K, Bellenger NG, Anderson L, et al. The role of cardiovascular magnetic resonance in heart failure. Eur J Heart Fail 2000;2(3):241–52.

11. Reiter TT, Ritter OO, Prince MR, et al. Minimizing risk of nephrogenic systemic fibrosis in cardiovascular magnetic resonance. J Cardiovasc Magn Reson 2012;14:31.

12. Arrighi JA, Dilsizian VV. Multimodality imaging for assessment of myocardial viability: nuclear, echocardiography, MR, and CT. Curr Cardiol Rep 2012;14(2):234–43.

13. Lin FY, Min JK. Assessment of cardiac volumes by multidetector computed tomography. J Cardiovasc Comput Tomogr 2008;2(4):256–62.

14. Mangalat D, Kalogeropoulos A, Georgiopoulou V, et al. Value of cardiac CT in patients with heart failure. Curr Cardiovasc Imaging Rep 2009;2(6):410–7.

15. Andreini D, Pontone G, Bartorelli AL, et al. Sixty-four-slice multidetector computed tomography: an accurate imaging modality for the evaluation of coronary arteries in dilated cardiomyopathy of unknown etiology. Circ Cardiovasc Imaging 2009; 2(3):199–205.

16. Allen LA, Rogers JG, Warnica JW, et al. High mortality without escape: the registry of heart failure patients receiving pulmonary artery catheters without randomization. J Card Fail 2008;14(8): 661–9.

17. Schrier RW, Abraham WT. Hormones and hemodynamics in heart failure. N Engl J Med 1999;341(8): 577–85.

18. Ky BB, French BB, Levy WC, et al. Multiple biomarkers for risk prediction in chronic heart failure. Circ Heart Fail 2012;5(2):183–90.

19. Morrison LK, Harrison A, Krishnaswamy P, et al. Utility of a rapid B-natriuretic peptide assay in differentiating congestive heart failure from lung disease in patients presenting with dyspnea. J Am Coll Cardiol 2002;39(2):202–9.

20. Hare JM, Walford GD, Hruban RH, et al. Ischemic cardiomyopathy: endomyocardial biopsy and ventriculographic evaluation of patients with congestive failure, dilated cardiomyopathy and coronary artery disease. J Am Coll Cardiol 1992;20(6): 1318–25.

21. Rahimtoola SH, Dilsizian V, Kramer CM, et al. Chronic ischemic left ventricular dysfunction. JACC Cardiovasc Imaging 2008;1(4):536–55.

22. Meluzin J, Černý J, Groch L, et al. Prognostic importance of the quantification of myocardial viability in revascularized patients with coronary artery disease and moderate-to-severe left ventricular dysfunction. Int J Cardiol 2003;90(1):23–31.

23. Pasquet A, Lauer MS, Williams MJ, et al. Prediction of global left ventricular function after bypass surgery in patients with severe left ventricular dysfunction. Impact of pre-operative myocardial function, perfusion, and metabolism. Eur Heart J 2000; 21(2):125–36.

24. Buckley O, Di Carli M. Predicting benefit from revascularization in patients with ischemic heart failure: imaging of myocardial ischemia and viability. Circulation 2011;123(4):444–50.

25. Allman KC, Shaw LJ, Hachamovitch R, et al. Myocardial viability testing and impact of revascularization on prognosis in patients with coronary artery disease and left ventricular dysfunction: a meta-analysis. J Am Coll Cardiol 2002;39(7): 1151–8.

26. Marwick TH, Zuchowski C, Lauer MS, et al. Functional status and quality of life in patients with heart failure undergoing coronary bypass surgery after assessment of myocardial viability. J Am Coll Cardiol 1999;33(3):750–8.

27. Braunwald E. Heart failure. Heart Failure 2013;1: 1–20.

28. Gandhi MS, Kamalov G, Shahbaz AU, et al. Cellular and molecular pathways to myocardial necrosis and replacement fibrosis. Heart Fail Rev 2011;16(1):23–34.

29. Mann DL. Heart failure: a companion to Braunwald's heart disease. St. Louis (MO): Elsevier Saunders; 2010.

30. Deschamps AM, Spinale FG. Pathways of matrix metalloproteinase induction in heart failure: bioactive molecules and transcriptional regulation. Cardiovasc Res 2006;69(3):666–76.

31. Yan AT, Yan RT, Spinale FG, et al. Relationships between plasma levels of matrix metalloproteinases and neurohormonal profile in patients with heart failure. Eur J Heart Fail 2008;10(2):125–8.

32. Li YY, McTiernan CF, Feldman AM. Interplay of matrix metalloproteinases, tissue inhibitors of met-alloproteinases and their regulators in cardiac matrix remodeling. Cardiovasc Res 2000;46(2):214–24.

33. Narula JJ, Haider NN, Virmani RR, et al. Apoptosis in myocytes in end-stage heart failure. N Engl J Med 1996;335(16):1182–9.

34. Fisher SA, Langille BL, Srivastava D. Apoptosis during cardiovascular development. Circ Res 2000;87(10):856–64.

35. Haudek SB, Taffet GE, Schneider MD, et al. TNF provokes cardiomyocyte apoptosis and cardiac re-modeling through activation of multiple cell death pathways. J Clin Invest 2007;117(9):2692–701.

36. Luo M, Anderson ME. Mechanisms of altered Ca^{2+} handling in heart failure. Circ Res 2013;113(6):690–708.

37. Papolos A, Frishman WH. Sarcoendoplasmic reticulum calcium transport ATPase 2a: a potential gene therapy target in heart failure. Cardiol Rev 2013;21:151–4.

38. Bers DM. CaMKII inhibition in heart failure makes jump to human. Circ Res 2010;107(9):1044–6.

39. Richardson PP, McKenna WW, Bristow MM, et al. Report of the 1995 World Health Organization/International Society and Federation of Cardiology Task Force on the Definition and Classification of Cardiomyopathies. Circulation 1996;93(5):841–2.

40. Hershberger RE, Siegfried JD. Update 2011: clinical and genetic issues in familial dilated cardiomyopathy. J Am Coll Cardiol 2011;57(16):1641–9.

41. Ackerman MJ, Priori SG, Willems S, et al. HRS/EHRA expert consensus statement on the state of genetic testing for the channelopathies and cardiomyopathies this document was developed as a partnership between the Heart Rhythm Society (HRS) and the European Heart Rhythm Association (EHRA). Heart Rhythm 2011;8:1308–39.

42. Miller EM, Wang Y, Ware SM. Uptake of cardiac screening and genetic testing among hypertrophic and dilated cardiomyopathy families. J Genet Couns 2013;22(2):258–67.

43. Hershberger RE, Lindenfeld J, Mestroni L, et al. Genetic evaluation of cardiomyopathy—a Heart Failure Society of America practice guideline. J Card Fail 2009;15(2):83–97.

44. West R, Ellis G, Brooks N, et al. Complications of diagnostic cardiac catheterisation: results from a confidential inquiry into cardiac catheter complications. Heart 2006;92(6):810–4.

45. Lindenfeld J, Albert NM, Boehmer JP, et al. Executive summary: HFSA 2010 comprehensive heart failure practice guideline. J Card Fail 2010;16(6):475–539.

46. Ten Kate G, Caliskan K, Dedic A, et al. Computed tomography coronary imaging as a gatekeeper for invasive coronary angiography in patients with newly diagnosed heart failure of unknown aetiology. Eur J Heart Fail 2013;15(9):1028–34.

47. Assomull RG, Shakespeare C, Kalra PR, et al. Role of cardiovascular magnetic resonance as a gatekeeper to invasive coronary angiography in patients presenting with heart failure of unknown etiology. Circulation 2011;124(12):1351–60.

48. Chen J, Einstein AJ, Fazel R, et al. Cumulative exposure to ionizing radiation from diagnostic and therapeutic cardiac imaging procedures: a population-based analysis. J Am Coll Cardiol 2010;56(9):702–11.

49. Gerber TC, Carr JJ, Arai AE, et al. Ionizing radiation in cardiac imaging: a science advisory from the American Heart Association Committee on Cardiac Imaging of the Council on Clinical Cardiology and Committee on Cardiovascular Imaging and Intervention of the Council on Cardiovascular Radiology and Intervention. Circulation 2009;119(7):1056–65.

50. Laskey WK, Feinendegen LE, Neumann RD, et al. Low-level ionizing radiation from noninvasive cardiac imaging: can we extrapolate estimated risks from epidemiologic data to the clinical setting? JACC Cardiovasc Imaging 2010;3(5):517–24.

51. Lloyd-Jones D, Adams R, Carnethon M, et al. Heart disease and stroke statistics—2009 update: a report from the American Heart Association Statistics Committee and Stroke Statistics Subcommittee. Circulation 2009;119(3):480–6.

52. Ward C. Clinical significance of the bicuspid aortic valve. Heart 2000;83(1):81–5.

53. Guy TS, Hill AC. Mitral valve prolapse. Annu Rev Med 2012;63:277–92.

54. Lindman BR, Bonow RO, Otto CM. Current management of calcific aortic stenosis. Circ Res 2013;113(2):223–37.

55. Hershberger RE, Cowan J, Morales A, et al. Progress with genetic cardiomyopathies: screening, counseling, and testing in dilated, hypertrophic, and arrhythmogenic right ventricular dysplasia/cardiomyopathy. Circ Heart Fail 2009;2(3):253–61.

56. Ackerman MJ, Mohler PJ. Defining a new paradigm for human arrhythmia syndromes: phenotypic manifestations of gene mutations in ion channel- and transporter-associated proteins. Circ Res 2010;107(4):457–65.

57. Kühl UU, Pauschinger MM, Seeberg BB, et al. Viral persistence in the myocardium is associated with progressive cardiac dysfunction. Circulation 2005;112(13):1965–70.

58. Blauwet LA, Cooper LT. Myocarditis. Prog Cardiovasc Dis 2010;52(4):274–88.

59. Caforio AL, Pankuweit S, Arbustini E, et al. Current state of knowledge on aetiology, diagnosis, management, and therapy of myocarditis: a position

statement of the European Society of Cardiology Working Group on Myocardial and Pericardial Diseases. Eur Heart J 2013;34(33):2636–48.

60. Frustaci A, Chimenti C, Calabrese F, et al. Immunosuppressive therapy for active lymphocytic myocarditis: virological and immunologic profile of responders versus nonresponders. Circulation 2003;107(6):857–63.

61. Cooper LT, Hare JM, Tazelaar HD, et al. Usefulness of immunosuppression for giant cell myocarditis. Am J Cardiol 2008;102(11):1535–9.

62. Cooper LT, Baughman KL, Feldman AM, et al. The role of endomyocardial biopsy in the management of cardiovascular disease: a scientific statement from the American Heart Association, the American College of Cardiology, and the European Society of Cardiology. Circulation 2007;116(19): 2216–33.

63. Berardi R, Caramanti M, Savini A, et al. State of the art for cardiotoxicity due to chemotherapy and to targeted therapies: a literature review. Crit Rev Oncol Hematol 2013;88(1):75–86.

The Renin-Angiotensin-Aldosterone System and Heart Failure

Gabriel Sayer, MD[a,b], Geetha Bhat, PhD, MD[a,b,*]

KEYWORDS

- Renin-angiotensin-aldosterone system • Neurohormonal • Heart failure • Aldosterone
- Angiotensin II • Angiotensin-converting enzyme inhibitors • Angiotensin-receptor blockers

KEY POINTS

- The renin-angiotensin-aldosterone system plays a critical role in the pathogenesis of chronic heart failure with a reduced ejection fraction by promoting adverse left ventricular remodeling.
- Blockade of the renin-angiotensin-aldosterone system has been achieved at multiple points, and can significantly reduce morbidity and mortality from heart failure.
- Angiotensin-converting enzyme inhibitors are the primary therapeutic agents for heart failure with reduced ejection fraction, regardless of cause or degree of symptoms.
- Additional inhibition of the renin-angiotensin-aldosterone system can be achieved by addition of an angiotensin-receptor blocker or an aldosterone antagonist.
- Aldosterone antagonists have an additional mortality benefit when added to an angiotensin-converting enzyme inhibitor, whereas angiotensin-receptor blockers only have a morbidity benefit.

INTRODUCTION

The development of the neurohormonal model of heart failure (HF) has underpinned a tremendous growth in basic and clinical investigations into HF physiology and clinical management. Through a strategy that has sequentially targeted individual neurohormonal systems, clinical trials have achieved incremental improvements in HF mortality during the past 25 years.[1,2] The renin-angiotensin-aldosterone system (RAAS) shown in **Fig. 1** was the first neurohormonal system to be studied in HF, because of its role in systemic vasoconstriction. Attempts to alleviate the symptoms of HF through the reduction of systemic vascular resistance (SVR) led to the pivotal finding that blockade of the RAAS significantly improves survival.[3] Further research has formed the basis of current professional guidelines, which uniformly recommend inhibition of RAAS with an angiotensin-converting enzyme (ACE) inhibitor as first-line therapy for symptomatic and asymptomatic HF.[4–6]

RAAS PHYSIOLOGY

Renin is an aspartyl protease produced in the juxtaglomerular cells of the renal afferent arteriole, where it is cleaved from its precursor, prorenin. Baroreceptors in the wall of the afferent arteriole respond to reduced perfusion pressure by stimulating the release of renin from secretory granules.[7] A decrease in systemic volume may also be sensed by arterial baroreceptors and the macula densa of the distal tubule, which initiate signaling pathways to promote further renin

The authors received no funding support and have nothing to disclose.
[a] Center for Heart Transplant and Assist Devices, Advocate Christ Medical Center, 4400 West 95th Street, Suite 407, Oak Lawn, IL 60453, USA; [b] University of Illinois at Chicago College of Medicine, Chicago, IL 60612, USA
* Corresponding author. Center for Heart Transplant and Assist Devices, Advocate Christ Medical Center, 4400 West 95th Street, Suite 407, Oak Lawn, IL 60453.
E-mail address: geetha.bhat@advocatehealth.com

Renin-Angiotensin-Aldosterone System

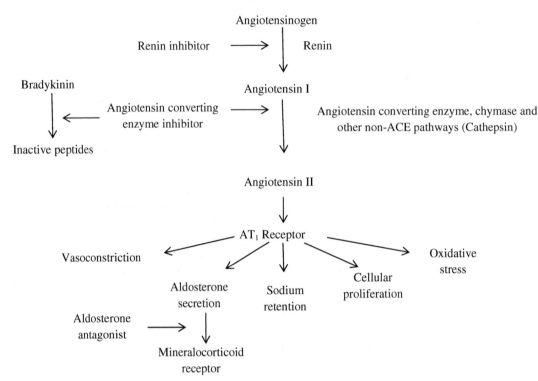

Fig. 1. Schematic depiction of the RAAS. ACE, angiotensin-converting enzyme.

release. The synthesis of prorenin is inhibited by conditions of increased renal perfusion, including elevated systemic blood pressure and volume overload. Additionally, there is a negative feedback mechanism in response to increased levels of circulating angiotensin II.

Renin cleaves 10 amino acids from angiotensinogen to form angiotensin I, which is subsequently cleaved by ACE to form angiotensin II. An alternative pathway for the conversion of angiotensin I to angiotensin II, involving the protease chymase, has also been identified.[8] Circulating angiotensin II is the primary mediator of the acute systemic response to volume depletion and hypotension after RAAS stimulation. However, local production of angiotensin II has been identified in numerous body tissues, including the heart.[9,10] Tissue-level production of angiotensin II may be responsible for the chronic maintenance of cardiovascular (CV) homeostasis, particularly in the setting of disease states, such as HF.[11]

Systemic Actions of Angiotensin II

Angiotensin II primarily acts through the AT$_1$ receptor, activating multiple CV and renal processes:

- Systemic arterial vasoconstriction
- Renal arteriolar vasoconstriction
- Stimulation of renal tubular reabsorption of sodium and water
- Vascular smooth muscle contraction
- Aldosterone release from the adrenal glands

The role of the AT$_2$ receptor is less well defined. In HF, the immediate result of angiotensin II formation is the maintenance of systemic blood pressure. An increase in plasma volume follows, through a direct augmentation of renal tubular sodium collection and as a secondary consequence of an increase in circulating aldosterone. In the kidney, increased efferent arteriolar resistance preserves the glomerular filtration rate in the setting of decreased renal perfusion. Angiotensin II also stimulates the release of prostaglandins, which prevent excess vasoconstriction in the systemic and renal circulation.[12]

Cardiac Actions of Angiotensin II and Aldosterone

In the myocyte, stimulation of the AT$_1$ receptor by angiotensin II produces cellular hypertrophy that is independent of the secondary effects of systemic vasoconstriction.[13,14] Angiotensin II also stimulates fibroblast hypertrophy and collagen deposition, ultimately promoting myocardial fibrosis.[15,16] Increased fibrosis and the expansion of the extracellular matrix are two of the hallmarks of the ventricular remodeling that is characteristic of chronic HF with a reduced ejection fraction (HFrEF). In a substudy of clinical trial patients, the role of RAAS activation in the development of HFrEF was confirmed by a strong correlation of renin levels with worsening degrees of ventricular function and more severe HF symptoms.[17]

In addition to adrenal production of aldosterone, angiotensin II may also stimulate myocardial generation of aldosterone. In the failing heart, aldosterone receptor density is upregulated, suggesting an increase in local production of aldosterone that is associated with activation of the RAAS.[18] Studies of cultured fibroblasts have demonstrated that aldosterone can stimulate collagen synthesis, and aldosterone may also increase the level of ACE in the heart, leading to increased production of angiotensin II.[19,20]

RAAS BLOCKADE WITH ACE INHIBITORS

In addition to blocking the generation of angiotensin II, ACE inhibitors also prevent bradykinin degradation, which increases the stimulation of nitric oxide and has positive effects on endothelial function.[21] By decreasing SVR, ACE-inhibitors lead to improvements in cardiac hemodynamics and exercise capacity.[22,23] However, their prominent role in the management of HFrEF stems from the finding of reduced mortality with ACE inhibitor treatment, a finding first noted in a rat model of myocardial infarction (MI) and subsequently confirmed in numerous human clinical studies.[3]

ACE Inhibitors and Cardiac Remodeling

ACE inhibitor administration was initially shown to reduce left ventricular (LV) size and maintain LV function after MI in animal studies.[24] These findings were translated to humans in a small randomized trial showing a reduction in indices of remodeling with captopril treatment after MI.[25] Subsequently, two large, randomized clinical investigations confirmed that the reverse remodeling benefits of ACE inhibition extended out to 1 year.[26,27] This effect was also demonstrated in patients with LV dysfunction but no symptoms of HF.[28]

ACE Inhibitors and CV Outcomes in Chronic HF

Selected trials that have demonstrated benefit of ACE inhibitors in chronic HFrEF are shown in **Table 1**.[29–35] The first trial to address outcomes was CONSENSUS, in which 253 patients with

New York Heart Association (NYHA) Class IV HF were randomized to enalapril or placebo.[29] Most patients had an ischemic cardiomyopathy. Because of a dramatic 40% reduction in 6-month mortality (26% with enalapril vs 44% with placebo), CONSENSUS was halted before full enrollment. In addition to the 6-month results, mortality was decreased by 31% at 1 year and death caused by progressive HF was reduced by 50%.

CONSENSUS was followed by the SOLVD trials, which evaluated the use of ACE inhibitors in mild to moderate HF (NYHA Class II–III) and asymptomatic LV dysfunction (NYHA Class I).[30,31] In the symptomatic HF trial, 2569 patients with a mean LVEF of 25% were followed for an average of 41 months. Enalapril lowered mortality from 40% to 35% (16% risk reduction) and lowered a composite of death and HF hospitalization from 57% to 48% (26% risk reduction). In the asymptomatic trial, 4228 patients with an LVEF less than or equal to 35% were followed for 3 years. There was no difference in mortality between the two arms ($P = .30$), but enalapril reduced the development of symptomatic HF by 37% and the risk of HF hospitalization by 44%.

ACE inhibition in the post-MI patient with low EF (**Table 1**) was studied in three large randomized trials.[32–34] SAVE and TRACE investigated the impact of ACE inhibitors in patients with asymptomatic LV dysfunction, whereas AIRE studied patients with symptomatic HF between 2 and 9 days after MI. ACE inhibitors produced a 19% reduction in mortality (20% vs 25%) in SAVE, and a 22% reduction in mortality (35% vs 42%) in TRACE. Both trials demonstrated significant decreases in the development of HF with treatment. AIRE enrolled 2006 patients with NYHA Class II to IV HF after an acute MI. At 15 months, mortality was reduced from 23% to 17% ($P = .002$), and progressive HF was reduced from 18% to 14%.

The only large trial to compare an ACE inhibitor with an active treatment was the VHeFT II, in which 806 men with symptomatic HF and an LVEF less than or equal to 45% were randomized to enalapril or the combination of hydralazine-isosorbide dinitrate.[35] After 2 years of follow-up, enalapril reduced mortality by 28% ($P = .016$), firmly establishing ACE inhibitors as superior to other vasodilator therapy used in HF at that time. The question of whether ACE inhibitor dose is important was answered by the ATLAS trial.[36] Low-dose lisinopril (2.5–5 mg) was compared with high-dose lisinopril (32.5–35 mg) in 3164 patients with symptomatic HF and LVEF less than or equal to 30%. Higher doses of lisinopril did not improve mortality, but did reduce a composite end point including mortality and HF hospitalization by

Table 1
Selected ACE inhibitor clinical trials

Trial Name	Study Details	Mean Duration of Follow-up	Primary Conclusion
Heart failure			
CONSENSUS I[29]	NYHA Class IV HF Enalapril (N = 127) Placebo (N = 126)	188 d	Mortality at 6 mo Enalapril 26% vs Placebo 44% (RRR = 40%; P = .002)
SOLVD (treatment)[30]	NYHA Class II–III HF Enalapril (N = 1285) Placebo (N = 1284)	3.5 y	Total mortality Enalapril 35% vs Placebo 39.7% (RRR = 16%; P<.0036)
SOLVD (prevention)[31]	Enalapril up to 10 mg twice daily (N = 2111) vs placebo (N = 2117) LVEF ≤35% No CHF treatment	3.1 y	All-cause mortality 14.8% in enalapril vs 15.8% in placebo (RR = 0.94; 95% CI, 0.82–1.08)
V-HeFT II[35]	Chronic HF, CT ratio >0.55 LVEF <45% Enalapril (N = 403) 20 mg daily vs Hydralazine + ISDN 160 mg daily (N = 401)	2.5 y	Average 2-y mortality with enalapril (18%) was lower than with hydralazine + ISDN (25%) P = .016, but the nonspecific vasodilator combination showed significantly more improvement in exercise performance and LV function
Postmyocardial infarction			
SAVE[32]	LVEF ≤40%, 3–16 d post-MI Captopril (N = 1115) Placebo (N = 1116)	3.5 y	Mortality Captopril 20% vs Placebo 25% (RRR = 19%; P≤.019)
AIRE[33]	LVEF 3–10 d post-MI Ramipril (N = 1014) vs Placebo (N = 992)	1.3 y	Mortality Ramipril 17% Placebo 23% (RRR = 27%; P = .002)
TRACE[34]	3–7 d Post-MI Trandolapril (N = 876) Placebo (N = 873)	2 y	Mortality Trandolapril 34.7% vs Placebo 42.3% (RR = 0.78; CI, 0.67–0.91; P = .001)

Abbreviations: CHF, congestive heart failure; CI, confidence interval; NYHA, New York Heart Association; RR, relative risk; RRR, relative risk reduction.

15% (P<.001). This finding was primarily because of a 24% decrease in HF hospitalizations.

ACE Inhibitors and the Prevention of HF

Three trials have explored the effects of ACE inhibitors in patients with stable CV disease but no evidence of LV dysfunction or HF (**Table 2**).[37–39] In the HOPE trial, which included 9297 patients, ramipril reduced the incidence of HF by 23% (P<.001).[37] Perindopril reduced HF hospitalization by 39% in the EUROPA trial, although the absolute risk reduction was only 0.7% because of the low risk of the trial cohort.[38] Finally, in the PEACE trial,

treatment with trandolapril reduced HF hospitalization by 23%, although this was a post hoc analysis and there was no difference in the primary outcome between treatment arms, limiting the interpretation of secondary end points.[39] A meta-analysis of these three trials did show a modest but highly significant reduction in the development of HF (2.1% vs 2.7%; P = .0007).[40]

RAAS BLOCKADE WITH ANGIOTENSIN-RECEPTOR BLOCKERS

Angiotensin receptor blockers (ARBs) selectively bind to the AT_1 receptor and prevent its activation.

Table 2
ACE inhibitor clinical trials in increased cardiovascular risk patients

Trial Name	Study Details	Mean Duration of Follow-up	Primary Conclusion
HOPE[37]	N = 9297 >55 y old with vascular disease or diabetes plus one other cardiovascular risk factor LVEF <40% Ramipril 10 mg daily vs placebo Follow up 5 y	5 y	Primary outcome of MI, stroke, or death from cardiovascular causes occurred in 14% of ramipril group vs 17.8% in placebo group (RR = 0.78; 95% CI, 0.70–0.86; $P<.001$)
EUROPA[38]	N = 12,218 Stable CAD, no heart failure Perindopril 8 mg daily vs placebo Mean follow-up 4.2 y	4.2 y	Primary end point of cardiovascular death, MI, or cardiac arrest occurred in 8% perindopril group vs 10% in placebo group (RRR = 20%; 95% CI, 9–29; $P = .003$)
PEACE[39]	Trandolapril (N = 4157) vs placebo (N = 4132) Trandolapril 4 mg daily mean LVEF 58 ± 9%	4.8 y	Primary outcome of death from cardiovascular causes, MI, or coronary revascularization was 21.9% in trandolapril group vs 22.5% in placebo group

Abbreviations: CAD, coronary artery disease; CI, confidence interval; RR, relative risk; RRR, relative risk reduction.

A theoretical advantage of ARBs is the ability to block angiotensin II that is formed by non-ACE pathways, and thus offer a more complete inhibition of RAAS activity. Furthermore, ARBs do not prevent bradykinin degradation, and are less likely than ACE inhibitors to produce cough. Like ACE inhibitors, ARBs produce immediate decreases in cardiac filling pressures and SVR, and have similar beneficial effects on exercise capacity.[41,42]

ARBs and CV Outcomes in Chronic HF

Selected studies evaluating the use of ARBs in the treatment of HFrEF are shown in **Table 3**.[43–50] The ELITE II trial randomized 3152 patients to losartan or captopril.[43] Neither medication was superior in terms of mortality or any of the other end points, including HF hospitalizations. However, losartan was better tolerated than captopril, with fewer study withdrawals in the losartan arm, and a significantly reduced incidence of cough. OPTIMAAL compared losartan and captopril in 5447 patients with acute MI with evidence of HF.[44] There was no significant difference in outcomes between the two groups, although there was a strong trend favoring captopril in terms of mortality, sudden cardiac death, and HF hospitalizations. The VALIANT trial was a larger investigation of 14,703 patients with acute MI with HF or LV dysfunction that had three study groups: valsartan, captopril, or a combination of the two therapies.[45] In a comparison of just the captopril and valsartan arms, there was no difference in mortality or HF hospitalization.

Because of the well-established benefits of ACE-inhibitors in HFrEF, ethical considerations precluded the use of placebo comparisons for most studies of ARBs. The CHARM-Alternative trial was able to use a placebo control by evaluating candesartan in patients with HFrEF who were intolerant of ACE inhibitors.[46] In 2028 patients with an LVEF less than or equal to 40%, candesartan reduced CV death from 25% to 22% (15% risk reduction) and HF hospitalizations from 28% to 20% (32% risk reduction). The effect size is similar to those seen in ACE inhibitor trials, and the use of ARBs in patients intolerant to ACE inhibitors is a Class I recommendation in HF guidelines.[4–6]

Most studies with losartan used a dose of 50 mg, which is considered suboptimal. The HEAAL trial compared high-dose losartan (150 mg) with low-dose losartan (50 mg) in patients with HFrEF who were intolerant to ACE inhibitors.[47] A combined end point of CV death or HF hospitalization was reduced in the high-dose group from 46% to 43%, mostly driven by a reduction in HF hospitalizations from 26% to 23% ($P = .025$). An increase in renal dysfunction, hypotension, and hyperkalemia was seen with high-dose losartan, but there was no difference in medication discontinuation between the two groups.

Table 3
Angiotensin-receptor blocker clinical trials

Trial Name	Study Details	Duration of Follow-up	Primary Conclusion
Heart failure			
ELITE II[43]	N = 3152, NYHA Class II–IV LVEF ≤40% Losartan 50 mg daily vs captopril 50 mg TID	1.5 y (median)	Mortality 17.1% in losartan vs 15.9% captopril (HR, 1.13; 95% CI, 0.95–1.35; P = .16)
HEAAL[47]	N = 3846, NYHA Class II–IV LVEF ≤40% Intolerance to ACE I Losartan 150 mg vs 50 mg daily	4.7 y (median)	Mortality 43% in the 150-mg losartan vs 46% in the 50-mg losartan group died or were admitted for HF (HR, 0.90; 95% CI, 0.82–0.99; P = .027)
Val-HeFT[48]	N = 5010, NYHA Class II–IV LVEF ≤40% Valsartan 160 mg BID vs placebo	1.9 y (mean)	Combined end point of mortality and morbidity experienced by 28.8% on valsartan vs 32.1% on placebo (RR = 0.87; 97.5% CI, 0.77–0.97; P = .009)
CHARM-ALTERNATIVE[46]	N = 2028, HF, LVEF ≤40% ACE I, intolerant Candesartan 32 mg daily vs placebo	2.8 y (median)	33% of candesartan vs 40% placebo experienced composite end point of CV death or HF hospitalization (unadjusted HR, 0.77; 95%, CI, 0.67–0.89; P = .0004)
CHARM-ADDED[49]	N = 2548, HF, Class II–IV LVEF ≤40% Candesartan 32 mg daily vs placebo added to ACE I	3.4 y (median)	37.9% of candesartan vs 42.3% of placebo experienced composite end point of CV death or HF hospitalization (unadjusted HR, 0.85; 95% CI, 0.75–0.96; P = .011)
CHARM-PRESERVED[50]	N = 3023, NYHA Class II–IV LVEF ≥40% Candesartan 32 mg daily vs placebo	3 y (median)	22% of candesartan vs 24.3% placebo experienced composite end point of CV death or HF hospitalization (unadjusted HR, 0.89; 95% CI, 0.77–1.03; P = .118)
Postmyocardial infarction			
OPTIMAAL[44]	N = 5477, acute MI and HF Losartan (target 50 mg daily) vs captopril (target 50 mg TID)	2.7 y (mean)	All-cause mortality rate was 18% in the losartan group and 16% in the captopril group (RR = 1.13; 95% CI, 0.99–1.28; P = .07)
VALIANT[45]	N = 14,703 post-MI Complicated by LVSD, HF valsartan vs valsartan plus captopril vs captopril	2 y (mean)	All-cause mortality rates in valsartan, captopril, and combination therapy groups were 19.9%, 19.5%, and 19.3%, respectively

Abbreviations: CI, confidence interval; HR, hazard ratio; RR, relative risk.

CV Outcomes of Combination Therapy with ACE Inhibitors and ARBs

ACE inhibitors do not completely suppress the RAAS because of the generation of angiotensin II through alternative pathways, and the disassociation of ACE inhibitors from ACE in between doses. Adding an ARB to an ACE inhibitor can more thoroughly shut down the RAAS, and the combination has been shown to have an additive effect on the reversal of myocardial remodeling in animal studies.[51] Preliminary studies in humans showed an improvement in hemodynamics and exercise capacity with combined therapy compared with monotherapy.[52,53]

Three large randomized trials have explored the additive benefits of ACE inhibitors and ARBs (see Table 3).[45,48,49] In the VAL-HeFT trial, the addition of valsartan to background therapy, which included an ACE inhibitor in 93% of patients, had no effect on mortality ($P = .80$) but did produce a 23% reduction in HF hospitalization compared with placebo.[48] The VALIANT trial showed similar mortality in all three of its groups, including the combined therapy arm ($P = .95$).[45] The CHARM-Added trial investigated the addition of candesartan or placebo to stable HF therapy, including an ACE-inhibitor.[49] After more than 3 years of follow-up, there was no difference in mortality, but a 15% reduction in a composite of CV death and hospitalizations, driven mostly by a reduction in HF hospitalizations. The most recent guidelines only recommend consideration of combination therapy with an ACE inhibitor and an ARB in persistently symptomatic patients who cannot tolerate an aldosterone antagonist, because of the superior outcomes data with the latter.[4,5]

A greater degree of RAAS inhibition causes more side effects than monotherapy. In the CHARM-added trial, there was a significant increase in adverse events with combination therapy.[49] This has been confirmed by a meta-analysis that included nine trials and 18,601 patients with safety end points.[54] Hypotension and impaired renal function were twice as likely in the combination therapy group, whereas hyperkalemia was four times as likely.

RAAS BLOCKADE WITH ALDOSTERONE ANTAGONISTS

Two benefits of aldosterone antagonism in chronic HF have been proposed: reduced risk of arrhythmia because of higher serum potassium levels, and reduction in LV remodeling and fibrosis. In animal studies, aldosterone antagonists ameliorated the remodeling process after the development of HF.[55,56] Administration of eplerenone after MI led to improved LV function, decreased LV volume, and a reduction in collagen production in a small human study.[57] A substudy of the RALES trial also showed that spironolactone reduced markers of collagen synthesis, suggesting that this therapeutic approach may reduce the fibrosis seen with ventricular remodeling.[58]

Aldosterone Antagonists in CV Outcomes Trials

Trials of aldosterone antagonists in chronic HFrEF are shown in **Table 4**.[59-61] The RALES trial investigated the use of spironolactone in 1663 patients with severe HF (NYHA Class III–IV, mean LVEF 25%).[59] Almost all patients were taking an ACE inhibitor, but only 11% were on a β-blocker. Spironolactone resulted in an absolute 11% reduction in the risk of mortality, and a relative risk reduction of 30% over 36 months. Both HF deaths and sudden cardiac deaths were decreased, as was HF hospitalization (by 35%). EPHESUS extended these findings to the post-MI population.[60] A total of 6642 patients with an LVEF less than or equal to 40% after a recent MI and symptomatic HF or diabetes were randomized to eplerenone or placebo. At 16 months, there was a 17% reduction in CV death and a 15% reduction in HF hospitalizations.

The EMPHASIS-HF trial extended the findings of RALES to less severe HF.[61] A total of 2737 patients with LVEF less than or equal to 30%, NYHA Class II symptoms and an elevated B-type natriuretic peptide (BNP), or a recent hospitalization were enrolled. Patients receiving eplerenone had a significant improvement in the combined end point of CV death or HF hospitalization (18.3% vs 25.9%), and all-cause mortality (12.5% vs 15.5%). EPHESUS and EMPHASIS-HF had high rates of ACE inhibitor use (87% and 94% of study population, respectively) and β-blocker use (75% and 87% of study population).[60,61] Following these publications, aldosterone antagonists have received a Class I indication for all patients with HF that meet the study criteria in the most recent HF guidelines.[4]

All three aldosterone antagonist trials excluded patients with significant renal dysfunction (serum creatinine >2.5 mg/dL in men or >2 mg/dL in women or glomerular filtration rate <30 ml/min/1.73 m²) and/or hyperkalemia (>5 mmol/L). The treatment groups had higher rates of hyperkalemia, with absolute rates of potassium levels greater than 5.5 mmol/L ranging from 5% to 12%.[59-61] After the publication of RALES, there was a significant increase in the rate of hyperkalemia in Canada,

Table 4
Aldosterone antagonist clinical trials

Trial Name	Study Details	Duration of Follow-up	Primary Conclusion
Heart failure			
RALES[59]	N = 1663 NYHA Class III–IV LVEF ≤35% on ACE I Spironolactone 25–50 mg daily vs placebo	2 y (mean)	All-cause mortality rate 35% in Spironolactone group vs 46% in placebo group (RR = 0.70; 95% CI, 0.60–0.82; $P \leq .001$)
EPHESUS[60]	N = 6632, acute MI Complicated by LVSD and HF Eplerenone 25–50 mg daily vs placebo	1.3 y (mean)	Primary end point of death from any cause and death from CV causes or hospitalization for CV causes occurred in 14.4% of eplerenone group vs 16.7% of placebo group (RR = 0.85; 95% CI, 0.75–0.96; $P = .0008$) and 26.7% of eplerenone group vs 30% of placebo group (RR = 0.87; 95% CI, 0.79–0.95; $P = .002$ respectively)
EMPHASIS[61]	N = 2737 NYHA Class II, LVEF ≤35% Eplerenone (up to 50 mg daily) vs placebo	1.8 y (median)	Composite end point of death from cardiovascular causes or hospitalization for HF occurred in 18.3% of eplerenone group vs 25.9% in placebo group (HR, 0.63; 95% CI, 0.54–0.74; $P < .001$)

Abbreviations: CI, confidence interval; HR, hazard ratio; RR, relative risk.

suggesting the need for caution when applying additional RAAS blockade outside of a trial.[62] The American College of Cardiology/American Heart Association Heart Failure Guidelines recommend against the use of all three RAAS inhibiting agents (ACE inhibitors, ARBs, and aldosterone antagonists) concomitantly and consider it a Class III indication. Only two of three classes of agents should be used together.[4]

RAAS BLOCKADE WITH A DIRECT RENIN INHIBITOR

Alsikiren, the first orally active direct renin inhibitor, blocks the initiation of the RAAS cascade, reducing levels of renin and angiotensin. Initial enthusiasm for this therapy was based on its ability to lower neurohormone levels in patients already on optimal therapy.[63] However, larger studies have shown potential harm from adding alsikiren to pre-existing ACE inhibitor treatment. In ALTITUDE, alsikiren increased the rate of CV death compared with placebo in a cohort of 8561 patients with diabetes and either kidney disease or known CV disease.[64] In ASPIRE, the use of alsikiren in patients after MI did not have additional effects on LV remodeling and increased the incidence of adverse effects, including hypotension, renal dysfunction, and hyperkalemia.[65] Finally, the recently reported ASTRONAUT trial added alsikiren to standard HF

therapy in patients admitted with decompensated HF. Despite a significant decrease in N-terminal pro-BNP with alsikiren, there was no difference in CV deaths or HF hospitalization between the two groups, and there was an increase in adverse events with alsikiren.[66] Currently, there are no recommendations regarding direct renin inhibitors in professional guidelines.

RAAS BLOCKADE IN HF WITH PRESERVED EF

The physiology of HF with preserved EF (HFpEF) is not well elucidated, and no therapy has been shown to alter mortality in this population. In the CHARM-Preserved trial, candesartan was compared with placebo in 3023 patients with an LVEF greater than 40% and symptoms of HF.[50] No difference was seen in the primary outcome of CV death or hospitalization but candesartan did result in a marginally significant reduction in HF hospitalization ($P = .047$). Perindopril did not reduce its primary end point (CV death or HF hospitalization) in the PEP-CHF trial, which was significantly underpowered because of poor enrollment and high dropout rates.[67] During the first year of follow-up, when more patients remained on trial medication, there was a functional improvement (based on 6-minute walk) and a reduction in HF hospitalizations in the perindopril group. I-PRESERVE was a comparison of irbesartan and placebo in 4128 patients with symptomatic HF and LVEF greater than 45%.[68] After 4 years of follow-up, there was no difference in a composite end point of death or CV hospitalization.

Only one trial has looked at aldosterone antagonism in HFpEF to date. In ALDO-DHF, 422 patients with LVEF greater than 50% and evidence of diastolic dysfunction and mild to moderate HF symptoms were enrolled.[69] After 1 year, spironolactone reduced LV mass and N-terminal pro-BNP levels, but had an adverse effect 6-minute walk time, and no impact on HF symptoms or quality of life measures. The Treatment of Preserved Cardiac Function Heart Failure with an Aldosterone Antagonist (TOPCAT) study is an ongoing large, randomized trial funded by the National Institutes of Health that will be adequately powered to determine if spironolactone can improve CV outcomes in HFpEF.

SUMMARY

Understanding the pathophysiology of the RAAS and its role in chronic HFrEF has been critical in the development of highly effective therapies that have dramatically altered the natural history of this disease. ACE inhibitors are now firmly established as the primary therapy for HFrEF, regardless of cause, degree of LV dysfunction, or symptomatology. ARBs primary role is as a replacement for ACE inhibitors in those who are intolerant. The initial excitement for combination therapy with an ACE inhibitor and an ARB has been eclipsed by the superior outcomes achieved by the addition of an aldosterone antagonist to an ACE inhibitor. Attempts to interrupt other portions of the RAAS have thus far proved disappointing, as have attempts to inhibit RAAS in patients with HFpEF.

REFERENCES

1. Garg R, Yusuf S. Overview of randomized trials of angiotensin-converting enzyme inhibitors on mortality and morbidity in patients with heart failure. JAMA 1995;273:1450–6.
2. Fauchier L, Pierre B, de Labriolle A, et al. Comparison of the beneficial effect of beta-blockers on mortality in patients with ischaemic or non-ischaemic systolic heart failure: a meta-analysis of randomized controlled trials. Eur J Heart Fail 2007;9:1136–9.
3. Pfeffer MA, Pfeffer JM, Steinberg C, et al. Survival after an experimental myocardial infarction: beneficial effects of long-term therapy with captopril. Circulation 1985;72(2):406–12.
4. Yancy CW, Jessup M, Bozkurt B, et al. 2013 ACCF/AHA guideline for the management of heart failure. J Am Coll Cardiol 2013. http://dx.doi.org/10.1016/j.jacc.2013.05.019.
5. McMurray JJ, Adamopoulos S, Anker SD, et al. ESC Guidelines for the diagnosis and treatment of acute and chronic heart failure 2012. Eur Heart J 2012;33:1787–847.
6. Lindenfeld J, Albert NM, Boehmer JP, et al. HFSA 2010 Comprehensive Heart Failure Practice Guideline. J Card Fail 2010;16:e1–194.
7. Bock HA, Hermle M, Brunner FP, et al. Pressure dependent modulation of renin release in isolated perfused glomeruli. Kidney Int 1992;41:275–80.
8. Urata H, Healy B, Stewart RW, et al. Angiotensin II-forming pathways in normal and failing human hearts. Circ Res 1990;66:883–90.
9. Seikaly MG, Arant BS Jr, Seney FD Jr. Endogenous angiotensin concentrations in specific intrarenal fluid compartments of the rat. J Clin Invest 1990;86:1352–7.
10. van Kats JP, Danser AH, van Meegen JR, et al. Angiotensin production by the heart: a quantitative study in pigs with the use of radiolabeled angiotensin infusions. Circulation 1998;98:73–81.
11. Dzau VJ. Tissue renin-angiotensin system in myocardial hypertrophy and failure. Arch Intern Med 1993;153:937–42.
12. Vallotton MB, Gerber-Wicht C, Dolci W, et al. Interaction of vasopressin and angiotensin II in stimulation of prostacyclin synthesis in vascular smooth muscle cells. Am J Physiol 1989;257:E617–24.
13. Baker KM, Aceto JF. Angiotensin II stimulation of protein synthesis and cell growth in chick heart cells. Am J Physiol 1990;259:H610–8.
14. Harrap SB, Dominiczak AF, Fraser R, et al. Plasma angiotensin II, predisposition to hypertension, and left ventricular size in healthy young adults. Circulation 1996;93:1148–54.
15. Peng J, Gurantz D, Tran V, et al. Tumor necrosis factor-alpha-induced AT1 receptor upregulation enhances angiotensin II-mediated cardiac fibroblast responses that favor fibrosis. Circ Res 2002;91:1119–26.
16. Weber KT. Extracellular matrix remodeling in heart failure: a role for de novo angiotensin II generation. Circulation 1997;96:4065–82.
17. Francis GS, Benedict C, Johnstone DE, et al. Comparison of neuroendocrine activation in patients with left ventricular dysfunction with and without congestive heart failure. A substudy of the Studies of Left Ventricular Dysfunction (SOLVD). Circulation 1990;82:1724–9.
18. Yoshida M, Ma J, Tomita T, et al. Mineralocorticoid receptor is overexpressed in cardiomyocytes of patients with congestive heart failure. Congest Heart Fail 2005;11:12–6.

19. Brilla CG, Zhou G, Matsubara L, et al. Collagen metabolism in cultured adult rat cardiac fibroblasts: response to angiotensin II and aldosterone. J Mol Cell Cardiol 1994;26:809–20.

20. Harada E, Yoshimura M, Yasue H, et al. Aldosterone induces angiotensin-converting-enzyme gene expression in cultured neonatal rat cardiocytes. Circulation 2001;104:137–9.

21. Hornig B, Kohler C, Drexler H. Role of bradykinin in mediating vascular effects of angiotensin-converting enzyme inhibitors in humans. Circulation 1997;95:1115–8.

22. Levine TB, Olivari MT, Garberg V, et al. Hemodynamic and clinical response to enalapril, a long-acting converting-enzyme inhibitor, in patients with congestive heart failure. Circulation 1984;69:548–53.

23. Uretsky BF, Shaver JA, Liang CS, et al. Modulation of hemodynamic effects with a converting enzyme inhibitor: acute hemodynamic dose-response relationship of a new angiotensin converting enzyme inhibitor, lisinopril, with observations on long-term clinical, functional, and biochemical responses. Am Heart J 1988;116:480–8.

24. Pfeffer JM, Pfeffer MA, Braunwald E. Influence of chronic captopril therapy on the infarcted left ventricle of the rat. Circ Res 1985;57:84–95.

25. Sharpe N, Smith H, Murphy J, et al. Early prevention of left ventricular dysfunction after myocardial infarction with angiotensin-converting-enzyme inhibition. Lancet 1991;337:872–6.

26. St John Sutton M, Pfeffer MA, Plappert T, et al. Quantitative two-dimensional echocardiographic measurements are major predictors of adverse cardiovascular events after acute myocardial infarction. The protective effects of captopril. Circulation 1994;89:68–75.

27. Konstam MA, Rousseau MF, Kronenberg MW, et al. Effects of the angiotensin converting enzyme inhibitor enalapril on the long-term progression of left ventricular dysfunction in patients with heart failure. Circulation 1992;86:431–8.

28. Konstam MA, Kronenberg MW, Rousseau MF, et al. Effects of the angiotensin converting enzyme inhibitor enalapril on the long-term progression of left ventricular dilatation in patients with asymptomatic systolic dysfunction. Circulation 1993;88:2277–83.

29. Enalapril for congestive heart failure. N Engl J Med 1987;317:1349–51.

30. Effect of enalapril on survival in patients with reduced left ventricular ejection fractions and congestive heart failure. N Engl J Med 1991;325:293–302.

31. Effect of enalapril on mortality and the development of heart failure in asymptomatic patients with reduced left ventricular ejection fractions. N Engl J Med 1992;327:685–91.

32. Pfeffer MA, Braunwald E, Moye LA, et al. Effect of captopril on mortality and morbidity in patients with left ventricular dysfunction after myocardial infarction. Results of the survival and ventricular enlargement trial. N Engl J Med 1992;327:669–77.

33. Effect of ramipril on mortality and morbidity of survivors of acute myocardial infarction with clinical evidence of heart failure. Lancet 1993;342:821–8.

34. Kober L, Torp-Pedersen C, Carlsen JE, et al. A clinical trial of the angiotensin-converting-enzyme inhibitor trandolapril in patients with left ventricular dysfunction after myocardial infarction. N Engl J Med 1995;333:1670–6.

35. Cohn JN, Johnson G, Ziesche S, et al. A comparison of enalapril with hydralazine-isosorbide dinitrate in the treatment of chronic congestive heart failure. N Engl J Med 1991;325:303–10.

36. Packer M, Poole-Wilson PA, Armstrong PW, et al. Comparative effects of low and high doses of the angiotensin-converting enzyme inhibitor, lisinopril, on morbidity and mortality in chronic heart failure. Circulation 1999;100:2312–8.

37. Yusuf S, Sleight P, Pogue J, et al. Effects of an angiotensin-converting-enzyme inhibitor, ramipril, on cardiovascular events in high-risk patients. N Engl J Med 2000;342:145–53.

38. Fox KM, EURopean trial On reduction of cardiac events with Perindopril in stable coronary Artery disease Investigators. Efficacy of perindopril in reduction of cardiovascular events among patients with stable coronary artery disease: randomized, double-blind, placebo-controlled, multicentre trial (the EUROPA study). Lancet 2003;362:782–8.

39. Braunwald E, Domanski MJ, Fowler SE, et al. Angiotensin-converting-enzyme inhibition in stable coronary artery disease. N Engl J Med 2004;351:2058–68.

40. Dagenais GR, Pogue J, Fox K, et al. Angiotensin-converting-enzyme inhibitors in stable vascular disease without left ventricular systolic dysfunction or heart failure: a combined analysis of three trials. Lancet 2006;368:581–8.

41. Havranek EP, Thomas I, Smith WB, et al. Dose-related beneficial long-term hemodynamic and clinical efficacy of irbesartan in heart failure. J Am Coll Cardiol 1999;33:1174–81.

42. Lang RM, Elkayam U, Yellen LG, et al. Comparative effects of losartan and enalapril on exercise capacity and clinical status in patients with heart failure. J Am Coll Cardiol 1997;30:983–91.

43. Pitt B, Poole-Wilson PA, Segal R, et al. Effect of losartan compared with captopril on mortality in patients with symptomatic heart failure: randomised trial–the Losartan Heart Failure Survival Study ELITE II. Lancet 2000;355:1582–7.

44. Dickstein K, Kjekshus J, OPTIMAAL Steering Committee of the OPTIMAAL Study Group. Effects of

losartan and captopril on mortality and morbidity in high-risk patients after acute myocardial infarction: the OPTIMAAL randomised trial. Lancet 2002;360: 752–60.

45. Pfeffer MA, McMurray JJ, Velazquez EJ, et al. Valsartan, captopril, or both in myocardial infarction complicated by heart failure, left ventricular dysfunction, or both. N Engl J Med 2003;349:1893–906.

46. Granger CB, McMurray JJ, Yusuf S, et al. Effects of candesartan in patients with chronic heart failure and reduced left-ventricular systolic function intolerant to angiotensin-converting-enzyme inhibitors: the CHARM-Alternative trial. Lancet 2003;362: 772–6.

47. Konstam MA, Neaton JD, Dickstein K, et al. Effects of high-dose versus low-dose losartan on clinical outcomes in patients with heart failure (HEAAL study): a randomised, double-blind trial. Lancet 2009;374:1840–8.

48. Cohn JN, Tognoni G, Valsartan Heart Failure Trial Investigators. A randomized trial of the angiotensin-receptor blocker valsartan in chronic heart failure. N Engl J Med 2001;345:1667–75.

49. McMurray JJ, Ostergren J, Swedberg K, et al. Effects of candesartan in patients with chronic heart failure and reduced left-ventricular systolic function taking angiotensin-converting-enzyme inhibitors: the CHARM-Added trial. Lancet 2003;362: 767–71.

50. Yusuf S, Pfeffer MA, Swedberg K, et al. Effects of candesartan in patients with chronic heart failure and preserved left-ventricular ejection fraction: the CHARM-Preserved Trial. Lancet 2003;362: 777–81.

51. Kim S, Yoshiyama M, Izumi Y, et al. Effects of combination of ACE inhibitor and angiotensin receptor blocker on cardiac remodeling, cardiac function, and survival in rat heart failure. Circulation 2001; 103:148–54.

52. Baruch L, Anand I, Cohen IS, et al. Augmented short- and long-term hemodynamic and hormonal effects of an angiotensin receptor blocker added to angiotensin converting enzyme inhibitor therapy in patients with heart failure. Circulation 1999;99: 2658–64.

53. Hamroff G, Katz SD, Mancini D, et al. Addition of angiotensin II receptor blockade to maximal angiotensin-converting enzyme inhibition improves exercise capacity in patients with severe congestive heart failure. Circulation 1999;99:990–2.

54. Lakhdar R, Al-Mallah MH, Lanfear DE. Safety and tolerability of angiotensin-converting enzyme inhibitor versus the combination of angiotensin-converting enzyme inhibitor and angiotensin receptor blocker in patients with left ventricular dysfunction: a systematic review and meta-analysis of randomized controlled trials. J Card Fail 2008;14:181–8.

55. Fraccarollo D, Galuppo P, Hildemann S, et al. Additive improvement of left ventricular remodeling and neurohormonal activation by aldosterone receptor blockade with eplerenone and ACE inhibition in rats with myocardial infarction. J Am Coll Cardiol 2003;42:1666–73.

56. Suzuki G, Morita H, Mishima T, et al. Effects of long-term monotherapy with eplerenone, a novel aldosterone blocker, on progression of left ventricular dysfunction and remodeling in dogs with heart failure. Circulation 2002;106:2967–72.

57. Hayashi M, Tsutamoto T, Wada A, et al. Immediate administration of mineralocorticoid receptor antagonist spironolactone prevents post-infarct left ventricular remodeling associated with suppression of a marker of myocardial collagen synthesis in patients with first anterior acute myocardial infarction. Circulation 2003;107: 2559–65.

58. Zannad F, Alla F, Dousset B, et al. Limitation of excessive extracellular matrix turnover may contribute to survival benefit of spironolactone therapy in patients with congestive heart failure: insights from the randomized aldactone evaluation study (RALES). Circulation 2000;102:2700–6.

59. Pitt B, Zannad F, Remme WJ, et al. The effect of spironolactone on morbidity and mortality in patients with severe heart failure. N Engl J Med 1999;341:709–17.

60. Pitt B, Remme W, Zannad F, et al. Eplerenone, a selective aldosterone blocker, in patients with left ventricular dysfunction after myocardial infarction. N Engl J Med 2003;348:1309–21.

61. Zannad F, McMurray JJ, Krum H, et al. Eplerenone in patients with systolic heart failure and mild symptoms. N Engl J Med 2011;364:11–21.

62. Juurlink DN, Mamdani MM, Lee DS, et al. Rates of hyperkalemia after publication of the Randomized Aldactone Evaluation Study. N Engl J Med 2004; 351:543–51.

63. McMurray JJ, Pitt B, Latini R, et al. Effects of the oral direct renin inhibitor aliskiren in patients with symptomatic heart failure. Circ Heart Fail 2008;1: 17–24.

64. Parving HH, Brenner BM, McMurray JJ, et al. Cardiorenal end points in a trial of aliskiren for type 2 diabetes. N Engl J Med 2012;367:2204–13.

65. Solomon SD, Shin SH, Shah A, et al. Effect of the direct renin inhibitor aliskiren on left ventricular remodeling following myocardial infarction with systolic dysfunction. Eur Heart J 2011;32: 1227–34.

66. Gheorghiade M, Bohm M, Greene SJ, et al. Effect of aliskiren on postdischarge mortality and heart failure readmissions among patients hospitalized for heart failure: the ASTRONAUT randomized trial. JAMA 2013;309:1125–35.

67. Cleland JG, Tendera M, Adamus J, et al. The perindopril in elderly people with chronic heart failure (PEP-CHF) study. Eur Heart J 2006;27:2338–45.

68. Massie BM, Carson PE, McMurray JJ, et al. Irbesartan in patients with heart failure and preserved ejection fraction. N Engl J Med 2008;359:2456–67.

69. Edelmann F, Wachter R, Schmidt AG, et al. Effect of spironolactone on diastolic function and exercise capacity in patients with heart failure with preserved ejection fraction: the Aldo-DHF randomized controlled trial. JAMA 2013;309: 781–91.

The Sympathetic Nervous System and Heart Failure

David Y. Zhang, MD, PhD[a], Allen S. Anderson, MD[b],*

KEYWORDS

- Heart failure • Sympathetic nervous system • Neurohormone • Renin-angiotensin-aldosterone

KEY POINTS

- Heart failure is a syndrome characterized by upregulation of the sympathetic nervous system and abnormal responsiveness of the parasympathetic nervous system.
- Hyperactivity of the sympathetic nervous system is triggered by both central and peripheral pathways that are associated with abnormal cardiovascular reflexes observed in a variety of disease states such as cardiac ischemia, ventricular dysfunction, renal failure, and obstructive sleep apnea.
- The renin-angiotensin aldosterone axis is the major regulator of the sympathetic nervous system in the brain.
- Sympathetic hyperactivity in heart failure leads to specific adverse effects which worsen the disease process including adverse remodeling, alteration of the beta adrenergic receptor system, and skeletal muscle abnormalities.
- The parasympathetic nervous system is also altered in heart failure with resulting adverse effects.

INTRODUCTION

Heart failure (HF) is a syndrome characterized by upregulation of the sympathetic nervous system and abnormal responsiveness of the parasympathetic nervous system.[1] Evidence for this dysregulation has included the demonstration of abnormalities in HF patients, including increased urinary catecholamine levels, increased plasma norepinephrine, increased sympathetic tone, and abnormalities in cardiovascular reflexes. Later studies showed that the degree of sympathetic activation as measured by plasma norepinephrine levels correlated with New York Heart Association (NYHA) functional capacity and prognosis, with higher levels portending a worse outcome and NYHA class.[2] The 1980s and 1990s witnessed the development of the neurohormonal hypothesis of HF, and the demonstration that inhibition of the renin-angiotensin-aldosterone system with angiotensin-converting enzyme inhibitors improved symptoms and mortality in HF resulting from systolic dysfunction. These events shifted the paradigm of treating HF and provided a framework to consider the use of β-blockers for HF therapy, contrary to the prevailing wisdom of the time. Against this backdrop, this article reviews the contemporary understanding of the sympathetic nervous system and the failing heart.

THE AUTONOMIC NERVOUS SYSTEM AND THE HEART

The sympathetic nervous system (SNS) has a wide variety of cardiovascular effects, including heart-rate acceleration, increased cardiac contractility, reduced venous capacitance, and peripheral vasoconstriction.[1,3] Conversely, the parasympathetic nervous system affects the cardiovascular system by slowing the heart rate through vagal innervation.[4]

The authors have nothing to disclose.
a Section of Cardiology, Department of Medicine, University of Chicago, 5841 S. Maryland Ave, Chicago, IL 60637, USA; b Center for Heart Failure, Bluhm Cardiovascular Institute, Feinberg School of Medicine, Northwestern University, 676 North Saint Clair Street, Suite 600, Chicago, IL 60611, USA
* Corresponding author.
E-mail address: aanderso@nmff.org

Cardiol Clin 32 (2014) 33–45
http://dx.doi.org/10.1016/j.ccl.2013.09.010

cardiology.theclinics.com

Anatomy

Cardiac sympathetic nerve fibers travel along coronary arteries at the subepicardial level, predominantly in the ventricles.[3] The cardiac parasympathetic nerve fibers run with the vagal nerve subendocardially after crossing the atrioventricular groove, and are abundant mainly in atrial myocardium and less so in the ventricle myocardium.[5]

Physiology

Four categories of the physiologic effects are observed after SNS activation.[6] (1) Norepinephrine (NE) released from neurons via the left stellate ganglions reaches the left ventricles, leading to an increase in contractile strength and blood pressure; NE released from neurons via the right stellate ganglion increases heart rate and shortens atrioventricular conduction via the sinus and atrioventricular nodes. (2) Epinephrine released into circulation by the adrenal cortex exerts effects on both the myocardium and peripheral vessels. (3) Locally released epinephrine and NE have direct effects on peripheral vessels. (4) Circulating norepinephrine acts in multiple locations, such as to increase heart rate during exercise of heart-transplant recipients who lack adrenergic innervation to the cardiac allograft.

Receptors

Norepinephrine and epinephrine released by components of the sympathetic nerve system bind to specific adrenergic receptors (ARs). All ARs are proteins embedded in the cell membrane with 7 transmembrane structures, coupling to heterotrimeric G proteins (**Fig. 1**). β-Receptor density displays a gradient, greatest at the apex and decreasing toward the base. There are a total of 9 different AR subtypes including 3 α1-receptors, 3 α2-receptors, and 3 β-receptors (β1, β2, and β3).[7] The human heart contains mainly β1, β2, and β3 receptors.[7] Activation of β1- and β2-ARs is the most powerful physiologic mechanism to acutely increase cardiac performance via positive inotropic, dromotropic, and chronotropic effects. β1-ARs activate G_s proteins, whereas β2-ARs couple both G_i and G_s proteins. G_s signaling acts as a "receptor accelerator" and G_i signaling acts as a "receptor brake."[8] The human heart also expresses α1-ARs at low levels (about 20%), but its role in physiologic conditions is unknown.[9]

REFLEX MECHANISM OF SYMPATHETIC HYPERACTIVITY IN HEART FAILURE
Afferent Pathways

Our present understanding of the complex mechanisms engaged by HF arises primarily from the application of NE kinetic methods, which quantify the spillover into plasma from total body, cardiac, renal, brain, or forearm NE production, and from microneurographic recordings obtained from sympathetic fibers innervating muscle or cutaneous vascular beds.[3,10,11] The latter technology refers to muscle sympathetic nerve activity (MSNA), which is a real-time measure of sympathetic nerve activity characterized by inserting a tungsten microelectrode into the muscle fascicle of the innervating peripheral nerve. Based on animal and human studies, the main reflex responses originate from the following afferent pathways (**Fig. 2**):

- Aortic arch and carotid baroreceptors (SNS inhibition)

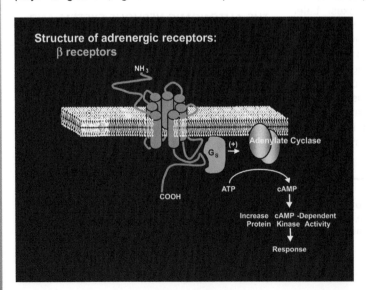

Fig. 1. β-Receptors are G-protein–coupled receptors, and they act by activating a G_s protein. G_s activates adenylyl cyclase, leading to an increase in levels of intracellular cyclic adenosine monophosphate (cAMP). Increased cAMP activates protein kinase A, which phosphorylates cellular proteins. ATP, adenosine triphosphate.

Structure of adrenergic receptors:
β receptors

NH₃

Adenylate Cyclase

G_s (+)

ATP   cAMP

COOH

Increase cAMP -Dependent
Protein Kinase Activity

Response

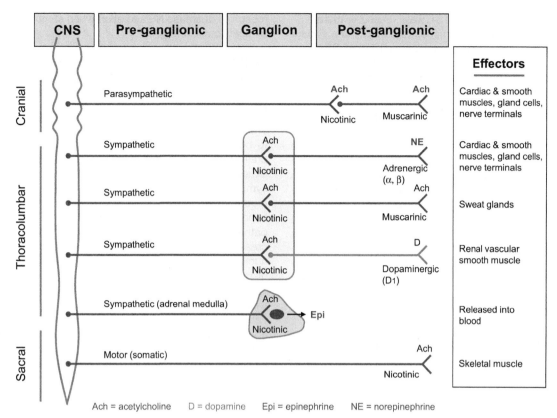

Fig. 2. Summary of sympathetic and parasympathetic autonomic neural outflows from the central nervous system (CNS) that regulate the cardiovascular system. There are 2 major sets of neurons serially connected to regulate peripheral target organs controlled by the motor outflow of the sympathetic nervous system. The first set, called preganglionic neurons, originates in the brainstem or the spinal cord. The postganglionic neurons are the second set, located in a group of nerve cells called sympathetic ganglia outside the central nervous system. The predominant neurotransmitter of the sympathetic preganglionic neurons is acetylcholine. On the other hand, the predominant neurotransmitter of most sympathetic postganglionic neurons is norepinephrine, with exceptions such as postganglionic neurons innervating sweat glands by releasing acetylcholine. (*Adapted from* Johnston TB, Whillis J. Gray's anatomy. 31st edition. London: Longmans; 1954.)

- Cardiopulmonary baroreceptors (diverse reflexes including the Bezold-Jarisch reflex, SNS inhibition)
- Cardiovascular-low threshold polymodal receptors (SNS activation)
- Peripheral chemoreceptors (SNS activation)[5]

In systolic HF, SNS hyperactivity is closely related to abnormalities observed in the cardiovascular reflexes.[1,3] The SNS inhibitory reflexes such as the arterial baroreceptor reflex are significantly suppressed, whereas the SNS excitatory reflexes such as the peripheral chemoreceptor reflex are augmented.[12] In asymptomatic patients with left ventricular dysfunction, SNS activation precedes the development of symptoms and is related to poor survival.[13] Of interest, decreased parasympathetic tone is noted to precede sympathetic activation in a canine model of nonischemic HF.[14] It has long been considered that a generalized activation of the SNS in left ventricular systolic dysfunction leads to alterations of cardiac and peripheral hemodynamics, which are initially appropriate but eventually pathologic.[15] However, the time course and magnitude of SNS activation are now recognized to be organ-specific and independent of ventricular systolic dysfunction.[3]

Obstructive sleep apnea
Among HF patients, approximately one-third have obstructive sleep apnea (OSA) and one-third have central sleep apnea.[16] It has been demonstrated that each pause in breathing during sleep elicits profound increases in MSNA in humans with OSA.[17] Compared with HF patients without sleep apnea, MSNA was 11 bursts per 100 heartbeats higher in those with existing OSA.[18] In a subset study of a randomized controlled trial, MSNA in patients was decreased by 12 bursts per 100 heartbeats after they received successful

continuous positive airway pressure therapy.[19] These data have demonstrated that 2 independent sympathoexcitatory processes (HF and OSA) can increase MSNA via an additive summation effect. Sleep-related breathing disorders provide a potent stimulus for adrenergic upregulation.

Myocardial ischemia and infarction

One study followed patients with relatively preserved ejection fraction (mean 52%) 6 months after myocardial infarction. These subjects were noted to have higher MSNA burst incidence in comparison with patients with coronary artery disease or healthy control subjects.[20] Compared with patients with nonischemic cardiomyopathy and a low left ventricular ejection fraction, MSNA was significantly higher in those with ischemic cardiomyopathy.[21] Myocardial ischemia and prior infarction have adverse effects on sympathetic outflow, both additive and independent of magnitude of ejection fraction.[3]

Reflex from skeletal muscle

Skeletal muscles have the capacity to increase the set point of central sympathetic outflow in HF at rest or during exercise. This reset can be achieved by an adenosine/angiotensin-mediated sympathoexcitatory reflex, activation of a muscle mechanoreflex elicited by passive exercise, or a muscle metaboreflex activated by handgrip.[22–24]

Renal failure

MSNA stimulation is noted in patients with chronic renal failure.[25] Similar activation in milder renal insufficiency or the cardiorenal syndrome may lead to increased adrenergic stimulation.

Efferent Pathways

Coordination of sympathetic outflow from the brain begins in the dorsolateral reticular formation of the medulla, and is modulated by the hypothalamus. Two sets of motor neurons conduct signals to the periphery, preganglionic and postganglionic. The preganglionic fibers originate from the brainstem or the lateral horns of thoracolumbar spinal cord segments. These short, myelinated fibers use acetylcholine as a neurotransmitter, and synapse either with chromaffin cells in the adrenal medulla or with postganglionic fibers in either paravertebral or prevertebral (also known as preaortic) ganglia. These fibers travel along blood vessels in the periphery or in the heart. Norepinephrine is the principal neurotransmitter distally. NE uptake and release into the synaptic junction may be inhibited by presynaptic α2-receptor antagonists and increased by β2-receptor stimulation with epinephrine. Terminal muscarinic

receptors decrease NE secretion when stimulated by acetylcholine (**Fig. 3**).[1,3]

CENTRAL MECHANISM OF SYMPATHETIC HYPERACTIVITY IN HEART FAILURE
Coupling of Renin-Angiotensin System and Reactive Oxidative Stress in Brain

The renin-angiotensin system (RAS) is considered to be the main system of regulating SNS in the brain.[26] The brain RAS system is activated in experimental chronic systolic HF with enhanced sympathetic outflow.[27] Angiotensin II type 1 (AT1) receptors are expressed at high levels in areas of hypothalamus and medulla, which regulate sympathetic outflow.[28] In addition, aldosterone can increase AT1 receptor levels in the paraventricular nucleus (PVN) of the hypothalamus.[29] The mechanism of RAS causing sympathetic excitation is involved with brain reactive oxidative stress. It is well established that activation of the AT1 receptor can induce oxidative stress in the rostral ventrolateral medulla (RVLM), known as the vasomotor center.[27] In animal models of chronic HF, microinjection of angiotensin II into the RVLM results in sympathoexcitation, whereas microinjection of AT1 receptor blockers into the RVLM causes sympathoinhibition.[27]

Brain Inflammatory Mediators

Nuclear factor κB (NF-κB) exhibits cross-talk between proinflammatory cytokines and brain RAS in rats with chronic systolic HF.[30] Nitric oxide (NO) causes sympathoinhibition in the brain, probably through the mechanism of counteracting oxidative stress.[31] Overexpression of NO synthase in the brain can attenuate abnormal sympathoexcitation in mice with HF. Of note, small G-protein Rho/Rho kinase pathway, mineralocorticoid receptors, Na sensitivity, or toll-like receptor 4 in the brain each can cause sympathoexcitation in a rat model of systolic HF.

In 2009, Floras[3] proposed a new model of SNS activation in systolic HF that characterized a balance between normal compensatory reflexes and excessive responses in the setting of increased adrenergic output attributable to a higher central adrenergic set point (see **Fig. 1**). Critical components of this model included: (1) impaired vagally mediated arterial baroreceptor reflex regulation of heart rate; (2) MSNA regulated by an arterial baroreflex that rapidly responds to changes in diastolic blood pressure, modulates generalized sympathetic discharge, and responds to diminished pulsatile arterial mechanoreceptor stretch by adjusting, as required, a centrally established set point for sympathetic outflow; (3) pulmonary

Diagram of the adrenergic synapse

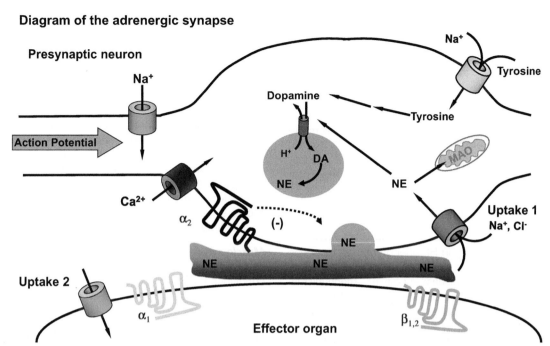

Fig. 3. Adrenergic receptors and norepinephrine (NE) transport in the cardiac presynaptic nerve terminal. Thick solid black arrows indicate processes that facilitate NE transport to and from the synaptic cleft. Dashed black arrow shows negative feedback mechanisms that affect secretion. NE is stored within vesicles at the sympathetic nerve terminal. Sympathetic nerve activity results in release of NE from the storage vesicles in the synaptic cleft, where it is available to attach to postsynaptic α1-, β1-, and β2-adrenergic receptors, as well as presynaptic adrenergic receptors. In addition to these postsynaptic adrenergic receptors, there are presynaptic α2-adrenergic receptors located on the sympathetic nerve terminal. Activation of the α2 presynaptic receptor by an agonist reduces release of NE from the sympathetic nerve terminal, decreasing NE in the cleft and decreasing adrenergic activation of the cardiomyocyte. MAO, monoamine oxidase.

mechanoreceptor-mediated entrainment of sympathetic outflow; (4) blunted inhibitory ventricular baroreceptor reflex control of MSNA; and (5) increased cardiac norepinephrine spillover early in the course of HF caused by a cardiac-specific sympathoexcitatory reflex stimulated in the setting of elevated left ventricular diastolic filling pressures.

EFFECT OF SYMPATHETIC HYPERACTIVITY ON HEART FAILURE
NE Spillover

In systolic HF, sympathetic hyperactivity is evidenced by increased plasma NE levels, central sympathetic outflow, and NE plasma spillover from activated sympathetic nerve fibers.[1] While NE clearance is reduced in patients with HF, it does not account for the increased NE measured. The use of isotope dilution methods to measure cardiac NE plasma release have indicated as much as a 50-fold increased cardiac NE spillover in untreated systolic HF.[1] In addition, systolic HF patients may have decreased NE concentrations

in the cardiomyocytes and/or reduced postsynaptic β-receptor density.[1]

Cardiac Remodeling

In HF, the cardiac neuronal hierarchy undergoes a pathologic remodeling process. Spatially organized reflexes acting in isolation may destabilize efferent neuronal control of regional cardiac mechanical and/or electrical events.[1] For example, angiotensin II can initiate a positive feedback mechanism, leading to upregulated AT1 receptors, NO inhibition, and increasing oxidative stress by increased production of superoxide anion.[32] This pathway can lead to further increases in sympathetic outflow and disease progression.

Receptor Level Changes

Prolonged SNS activation can adversely affect excitation-contraction coupling and enhance the apoptotic pathways, playing a central role in the disease progression of chronic HF.[33] A striking characteristic of HF is the set of molecular events in the β-AR signaling pathway, including a decrease in β1-AR density, uncoupling of β1-ARs from G_s, increased G_i protein, and impaired compartmentalization of cyclic adenosine monophosphate/protein kinase A signaling.[34] The role of β2-AR in HF has not been described clearly. There is no significant change in the levels of β2-ARs in the failing heart.[35] The role of β3-ARs in HF has not been elucidated. Recently it has been demonstrated that β-AR desensitization by tumor necrosis factor α is mediated by G-protein–coupled receptor kinase 2 and is agonist independent, suggesting a novel mechanism for inflammatory modulation of β-receptor response.[36]

Impact of β-Adrenergic Receptor Polymorphism

Marked variability in HF phenotype and response to therapy implies complex interactions of genetic variations and disease-modifying mechanisms. Polymorphisms in adrenergic receptor genes have been associated with variable clinical response to β-blocker therapy through the study of pharmacogenomics. A substudy of BEST (Beta Blocker Evaluation of Survival Trial), a bucindolol versus placebo HF trial, demonstrated drug response variability that was dependent on 2 coding AR polymorphisms: the Arg389Gly of the β1-AR, and a position 322-325 4-amino-acid deletion (Del) in the prejunctional sympathetic nerve terminal α2C-AR.[37] Subpopulations with enhanced (β(1)389 Arg homozygotes), intermediate (β(1)389 Gly carriers + α(2C)322-325 Wt homozygotes), and no (β(1)389 Gly carriers + α(2C)322-325 Del carriers) efficacy were identified.[38] A substudy of HF-ACTION (Heart Failure: A Controlled Trial Investigating Outcomes of Exercise TraiNing) patients with the ADRβ1-389 Arg/Arg genotype receiving low-dose β-blockers had a 2-fold increase in the risk of death compared with those receiving a high dose (hazard ratio 2.09; $P = .015$), which was not conferred in Gly carriers.[39] There was a gene-dose interaction with the ADRβ1-389 Arg/Arg versus Gly carrier genotype and β-blocker dose, suggesting that patients with the Arg/Arg genotype might require a higher dose of β-blockade to achieve a treatment response similar to that of Gly carriers.

ROLE OF PARASYMPATHETIC DYSFUNCTION IN HEART FAILURE

The sensory endings of both vagal and sympathetic afferent fibers in the heart are mechanoreceptors, thereby stimulated by the mechanical stretching associated with cardiac dilatation in HF. In HF with chamber dilatation, both vagal and sympathetic afferent cardiac fibers increase firing, as a result of

which the afferent sympathetic excitation leads to tonic and reflex inhibition of cardiac vagal efferent activity.[5] In cases of diastolic dysfunction with no dilatation of heart, the mechanism of reduced vagal activity has not been fully determined.[15]

Translation into Heart Failure: Diagnostic Implications

Two state-of-the-art techniques can be used to quantify sympathetic nerve activity with potential diagnostic values: the radiotracer measurement of regional NE spillover and microneurography (microelectrode direct measurement of postganglionic sympathetic nerve activity: the proximate neural stimulus to NE release).

Muscle sympathetic nerve activity

Excessive sympathetic activation under resting conditions has been shown to increase from the early stages of systolic HF, and is related to prognosis. Direct recording of multiunit efferent MSNA by microneurography is the best method for quantifying sympathetic nerve activity in humans.[40] To date, this technique has been used to evaluate the actual central sympathetic outflow to the periphery in HF patients at rest and during exercise. However, because the firing occurrence of sympathetic activation is mainly synchronized by pulse pressure, multiunit MSNA, expressed as burst frequency (bursts/min) and burst incidence (bursts/100 heartbeats), may have limitations for the quantification of sympathetic nerve activity.[40] In HF, multiunit MSNA is near the maximum level, and cannot increase more than the heartbeat. Although single-unit MSNA analysis in humans is technically demanding, it provides more detailed information regarding central sympathetic firing.

Nuclear imaging

Cardiac neuronal distribution and function can be imaged using radiolabeled analogues of NE with standard gamma cameras and positron emission tomography (PET). In addition, postsynaptic β-AR distribution and density can also be determined by PET. An analogue of NE, ^{123}I-metaiodobenzylguanidine (MIBG), can be used to measure cardiac sympathetic neuronal activity noninvasively, as well as other semiquantitative parameters including early heart-to-mediastinum ratio, late heart-to-mediastinum ratio, and myocardial washout. Decreased late heart-to-mediastinum ratio or increased myocardial MIBG washout is associated with a worse prognosis in comparison with those patients having normal myocardial MIBG parameters.[41] β-Blockade and renin-angiotensin-aldosterone inhibition are associated with an increase in MIBG uptake and a reduced washout.[1] The ADMIRE-HF (AdreView Myocardial Imaging for Risk Evaluation in Heart Failure) trial demonstrated that MIBG cardiac imaging can provide independent prognostic information for risk-stratifying patients with HF, in additional to commonly used markers such as left ventricular ejection fraction and B-type natriuretic pepetide.[42] The survival data from 961 patients of NYHA class II to III in the ADMIRE-HF trial were analyzed using the Seattle Heart Failure Model (SHFM). The addition of MIBG imaging to the SHFM improves risk stratification, especially in higher-risk patients. MIBG may have clinical utility in higher-risk patients who are being considered for therapy such as implantable cardioverter-defibrillators, cardiac resynchronization devices, left ventricular assist devices (LVADs), and cardiac transplantation.[43]

Other measurements

The measurement of plasma NE can only be used as a crude guide to assess SNS activity, because it depends on the rate of immediate NE reuptake and NE clearance from circulation.[1] Also, the technique for measuring serum levels is somewhat complicated. Nevertheless, elevated plasma NE levels have been correlated with NYHA functional capacity and prognosis in patients with left ventricular systolic HF. Heart-rate variability (HRV), an easily performed noninvasive methodology, does have prognostic significance (ie, decreased HRV is a negative prognosticator) but practical limitations, given that a high percentage of the HF subjects have atrial fibrillation, paced rhythm, or are diabetic (associated with autonomic dysfunction and decreased HRV).[1]

THE SYMPATHETIC NERVOUS SYSTEM IN HEART FAILURE: THERAPEUTIC IMPLICATIONS
β-Blockers

β-Blockers can be broadly classified into 3 generations based on receptor-level activity:

1. First generation, which are nonselective and competitively block both the β1- and β2-receptors (propranolol, nadolol, timolol)
2. Second generation, with much higher affinity for the β1- than for the β2-receptor (atenolol, metoprolol, bisoprolol)
3. Third generation, which may be selective (celiprolol, nebivolol) or nonselective (bucindolol, carvedilol, labetalol), but all causing peripheral vasodilatation mediated via either α1-receptor blockade (bucindolol, carvedilol, labetalol), β2-receptor agonism (celiprolol), or NO synthesis (nebivolol).[44]

Among all β-blockers, bisoprolol (except in the United States), carvedilol, and metoprolol succinate (except in Canada) are almost universally approved for the treatment of chronic systolic HF (**Table 1**).[1] Carvedilol was the first β-blocker with demonstrated efficacy in chronic systolic HF. The US Carvedilol Trials program demonstrated that administration of the β-blocker to a population of predominantly NYHA Class II and III patients who were stable on a background regimen of angiotensin-converting enzyme (ACE) inhibitors, diuretics, and digoxin reduced all-cause mortality by 65% and the risk of death or hospitalization for cardiovascular reasons by 35%. Of note, the trial was stopped early by the trial's Data Safety and Monitoring Board because of the drug's observed favorable effect on mortality.[45] The Carvedilol Prospective Randomized Cumulative Survival Study Group (COPERNICUS) Study in 1997 extended the evidence of efficacy to a sicker HF population, and included patients who were recently NYHA Class IV and hospitalized patients.[46] Subsequently, similar beneficial results were observed with metoprolol succinate (Metoprolol CR/XL Randomized Intervention Trial in Congestive Heart Failure [MERIT-HF]) and bisoprolol (The Cardiac Insufficiency Bisoprolol Study II [CIBIS-II]).[47,48] Clearly, however, not all β-blockers are efficacious in chronic HF. Bucindolol, a nonselective β-blocker with α-blocking effects, failed to demonstrate a survival benefit, and metoprolol tartrate, a selective β-blocker, at a relatively low dose of 50 mg twice daily, was inferior to carvedilol.[49,50] Extensive clinical studies have established that chronic β-blocker therapy with carvedilol, metoprolol succinate, or bisoprolol improves left ventricular performance and reverses left ventricular remodeling, reduces the risk of hospitalization, and improves survival.[1] However, the exact mechanism(s) for these laudatory effects are not clearly defined.

α-Blockers

As potent arteriolar vasodilators, this class of drugs was initially thought to have promise as HF therapy. Prazosin was compared with hydralazine and isosorbide dinitrate originally in the Veterans Administration Cooperative Study (V-HeFT). However, patients in the prazosin arm experienced worse outcomes than those receiving the combined vasodilator therapy of hydralazine and isosorbide dinitrate.[51] The underlying mechanism for this observed adverse effect could be sympathetic upregulation as indicated by increased catecholamine levels after chronic use of prazosin, counteracting any potentially beneficial action mediated through inhibition of the α1-receptor.

Table 1
Large randomized trials with β-blockers and the American College of Cardiology/American Heart Association guidelines on recommended doses

β-Blocker	Trial	Year	n	Benefit	Initial Daily Dose	Maximum Daily Dose
Metoprolol	MDC	1993	383	All-cause mortality or morbidity was 34% lower in the metoprolol than in the placebo group (HR: 0.66; 95% CI: 0.62 to 1.06; $P = .058$). The change in LVEF from baseline to 12 mo was significantly greater with metoprolol than with placebo (0.13 vs 0.06; $P<.0001$)	5–10 mg twice daily	100 mg twice daily
Metoprolol CR/XL	MERIT-HF	1999	3991	All-cause mortality was 34% lower in the metoprolol CR/XL group than in the placebo group (7.2% vs 11.0%; HR: 0.66; 95% CI: 0.53 to 0.81; $P = .00009$)	12.5–25 mg once daily	200 mg once daily
Carvedilol	US Carvedilol HF Study Group	1996	1094	All-cause mortality was 65% lower in the carvedilol than in the placebo group (3.2% vs 7.8%; HR: 0.65; 95% CI: 0.39 to 0.80; $P<.001$)	3.125 mg twice daily	25 mg twice daily
	Australia/New Zealand HF Research Collaborative Group	1997	415	All-cause mortality or morbidity was 26% lower in the carvedilol than in the placebo group (104% vs 131%; HR: 0.74; 95% CI: 0.57–0.95)	—	—
	CAPRICORN	2001	1959	All-cause mortality was lower in the carvedilol than in the placebo group (12% vs 15%; HR: 0.77; 95% CI: 0.60 to 0.98; $P = .03$)	—	—
	COPERNICUS	2001	2289	Carvedilol reduced the combined risk of death or hospitalization for a cardiovascular reason by 27% ($P = .00002$) and the combined risk of death or HF hospitalization by 31% ($P = .000004$)	—	—
	COMET	2003	3029	All-cause mortality was lower in the carvedilol than in the metoprolol group (34% vs 40%; HR: 0.83; 95% CI: 0.74–0.93; $P = .0017$)	—	—
Bisoprolol	CIBIS	1994	641	All-cause mortality did not reach statistical significance: 67 patients died on placebo, 53 on bisoprolol (HR: 0.80; 95% CI: 0.56–1.15; $P = .22$). Bisoprolol reduced HF hospitalization ($P<.01$) and improved the functional status	—	—
	CIBIS-II	1999	2647	All-cause mortality was 34% lower with bisoprolol than on placebo (11.8% vs 17.3%; HR: 0.66; 95% CI: 0.54–0.81; $P<.0001$)	1.25 mg once daily	10 mg once daily
	CIBIS-III	2005	1010	This study demonstrated that it may be as safe and efficacious to initiate treatment of CHF with bisoprolol as with enalapril	—	—
Nebivolol	SENIORS	2005	2128	All-cause mortality or cardiovascular hospital admission occurred in 332 patients (31.1%) on nebivolol compared with 375 (35.3%) on placebo (HR: 0.86; 95% CI: 0.74 to 0.99; $P = .039$)	1.25 mg once daily	10 mg once daily

Abbreviations: CHF, congestive heart failure; CI, confidence interval; HR, hazard ratio; LVEF, left ventricular ejection fraction.

Data from Triposkiadis F, Karayannis G, Giamouzis G, et al. The sympathetic nervous system in heart failure: physiology, pathophysiology, and clinical implications. J Am Coll Cardiol 2009;54(19):1747–62; and Jessup M, Abraham WT, Casey DE, et al. 2009 focused update: ACCF/AHA guidelines for the diagnosis and management of heart failure in adults: a report of the American College of Cardiology Foundation/American Heart Association Task Force on Practice Guidelines: developed in collaboration with the International Society for Heart and Lung Transplantation. Circulation 2009;119(14):1977–2016.

Later, in the ALLHAT (Antihypertensive and Lipid-Lowering Treatment to Prevent Heart Attack Trial) study (ALLHAT collaborative), the study of another α1-blocker, doxazosin, was terminated early because of a higher HF incidence in subjects taking the drug.[15]

Centrally-Acting α2-Blockers

In the past decade, more experiments have revealed that the central nervous system (CNS) plays a key role in the sympathoexcitation noted in HF. Thus, the central α2-receptor has been considered as a possible target in the treatment of HF, because excitation of the central α2-receptor inhibits the activation of the SNS. Clonidine displays α2-agonist actions in the CNS. At modest doses, clonidine significantly attenuates cardiac and renal sympathetic tone in patients with HF.[15] Of interest, chronic clonidine administration exerted marked sympathoinhibitory effects without further clinical deterioration in a small, short-term clinical study.[15] Large clinical trials will be needed to evaluate potential benefits. However, in clinical trials of the centrally acting sympathoinhibitory agent, moxonidine (which acts through both α2- and imidazoline receptors), the drug was associated with an increased mortality.[15,36]

Renin-Angiotensin-Aldosterone Modulators

Angiotensin II and aldosterone production enhance the release and inhibit the uptake of norepinephrine at nerve endings, and thus modulate the adrenergic response in the periphery.[30] However, angiotensin and aldosterone also have targets of action centrally. High densities of AT1 receptors are present in brain regions both outside and inside the blood-brain barrier, thus providing a pathway whereby peripherally administered AT1 receptor blockers are able to exert centrally acting effects on sympathetic activity. Recent studies have suggested that systemically administered AT1 receptor blockers reduced blood pressure in hypertensive rats, by acting on CNS AT1 receptors.[31] Plasma aldosterone levels may be elevated as high as 20-fold in patients with HF, primarily because of increased production by the adrenal glands following stimulation by the high plasma angiotensin II concentrations. Two trials of aldosterone receptor blockers, RALES (Randomized Aldactone Evaluation Study) and EPHESUS (Eplerenone Post-Acute Myocardial Infarction Heart Failure Efficacy and Survival Study), demonstrated the benefit of aldosterone antagonists in HF patients.[52,53] Data have shown that these drugs decrease central sympathetic activity in rats and improve norepinephrine uptake in humans with HF.[15]

Digoxin

Digoxin is considered the oldest HF therapy still in use. Its utility in HF has been debated, but best evidence suggests that it may be an effective agent for improving symptoms and reducing hospitalizations while having a neutral effect on mortality. Digoxin acts via several mechanisms that may be helpful for treating HF, the most commonly acknowledged of which is to increase inotropy by indirectly increasing intracellular calcium available to the sarcoplasmic reticulum. However, digoxin also modulates sympathetic outflow by improving baroreceptor function, decreasing sympathetic tone, and increasing sympathetic tone.[54,55]

Exercise

Exercise intolerance is a hallmark of patients with chronic HF, and skeletal myopathy contributes to the limitation of functional capacity.[15] The activation of SNS and myogenic reflex engagement regulate the heart and muscle vasculature to maintain adequate blood pressure during exercise.[56] However, abnormal activation of the SNS contributes to the skeletal myopathy seen in HF, because SNS-mediated vasoconstriction at rest and during exercise restrains muscle blood flow, arteriolar dilation, and capillary recruitment, leading to underperfusion, ischemia, release of reactive oxygen species, and chronic inflammation.[41] HF-ACTION, the first large, randomized controlled trial to evaluate the effects of exercise training in HF patients, demonstrated that exercise training was safe and offered clinical benefits, although it did not meet its primary end point and was considered a negative trial.[43] Proposed mechanisms beneficial effects include: (1) improvement in arterial and chemoreflex control; (2) significant reduction in central sympathetic outflow; (3) correction of CNS abnormalities; (4) increase in peripheral blood flow; (5) reduction of circulating cytokines; and (6) increase in muscle mass. Experimental evidence suggests that the exercise training–induced beneficial effects on autonomic activity in HF may be due to an upregulation in central antioxidative mechanisms and suppressed central prooxidant mechanisms.[15]

NOVEL THERAPIES AND FUTURE PERSPECTIVES
New Centrally Acting Medications

Previous studies have shown AT1 receptor–induced oxidative stress in the brain, especially in the RVLM, to be a novel therapeutic target for chronic HF through the mechanism of SNS inhibition.[27] Central administration of antisense oligonucleotides targeted against mRNA of the AT1 receptor in a rat model of ischemic HF reduced both the resting sympathetic tone and the sympathetic reflex response.[57] Orally administered atorvastatin causes sympathoinhibition and improves baroreflex dysfunction through reduction of oxidative stress and upregulation of NO synthase in the brain of hypertensive rats.[15] Further clinical trials are necessary to clarify whether statins would have favorable modulatory effects on SNS hyperactivity in human systolic HF.

Parasympathetic stimulation

Research on the therapeutic modulation of cardiac autonomic tone by electrical stimulation has yielded encouraging early clinical results. Vagal nerve stimulation has reduced the rates of morbidity and sudden death from HF therapeutic vagus nerve stimulation is limited by side effects of hypotension and bradycardia.[58] Of interest, the recent Systolic HF trial of treatment with the I_f inhibitor ivabradine (SHIFT) evaluated the effects of ivabradine, a selective inhibitor of the I_f current in the sinoatrial node, without inotropic effects.[59] The results favored ivabradine over placebo regarding lower hospital admission rates due to HF. Sympathetic nerve stimulation implemented in the experiment may exacerbate the sympathetic-dominated autonomic imbalance. By contrast, concurrent stimulation of both sympathetic and parasympathetic cardiac nerves increases myocardial contractility without increasing heart rate.[58]

Renal sympathetic denervation

An ongoing trial of renal sympathetic denervation in patients with treatment-resistant hypertension (SIMPLICITY HTN) uses the strategy of sympathoinhibition to treat resistant hypertension via percutaneous renal sympathetic denervation.[60] Renal afferent nerves project directly into many areas within the CNS, controlling the SNS outflow activity.[61] Resistant hypertension with systolic HF was not an exclusion criterion for the SIMPLICITY trial.[62] Thus, future data from SIMPLICITY (subsets with HF) may demonstrate whether renal nerve ablation is a novel therapy for chronic HF.

Combined SNS inhibition and stimulation

Clenbuterol is a β-blocker with combined β1-inhibition/β2-stimulation effect, and has been proposed as a treatment modality to achieve sustained reversal of severe HF in select patients with LVADs.[63] The rationale for this approach was based on experimental studies demonstrating that clenbuterol treatment, alone or in combination with mechanical unloading, improved left ventricular function at the whole-heart and cellular levels by affecting cell morphology, excitation-contraction coupling, and myofilament sensitivity to calcium.[64]

In a substantial proportion of patients with nonpulsatile LVADs, the use of a combination of mechanical and pharmacologic therapy with β-blockers, ACE inhibitors, or angiotensin receptor blockers, and selective aldosterone receptor antagonists and clenbuterol, resulted in sustained improvement in left ventricular function after removal of the LVAD.[65]

Future perspectives

The mechanisms by which autonomic nervous system dysfunction occurs in HF have not been fully elucidated. In particular, the central abnormalities need further determination in clinical and basic research. How does the brain "recognize" the condition of "HF"? What is the input into the brain, neuronal, or humoral factors? The answers to these questions promise to contribute to a novel concept for the treatment of HF: "the brain is a major target in the treatment of HF through sympathoinhibition."

SPECIAL CATEGORIES IN HEART FAILURE
Diastolic Heart Failure

There is limited information regarding chronic SNS activation in HF with preserved left ventricular ejection fraction (diastolic HF).[66] However, the findings of a study by Grassi and colleagues[67] indicate that in patients with hypertension, SNS hyperactivity (increased muscle sympathetic nerve traffic) may contribute to the development of left ventricular diastolic dysfunction and account for the increased cardiovascular risk.

Left Ventricular Assist Devices

LVADs are now widely accepted as an option for patients with advanced HF. First-generation devices were pulsatile, but had poor longevity and durability. Newer-generation devices are nonpulsatile and more durable, but remain associated with an increased risk of stroke and infection. More importantly, little is understood about the physiologic effects of the chronic absence (or extreme reduction) of pulsatile flow in humans, especially on sympathetic activity. HF patients with continuous, nonpulsatile LVADs have marked sympathetic activation in comparison with healthy controls and patients with pulsatile devices, which at least in part is likely due to baroreceptor unloading.[68] Such chronic sympathetic activation may contribute to or worsen end-organ diseases, and reduce the possibility of ventricular recovery. Strategies to provide some degree of arterial pulsatility, even in continuous-flow LVADs, may be necessary to achieve optimal outcomes in these patients.

Right Heart Failure

There is lack of data evaluating the role of SNS activation in right HF. However, in patients with chronic renal failure, MSNA is stimulated by the afferent signals from the uremic kidney.[25] This reflex may become functionally important in patients with renal failure or right HF.

REFERENCES

1. Triposkiadis F, Karayannis G, Giamouzis G, et al. The sympathetic nervous system in heart failure: physiology, pathophysiology, and clinical implications. J Am Coll Cardiol 2009;54(19):1747–62.
2. Cohn JN, Pfeffer MA, Rouleau J, et al. Adverse mortality effect of central sympathetic inhibition with sustained-release moxonidine in patients with heart failure (MOXCON). Eur J Heart Fail 2003; 5(5):659–67.
3. Floras JS. Sympathetic nervous system activation in human heart failure: clinical implications of an updated model. J Am Coll Cardiol 2009;54(5):375–85.
4. Schwartz PJ. Vagal stimulation for heart diseases: from animals to men. An example of translational cardiology. Circ J 2011;75(1):20–7.
5. Schwartz PJ, De Ferrari GM. Sympathetic-parasympathetic interaction in health and disease: abnormalities and relevance in heart failure. Heart Fail Rev 2011;16(2):101–7.
6. Van Stee EW. Autonomic innervation of the heart. Environ Health Perspect 1978;26:151–8.
7. Bylund D, Bond R, Clarke D, et al. Adrenoceptors. In: Gidlestone, editor. The IUPHAR compendium of receptor characterization and classification. London: IUPHAR Media; 1998. p. 58–74.
8. Feldman DS, Elton TS, Benjmin S, et al. Mechanisms of disease: beta-adrenergic receptors—alterations in signal transduction and pharmacogenomics in heart failure. Nat Clin Pract Cardiovasc Med 2005; 2(9):475–83.
9. Woodcock EA, Du XJ, Reichelt ME, et al. Cardiac alpha 1-adrenergic drive in pathological remodelling. Cardiovasc Res 2008;77(3):452–62.
10. Al-Hesayen A, Parker JD. Impaired baroreceptor control of renal sympathetic activity in human chronic heart failure. Circulation 2004;109(23):2862–5.
11. Vallbo AB, Hagbarth KE, Wallin BG. Microneurography: how the technique developed and its role in the investigation of the sympathetic nervous system. J Appl Physiol 2004;96(4):1262–9.
12. Watson AM, Hood SG, May CN. Mechanisms of sympathetic activation in heart failure. Clin Exp Pharmacol Physiol 2006;33(12):1269–74.
13. Francis GS, Goldsmith SR, Levine TB, et al. The neurohumoral axis in congestive heart failure. Ann Intern Med 1984;101:370–7.
14. Ishise H, Asanoi H, Ishizaka S, et al. Time course of sympathovagal imbalance and left ventricular dysfunction in conscious dogs with heart failure. J Appl Physiol 1998;84(4):1234–41.
15. Kishi T. Heart failure as an autonomic nervous system dysfunction. J Cardiol 2012;59(2):117–22.
16. Wang H, Parker JD, Newton GE, et al. Influence of obstructive sleep apnea on mortality in patients with heart failure. J Am Coll Cardiol 2007;49(15): 1625–31.
17. Somers VK, Dyken ME, Clary MP, et al. Sympathetic neural mechanisms in obstructive sleep apnea. J Clin Invest 1995;96(4):1897–904.
18. Spaak J, Eqri ZJ, Kubo T, et al. Muscle sympathetic nerve activity during wakefulness in heart failure patients with and without sleep apnea. Hypertension 2005;46(6):1327–32.
19. Usui K, Douglas BT, Jonas S, et al. Inhibition of awake sympathetic nerve activity of heart failure patients with obstructive sleep apnea by nocturnal continuous positive airway pressure. J Am Coll Cardiol 2005;45(12):2008–11.
20. Graham LN, Smith PA, Stoker JB, et al. Time course of sympathetic neural hyperactivity after uncomplicated acute myocardial infarction. Circulation 2002;106(7):793–7.
21. Notarius CF, Spaak J, Morris BL, et al. Comparison of muscle sympathetic activity in ischemic and nonischemic heart failure. J Card Fail 2007;13(6): 470–5.
22. Middlekauff HR, Chiu J, Hamilton MA, et al. Muscle mechanoreceptor sensitivity in heart failure. Am J Physiol Heart Circ Physiol 2004;287(5): H1937–43.
23. Notarius CF, Atchison DJ, Rongen GA, et al. Effect of adenosine receptor blockade with caffeine on sympathetic response to handgrip exercise in heart failure. Am J Physiol Heart Circ Physiol 2001;281(3):H1312–8.
24. Rongen GA, Lambrou G, Smits P, et al. Angiotensin AT1 receptor blockade abolishes the reflex sympathoexcitatory response to adenosine. J Clin Invest 1998;101:769–76.
25. Hausberg M, Kosch M, Harmelink P, et al. Sympathetic nerve activity in end-stage renal disease. Circulation 2002;106(15):1974–9.
26. Jankowska EA, Ponikowski P, Piepoli MF, et al. Autonomic imbalance and immune activation in chronic heart failure—pathophysiological links. Cardiovasc Res 2006;70(3):434–45.
27. Zucker IH, Schultz HD, Patel KP, et al. Regulation of central angiotensin type 1 receptors and sympathetic outflow in heart failure. Am J Physiol Heart Circ Physiol 2009;297(5):H1557–66.
28. Fisher JP, Young CN, Fadel PJ. Central sympathetic overactivity: maladies and mechanisms. Auton Neurosci 2009;148(1–2):5–15.

29. Huang BS, Zheng H, Tan J, et al. Regulation of hypothalamic renin-angiotensin system and oxidative stress by aldosterone. Exp Physiol 2011;96(10): 1028–38.

30. Kang YM, Ma Y, Elks C, et al. Cross-talk between cytokines and renin-angiotensin in hypothalamic paraventricular nucleus in heart failure: role of nuclear factor-kappaB. Cardiovasc Res 2008;79(4): 671–8.

31. Hirooka Y, Sagara Y, Kishi T, et al. Oxidative stress and central cardiovascular regulation. Pathogenesis of hypertension and therapeutic aspects. Circ J 2010;74(5):827–35.

32. Garrido AM, Griendling KK. NADPH oxidases and angiotensin II receptor signaling. Mol Cell Endocrinol 2009;302(2):148–58.

33. Piacentino V 3rd, Weber CR, Chen X, et al. Cellular basis of abnormal calcium transients of failing human ventricular myocytes. Circ Res 2003;92(6): 651–8.

34. Dodge-Kafka KL, Soughaver J, Pare GC, et al. The protein kinase A anchoring protein mAKAP coordinates two integrated cAMP effector pathways. Nature 2005;437(7058):574–8.

35. Liggett SB, Tepe NM, Lorenz JN, et al. Early and delayed consequences of beta(2)-adrenergic receptor overexpression in mouse hearts: critical role for expression level. Circulation 2000;101(14): 1707–14.

36. Vasudevan NT, Mohan ML, Gupta MK, et al. Gβγ-independent recruitment of G-protein coupled receptor kinase 2 drives tumor necrosis factor α-induced cardiac β-adrenergic receptor dysfunction. Circulation 2013;128(4):377–87.

37. O'Connor CM, Anand I, Fiuzat M. Additive effects of beta-1 389 Arg/Gly and alpha-2c 322-325 wild-type/del genotype combinations on adjudicated hospitalizations and death in the Beta Blocker Evaluation of Survival Trial (BEST). J Card Fail 2008;14:S69.

38. O'Connor CM, Fiuzat M, Carson PE, et al. Combinatorial pharmacogenetic interactions of bucindolol and β1, α2C adrenergic receptor polymorphisms. PLoS One 2012;7(10):e44324.

39. Fiuzat M, Neely ML, Starr AZ, et al. Association between adrenergic receptor genotypes and beta-blocker dose in heart failure patients: analysis from the HF-Action DNA substudy. Eur J Heart Fail 2013;15(3):258–66.

40. Murai H, Takamura M, Kaneko S. Advantage of recording single-unit muscle sympathetic nerve activity in heart failure. Front Physiol 2012;3:109.

41. Verberne HJ, Brewster LM, Somsen GA, et al. Prognostic value of myocardial ^{123}I-metaiodobenzylguanidine (MIBG) parameters in patients with heart failure: a systematic review. Eur Heart J 2008;29(9):1147–59.

42. Jacobson AF, Lombard J, Banerjee G, et al. ^{123}I-mIBG scintigraphy to predict risk for adverse cardiac outcomes in heart failure patients: design of two prospective multicenter international trials. J Nucl Cardiol 2009;16(1):113–21.

43. Ketchum ES, Jacobcon AF, Caldwell JH, et al. Selective improvement in Seattle Heart Failure Model risk stratification using iodine-123 meta-iodobenzylguanidine imaging. J Nucl Cardiol 2012;19(5): 1007–16.

44. Lopez-Sendon J, Swedberg K, McMurray J, et al. Expert consensus document on beta-adrenergic receptor blockers. Eur Heart J 2004;25(15): 1341–62.

45. Packer M, Bristow MR, Cohn JN, et al. The effect of carvedilol on morbidity and mortality in patients with chronic heart failure. U.S. Carvedilol Heart Failure Study Group. N Engl J Med 1996;334(21): 1349–55.

46. Packer M, Coats A, Fowler MB, et al. Effect of carvedilol on survival in severe chronic heart failure. N Engl J Med 2001;344(22):1651–8.

47. Failure (MERIT-HF). Lancet 1999;353(9169):2001–7.

48. Study II (CIBIS-II): a randomised trial. Lancet 1999; 353(9146):9–13.

49. Beta-Blocker Evaluation of Survival Trial Investigators. A trial of the beta-blocker bucindolol in patients with advanced chronic heart failure. N Engl J Med 2001;344(22):1659–67.

50. Poole-Wilson PA, Swedberg K, Cleland JG, et al. Comparison of carvedilol and metoprolol on clinical outcomes in patients with chronic heart failure in the Carvedilol Or Metoprolol European Trial (COMET): randomised controlled trial. Lancet 2003;362(9377):7–13.

51. Cohn JN, Archibald DG, Ziesche S, et al. Effect of vasodilator therapy on mortality in chronic congestive heart failure. RESults of a Veterans Administration Cooperative Study. N Engl J Med 1886; 314(24):1547–52.

52. Pitt B, Zannad F, Remme WJ, et al. The effect of spironolactone on morbidity and mortality in patients with severe heart failure. Randomized Aldactone Evaluation Study Investigators. N Engl J Med 1999;341(10):709–17.

53. Pitt B, Remme W, Zannad F. Eplerenone, a selective aldosterone blocker, in patients with left ventricular dysfunction after myocardial infarction. N Engl J Med 2003;348(14):1309–21.

54. Thames MD, Miller BD, Abboud FM. Sensitization of vagal cardiopulmonary baroreflex by chronic digoxin. Am J Physiol 1982;243(5):H815–8.

55. Ferguson DW, Berg WJ, Sanders JS, et al. Sympathoinhibitory responses to digitalis glycosides in heart failure patients. Direct evidence from sympathetic neural recordings. Circulation 1989;80(1): 65–77.

56. Khan MH, Sinoway LI. Muscle reflex control of sympathetic nerve activity in heart failure: the role of exercise conditioning. Heart Fail Rev 2000;5(1):87–100.

57. Zhu GQ, Gao L, Li Y, et al. AT1 receptor mRNA antisense normalizes enhanced cardiac sympathetic afferent reflex in rats with chronic heart failure. Am J Physiol Heart Circ Physiol 2004;287(4):H1828–35.

58. Kobayashi M, Sakurai S, Takaseva T, et al. Effect of epivascular cardiac autonomic nerve stimulation on cardiac function. Ann Thorac Surg 2012;94(4):1150–6.

59. Swedberg K, Komajda M, Bohm M, et al. Ivabradine and outcomes in chronic heart failure (SHIFT): a randomised placebo-controlled study. Lancet 2010;376(9744):875–85.

60. Esler MD, Krum H, Schlaich M, et al. Renal sympathetic denervation for treatment of drug-resistant hypertension: one-year results from the Symplicity HTN-2 randomized, controlled trial. Circulation 2012;126(25):2976–82.

61. DiBona GF, Esler M. Translational medicine: the antihypertensive effect of renal denervation. Am J Physiol Regul Integr Comp Physiol 2010;298(2):R245–53.

62. Krum H, Schlaich M, Whitbourn R, et al. Catheter-based renal sympathetic denervation for resistant hypertension: a multicentre safety and proof-of-principle cohort study. Lancet 2009;373(9671):1275–81.

63. Birks EJ, Tansley PD, Hardy J, et al. Left ventricular assist device and drug therapy for the reversal of heart failure. N Engl J Med 2006;355(18):1873–84.

64. Soppa GK, Lee J, Staqq MA, et al. Role and possible mechanisms of clenbuterol in enhancing reverse remodelling during mechanical unloading in murine heart failure. Cardiovasc Res 2008;77(4):695–706.

65. Birks EJ, George RS, Hedqer M, et al. Reversal of severe heart failure with a continuous-flow left ventricular assist device and pharmacological therapy: a prospective study. Circulation 2011;123(4):381–90.

66. Hogg K, McMurray J. Neurohumoral pathways in heart failure with preserved systolic function. Prog Cardiovasc Dis 2005;47(6):357–66.

67. Grassi G, Seravalle G, Quarti-Trevano F, et al. Sympathetic and baroreflex cardiovascular control in hypertension-related left ventricular dysfunction. Hypertension 2009;53(2):205–9.

68. Markham DW, Fu Q, Palmer MD, et al. Sympathetic neural and hemodynamic responses to upright tilt in patients with pulsatile and nonpulsatile left ventricular assist devices. Circ Heart Fail 2013;6(2):293–9.

Evaluation of Patients with Heart Failure

Maria Patarroyo-Aponte, MD[a],
Monica Colvin-Adams, MD, MS, FAHA[b],*

KEYWORDS

- Heart failure • Evaluation • Risk factors • Cardiovascular disease

KEY POINTS

- Identification of risk factors for heart failure and its aggressive treatment are as important as early identification of heart failure.
- A complete patient history and a comprehensive physical examination can provide clues regarding the cause of heart failure and its severity.
- Echocardiogram is the most useful test during diagnosis of heart failure. A comprehensive echocardiogram gives the clinician information regarding ventricular function as well as causes of heart failure and its complications.
- Additional tests during evaluation of patients with heart failure must include routine laboratory tests and, in certain cases, specific laboratory tests and new imaging technologies, including cardiac magnetic resonance and computed tomography angiography.
- Noninvasive impedance cardiography could be helpful for evaluation of volume status in patients with heart failure and prevention of frequent hospitalizations caused by decompensated heart failure.

INTRODUCTION

Heart failure is one of the most prevalent cardiovascular diseases in the United States, and its incidence has been steadily increasing over the years. In 2010, the prevalence of heart failure in US adults was near 6.6 million. It is estimated that by 2030 the prevalence of heart failure will increase by 25%.[1] Data from the Framingham Health Study show that heart failure incidence is approximately 10 per 1000 in those older than 65 years of age.[2] Furthermore, despite the improvement in survival after diagnosis, the death rate associated with heart failure remains as high as 50% within 5 years of diagnosis.[3,4] Thus, the early identification of patients at risk of heart failure and prompt diagnosis

of those with heart failure symptoms is important to decrease mortality, hospital stay, and treatment costs.[5,6] This article reviews the appropriate evaluation of patients with heart failure, including clinical examination and diagnostic tools.

DEFINITION OF HEART FAILURE

Heart failure is characterized by abnormal cardiac structure or function that results in a failure of the heart to deliver oxygen to the organs at a rate that can fulfill their metabolic requirements.[7] Heart failure has been defined as a progressive syndrome caused by cardiac dysfunction (either systolic, diastolic, or mixed) that leads to neurohormonal and circulatory abnormalities resulting

The authors have nothing to disclose.
[a] Division of Cardiovascular Medicine, University of Minnesota Medical Center, Lillehei Heart Institute, University of Minnesota, 420 Delaware Street Southeast, MMC 508, Minneapolis, MN 55455, USA; [b] Section on Advanced Heart Failure, Transplant and Mechanical Circulatory Support, Cardiovascular Division, University of Minnesota Medical Center, Lillehei Heart Institute, University of Minnesota, 420 Delaware Street Southeast, MMC 508, Minneapolis, MN 55455, USA
* Corresponding author.
E-mail address: mcolvin1@umn.edu

in symptoms such fluid retention, shortness of breath, and fatigue.[7]

The physiology that underlies this syndrome includes neuroendocrine activation with increased production of norepinephrine, angiotensin II, and arginine vasopressin, which results in vasoconstriction, increase in left ventricular impedance, cardiac myocyte hypertrophy, and increase in myocardial collagen synthesis. In addition, there is increase in atrial natriuretic peptide, which counter-regulates vasoconstriction and remodeling of the heart.[8,9]

Heart failure is a progressive disease that has a preclinical phase characterized by the absence of symptoms compared with later phases, and by the presence of myocardial injury that triggers neuroendocrine activation and cardiac remodeling (stages A and B). This preclinical phase progresses to a clinical phase during which symptoms appear. In this symptomatic phase, the patient's symptoms can be controlled with medical treatment (stage C) or can be severe enough to require advanced therapies including mechanical circulatory support or heart transplant (stage D) (**Table 1**).[10] Patients with heart failure can present with a varied spectrum of symptoms and signs, with variations between patients and during the course of the disease. Although the disease is progressive, the symptoms can be stabilized with therapy.[11]

The heart failure syndrome may manifest clinically as:

- A syndrome of fluid retention. Patients present with peripheral edema or increase in abdominal girth.[10] Other signs of congestion include jugular venous distention, orthopnea, rales, and hepatojugular reflux.[12]
- A syndrome of decreased exercise tolerance. This syndrome is typically characterized by progressive fatigue or dyspnea with exertion.[10] Although these symptoms are common in patients with heart failure, they are also the most challenging for the clinician, given that they are not exclusive to patients with heart failure and can be present in other conditions, including pulmonary and muscular diseases.[13]
- Other cardiovascular symptoms/end-organ hypoperfusion. Patients with heart failure may present with signs and symptoms that may be related directly to cardiac dysfunction or compromise of other organs. Some of these symptoms include arrhythmias, acute myocardial infarction, or renal and hepatic failure.

Table 1
American College of Cardiology/American Heart Association Heart failure stages

Stage	Characteristics
Stage A	At risk for heart failure No structural heart disease or heart failure symptoms Examples: hypertension, diabetes, metabolic syndrome, family history of cardiomyopathy, cardiotoxin exposure
Stage B	Structural heart disease No signs or symptoms or heart failure Examples: patients with acute myocardial infarction, valvular heart disease, left ventricular hypertrophy
Stage C	Structural heart disease Prior or current heart failure symptoms
Stage D	Refractory heart failure requiring specialized interventions Example: marked symptoms at rest despite maximal medical therapy

Adapted from Yancy CW, Jessup M, Bozkurt B, et al. 2013 ACC/AHA Guidelines for the Management of Heart Failure: A Report of the American College of Cardiology Foundation/American Heart Association Task Force on Practice Guidelines. Circulation 2013;128(16):e240–319.

EVALUATION OF PATIENTS WITH HEART FAILURE

A thorough evaluation of heart failure seeks to determine cause, severity, and prognosis, and combine a thorough history and physical examination with appropriate diagnostic tests (**Box 1**).

The evaluation of patients with heart failure is based on a complete and comprehensive history, physical examination, and diagnostic studies. The importance of the history and physical examination is supported by a meta-analysis of 22 studies of patients who presented with dyspnea to the emergency department. Wang and colleagues,[14] showed that the overall clinical impression of the emergency room physician, based on several signs and symptoms as well as laboratory and imaging tests, significantly increased the probability of having heart failure (positive likelihood ratio [LR], 4.4; 95% confidence interval [CI], 1.8–10). The most useful features were prior history of heart failure (positive LR, 5.8; 95% CI, 4.1–8.0), presence of paroxysmal nocturnal dyspnea (positive LR, 2.6; 95% CI, 1.5–4.5), S3 gallop on examination (positive LR, 11; 95% CI, 4.9–25.0), chest radiograph showing

---

Box 1
Evaluation of patients with heart failure

Initial diagnosis of heart failure

- History and physical examination
- Echocardiogram
- Routine laboratory testing including serum electrolytes, renal function, thyroid and liver function test, lipid profile, glucose, and complete blood count
- Biomarkers: N-terminal pro–brain natriuretic peptide or brain natriuretic peptide, troponin
- Additional laboratory tests might include ferritin, human immunodeficiency virus, plasma metanephrins, protein electrophoresis, antinuclear antibodies (ANA), extractable nuclear antigens (ENA), uric acid
- Other imaging techniques: magnetic resonance imaging, nuclear medicine stress test, cardiac computed tomography
- Endomyocardial biopsy if giant cell myocarditis and necrotizing eosinophilic myocarditis are suspected

Chronic heart failure follow-up

- History: focus on duration and severity of symptoms
- Physical examination: weight, vital signs, and evaluation of signs of congestion and/or hypoperfusion
- Echocardiogram
- Routine laboratory testing: serum electrolytes, renal function, thyroid and liver function tests, lipid profile, glucose, and complete blood count
- Noninvasive impedance cardiography

Acute decompensated heart failure

- History and physical
- Hemodynamic evaluation with pulmonary artery catheter
- Routine laboratory tests: serum electrolytes, renal function test, liver function test

Prognostication

- Vital signs
- Laboratory test
- Cardiopulmonary stress test
- Six-minute walk test

---

pulmonary venous congestion (positive LR, 12.0; 95% CI, 6.8–21.0), and atrial fibrillation on electrocardiogram (positive LR, 3.8; 95% CI, 1.7–8.8).[14]

History and Physical Examination

History

A comprehensive history is the first step in the evaluation of patients with suspected or established heart failure. The personal history can provide important clues regarding risk factors for heart failure and aid interpretation of signs and symptoms that can lead to diagnosis of heart failure and determination of functional impairment and prognosis in patients with established heart failure.[10,15] Thus, the American Heart Association (AHA)/American College of Cardiology (ACC) heart failure guidelines

recommend a thorough history be obtained/performed in patients presenting with heart failure to identify disorders or behaviors that can cause or accelerate the development or progression of heart failure (class I indication; level of evidence, C).[10]

Some asymptomatic patients can be at risk for heart failure. These patients might have one or more risk factors for heart failure including hypertension, prior history of myocardial infarction, diabetes mellitus, valvular heart disease, family history of cardiomyopathy, congenital heart disease, sleep disorders, and exposure to cardiac toxins including chemotherapy agents and alcohol.[15] Once these risk factors are identified, they must be aggressively treated in order to prevent or delay development of heart failure symptoms. Identification of risk factors is recommended by the

AHA/ACC guidelines as a class I indication with level of evidence C.[10]

For patients with known or suspected heart failure, it is important to identify characteristic symptoms such as dyspnea, decreased exercise tolerance, edema, or ascites. Once identified, these symptoms must be well described, including duration and severity. Patients with chronic heart failure can adapt to their condition and may not recognize, or may minimize, the symptoms.[16] Documentation and grading of functional capacity, including the ability to perform routine daily activities and the New York Heart Association (NYHA) functional classification, is required (level of evidence, A) (**Table 2**).[15] Other symptoms that must be considered during evaluation of patients with heart failure include angina, syncope, lightheadedness, or symptoms of sleep disorders, specifically sleep apnea (**Box 2**).[15]

In addition, in patients with suspected familial cardiomyopathy, defined as 2 or more relatives with idiopathic dilated cardiomyopathy, a 3-generation family history should be obtained to aid in establishing the diagnosis of familial cardiomyopathy (class I indication; level of evidence, C).[10]

Physical examination

The AHA/ACC guidelines recommend that the evaluation of patients with heart failure include assessment of volume status, evidence of orthostatic blood pressure changes, and weight and height, with calculation of body mass index (class I; level of evidence, C).[10]

Box 2
Information that should be gathered during history
Presence of heart failure symptoms (including duration and severity)
• Decreased exercise tolerance and NYHA class
• Dyspnea of exertion
• Orthopnea
• Paroxysmal nocturnal dyspnea
• Edema
• Ascites
Other symptoms
• Angina
• Syncope
• Palpitations
• Symptoms of sleep disorder including daytime sleepiness, snoring, restless sleeping
Presence of risk factors for heart failure
• Prior history of myocardial infarction
• Hypertension
• Diabetes mellitus
• Dyslipidemia
• Thyroid disease
• Smoking
• Valvular heart disease
• Family history of cardiomyopathy, sudden cardiac death, coronary artery disease
• Congenital heart disease
• Sleep disorders
• Exposure to cardiac toxins including chemotherapy agents and alcohol

Table 2
NYHA functional class

NYHA Class	Criteria
I	No limitation of physical activity. The patient can perform the daily activities without symptoms of fatigue or dyspnea
II	Mild limitation. Usually the patient is asymptomatic at rest but gets fatigue or dyspnea with regular daily activities
III	IIIa: fatigue or dyspnea with less than regular daily activities; comfortable at rest IIIb: fatigue or dyspnea with minimal activity; comfortable at rest
IV	Patient symptomatic at rest, with worsening of the symptoms with minimal activity

The physical examination can provide clues regarding heart failure etiology and its severity based on volume status and perfusion state. This evaluation provides the clinician with a snapshot of the patient's hemodynamic profile, which may be useful in guiding treatment (**Table 3**). Physical examination should include:

• Vital signs. Vital signs provide important information including presence of orthostasis, low cardiac output states characterized by narrow pulse pressure and tachycardia, or hypotension that has been related to poor prognosis in patients with heart failure.[12,16,17] The presence of hypertension may provide information regarding cause.

Table 3
Hemodynamic profiles in patients with heart failure

Hemodynamic Profile (Forrester Classification)	Hemodynamic Profile Based on Clinical Evidence of Congestion and/or Hypoperfusion	Clinical Findings
Cardiac index >2.2 L/m/m², PCWP <18 mm Hg	A: warm and dry	Normal; no evidence of congestion or hypoperfusion
Cardiac index >2.2 L/m/m², PCWP >18 mm Hg	B: wet and warm	Evidence of congestion: S3, orthopnea, JVD, edema, ascites, hepatojugular reflux, rales (infrequent) Adequate perfusion Independent predictor of 1-y mortality (HR, 1.83)
Cardiac index <2.2 L/m/m², PCWP <18 mm Hg	L: cold and dry	Evidence of low perfusion: narrow pulse pressure, cool extremities, somnolent, obtunded, worsening renal failure, hypotension, and low sodium No clinical evidence of congestion
Cardiac index <2.2 L/m/m², PCWP >18 mm Hg	C: cold and wet	Evidence of congestion and hypoperfusion Independent predictor of 1-y mortality (HR, 2.48) Worse outcomes

Abbreviations: HR, hazard ratio; JVD, jugular venous distention; PCWP, pulmonary capillary wedge pressure.
   Data from Nohria A, Tsang SW, Fang JC, et al. Clinical assessment identifies hemodynamic profiles that predict outcomes in patients admitted with heart failure. J Am Coll Cardiol 2003;41(10):1797–804; and Forrester JS, Diamond G, Chatterjee K, et al. Medical therapy of acute myocardial infarction by application of hemodynamic subsets (first of two parts). N Engl J Med 1976;295(24):1356–62.

- Height and weight. Weight monitoring is an essential component to monitoring signs of heart failure.
- Complete cardiovascular examination, which must include presence of S3 or S4 gallop, increase of jugular venous pressure, and presence of murmurs that might provide clues regarding the cause of heart failure or presence of complications related to high filling pressures and left ventricular dilatation, such as severe mitral regurgitation and pulmonary hypertension. Drazner and colleagues,[18] showed in an analysis of studies of left ventricular dysfunction that presence of a third heart sound and increased jugular pressure were each independently associated with increased risk of hospitalization for heart failure, death, or hospitalization for heart failure, and death from pump failure.
- Pulmonary evaluation. The pulmonary vasculature can adapt to chronically increased filling pressures, and pulmonary edema may not be evident. However, the presence of other findings, such as pleural effusions and increased jugular venous pressure, may provide clues regarding volume status.
- Abdominal examination. The abdominal examination should include the presence of

ascites; organomegaly related to congestion and right ventricular failure; and hepatojugular reflux, which is a sensitive indicator of volume overload.
- Extremities. The clinician must look for signs of hypoperfusion, including cold extremities and signs of congestion as indicated by edema.
- Neurology. Mental status may be impaired in severe heart failure with low cardiac output.

Evaluation of Causes and Complications

Laboratories
Laboratory testing and imaging are also necessary to identify the structural abnormalities causing heart failure and to reveal the presence of disorders that can exacerbate heart failure. These tests can identify complications and end-organ damage related to heart failure.

Routine laboratory testing The AHA recommends the following laboratory tests to identify heart failure complications and to reveal the presence of disorders that can cause or exacerbate heart failure: serum electrolytes (including calcium and magnesium), renal function test (blood urea nitrogen and serum creatinine), glucose, lipid profile, complete blood count, serum albumin, liver function test, urinalysis, and thyroid function (indication class I; level of evidence, C).[10]

The presence of hyponatremia, usually caused by water retention or excessive diuresis from loop diuretics, is associated with poor prognosis.[17,19–23] Hypokalemia and hyperkalemia may be present, caused by diuretics, aldosterone antagonists, and angiotensin-converting enzyme inhibitors.[24–26]

Assessment of renal function may detect baseline renal impairment, prerenal state related to decreased cardiac output and excessive diuresis, or the presence of cardiorenal syndrome.[27–29] The urinalysis may identify abnormal urinary sediment related to glomerular disease and other signs of end-organ damage such as albuminuria. Hypoalbuminemia is common in patients with heart failure and is often associated with poor prognosis.[30–32]

Thyroid disorders may cause ventricular dysfunction or exacerbation of heart failure.[27,33–35] Abnormal thyroid function is related to increased hospitalizations and poor prognosis in patients with heart failure.[36–38] Ongoing cardiovascular risk assessment should continue as recommended by guidelines in order to prevent new onset and progression of cardiovascular disease; determination of lipids and glucose are key components of this assessment.

Uric acid increases oxidative stress, vasoconstriction, and endothelial dysfunction, and it has been associated with increased risk of developing heart failure.[39] Also, uric acid is a useful predictor of clinical events in patients with heart failure, including increased risk for atrial fibrillation, readmission for heart failure, and in-hospital and long-term mortality.[40–42] EXACT-HF (Xanthine Oxidase Inhibition for Hyperuricemic Heart Failure Patients) is a clinical trial assessing the effectiveness of allopurinol in relieving heart failure symptoms in patients with increased uric acid.

Supplemental laboratory assessments In addition to routine blood chemistries, complete blood count, and biomarkers, additional laboratory testing may be required to exclude specific causes of heart failure including hemochromatosis, human immunodeficiency virus (HIV), rheumatologic diseases, pheochromocytoma, and amyloidosis, and should be considered in patients presenting with new heart failure, depending on clinical presentation (class IIa indication; level of evidence, C).[10]

Biomarkers Biomarkers are proteins released in the blood as a consequence of activation of neurohormonal pathways related to hemodynamic changes in heart failure. These biomarkers include natriuretic peptides (atrial natriuretic peptide [ANP], brain natriuretic peptide [BNP], C-type natriuretic peptide [CNP]), endothelins, catecholamines

(noradrenaline), arginine vasopressin, cortisol, markers of renin-angiotensin-aldosterone system activity, and cortisol. There are also markers of cardiac injury (troponin), inflammatory markers (C-reactive protein, cytokines, interleukins, and growth differentiation factor), oxidative stress markers (myeloperoxidase and uric acid), and markers related to renal injury (cystatin C and neutrophil gelatinase-associated lipocalin) and cardiac fibrosis, such as galectin-3.[43,44]

BNP BNP, part of a group of peptides with natriuretic and diuretic properties, is probably the most commonly measured biomarker in the assessment of heart failure.[44,45] Produced by the ventricles, BNP is released as a prohormone in response to ventricular stretching. BNP is further degraded into N-terminal pro-BNP (NT-proBNP) and BNP.[45] Both the AHA/ACC heart failure guidelines and the Heart Failure Society of America guidelines recommend measurement of either BNP or NT-proBNP in patients presenting to the emergency department in whom the clinical diagnosis of heart failure is uncertain (class I indication; level of evidence, A).[10,15] In patients presenting to the emergency department with dyspnea, BNP greater than or equal to 100 pg/mL has a sensitivity of 90% and specificity of 73% of diagnosing heart failure,[46] with a diagnostic accuracy of 83% for levels greater than or equal to 100 pg/mL and a negative predictive value of 96% for levels less than or equal to 50 pg/mL.[47] The strength of BNP is its ability to exclude heart failure in cases in which there is low clinical suspicion and to enhance clinical judgment. A low BNP (<100 pg/mL) has a negative LR of 0.11 (95% CI, 0.07–0.16), meaning that heart failure is highly unlikely if the BNP is low.[14] N-terminal BNP or NT-proBNP, the prohormone, is highly sensitive and specific in diagnosing heart failure in patients presenting to the emergency department with dyspnea (negative predictive value of 99%).[48] NT-proBNP levels are up to 10 times higher than BNP in patients with heart failure because of potential differences in clearance mechanisms and cardiac secretion.[49] Lower values of NT-proBNP and BNP exclude heart failure. Although BNP and NT-proBNP levels improve with treatment in chronic heart failure and correlate with improved outcomes, randomized controlled trials to compare BNP-guided therapy with standard care without BNP measurements have been inconsistent.[50–57]

Both BNP and NT-proBNP levels increase with age. Thus, BNP values of 100 pg/mL have different specificity in older patients compared with younger patients.[58,59] The threshold for diagnosing heart failure varies with age; in patients younger than 50 years, NT-proBNP values higher than 450 pg/mL are diagnostic, whereas, in those 50 years or older, a level higher than 900 pg/mL is diagnostic.[48] BNP levels can be falsely increased in the setting of sepsis, acute coronary syndrome, renal dysfunction, and right ventricular failure secondary to pulmonary diseases like pulmonary embolism, and falsely low in the setting of obesity and pregnancy.

Although BNP and NT-proBNP have been deemed the biomarkers of heart failure, the clinician should consider the clinical settings and noncardiac conditions in which these tests are falsely affected. In addition, the ACCF/AHA guidelines recommend the measurement of BNP or NT-proBNP in both ambulatory and inpatient settings to support the diagnosis of heart failure, particularly in settings of diagnostic uncertainty (class I; level of evidence, A).[60]

Cardiac troponin High-sensitivity cardiac troponin T (hs-cTnT) is an independent predictor of death in patients with heart failure and correlates with left ventricular ejection fraction (LVEF), right ventricular tei index, and E/E′, the ratio of mitral peak velocity of early filling to early diastolic mitral annular velocity.[61–64] In a recent study, Arenja and colleagues,[65] showed that hs-cTnT is associated with in-hospital mortality and 1-year mortality in patients admitted with acute heart failure (adjusted odds ratio [OR], 1.03 for each increase of 0.1 mg L^{-1}; 95% CI, 1.02–1.05; $P<.001$). Cardiac troponin may be useful in establishing prognosis or disease severity in acutely decompensated heart failure.

Noninvasive assessment

Echocardiogram Echocardiogram is the most useful and one of the most commonly used diagnostic tests in patients with heart failure. Although ejection fraction is perhaps the most commonly assessed factor, atrial size, right ventricular size and function, Doppler assessment of valve function, and diastolic filling provide essential diagnostic and prognostic information.[10] In addition to the evaluation of diastolic function, left atrial and left ventricular filling pressures, pulmonary pressures, central venous pressure, and stroke volume can be estimated.[10,66] Severe stage 4 diastolic dysfunction (ie, restrictive filling pattern) is associated with worsening prognosis in heart failure.[67,68] Echocardiogram windows may be challenging in obese patients or those with chronic obstructive pulmonary disease. In these cases, radionuclide ventriculography or cardiac magnetic resonance imaging may be useful. Transesophageal echocardiogram and dobutamine stress echo are useful in additional evaluation of valvular abnormalities, the latter being

particularly helpful in assessing patients with left ventricular dysfunction and suspected severe aortic stenosis.[69] Initial evaluation with echo should be performed in all patients presenting with heart failure (class I; level of evidence, C).

Although routine evaluation of left ventricular function is not recommended in the absence of a change in clinical status or treatment interventions, repeat measurement of ejection fraction is recommended in patients who have had a significant change in clinical status, who have experienced or recovered from a clinical event, who have received treatment that may affect left ventricular function, or who may be candidates for device therapy (class I; level of evidence, C).

Chest radiograph A chest radiograph is useful in identifying pulmonary congestion, cardiomegaly, and other potential causes for dyspnea and should be performed in patients with suspected or new-onset heart failure (class I; level of evidence, C).

Additional imaging techniques Although many other imaging techniques provide information regarding the structure and function of the heart, most of them are still not widely used in patients with heart failure, mainly because of cost and the lack of availability and studies that support their use in clinical practice.

Cardiac magnetic resonance Although cardiac magnetic resonance (CMR) is not recommended in the routine evaluation of patients with heart failure, this technique has gained importance in the recent years because of its significantly enhanced resolution compared with echo, and its superiority in evaluating right ventricular size and function. CMR also provides morphologic and functional details, shunt assessment, and functional assessment of valves. CMR is particularly useful for identification and differentiation of several causes of heart failure, including infiltrative diseases (amyloidosis, hemochromatosis), ischemic versus nonischemic cardiomyopathy, and myocarditis (**Fig. 1**).[69] In addition, CMR provides highly accurate estimations of left and right ventricular volumes and ejection fraction, which is an advantage compared with other techniques, including echocardiogram.[69]

CMR using late gadolinium-enhanced imaging and coronary magnetic resonance angiogram has 100% sensitivity and 96% specificity for identification of ischemic causes of heart failure after comparison with invasive coronary angiography and clinical data,[70] and although its role in heart failure can has not been well established, CMR is helpful in identifying hemodynamically significant coronary artery disease with superior negative predictive value to adenosine single-photon

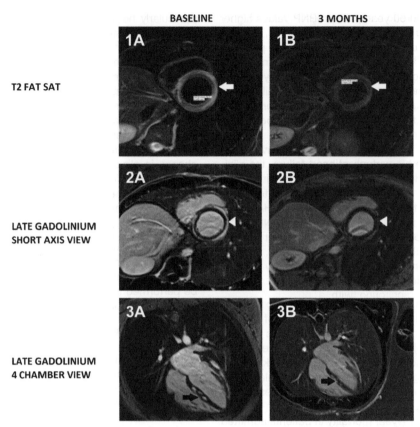

Fig. 1. CMR of a patient with acute myocarditis at baseline and 3 months after treatment. (*1A*) Diffuse myocardial edema (*white arrow*) with decrease in signal intensity after 3 months of treatment (*1B*). (*2A*) Late gadolinium enhancement shows diffuse pericardial edema (*arrowhead*) with significant improvement after 3 months (*2B*). (*3A*) Late gadolinium enhancement shows interventricular septum patchy myocardial edema (*black arrow*) that improved at 3 months (*3B*).

emission computed tomography (CT) perfusion imaging.[71] CMR is considered to be reasonable in assessing myocardial infiltrative processes and scar burden (class IIa; level of evidence, B).[60]

Nuclear imaging Nuclear imaging is used in patients with heart failure mainly for assessment of ischemia and/or viability. It is recommended for assessment of ischemia and viability in patients with known coronary artery disease who do not have angina, unless there is a contraindication to revascularization of any kind (indication, IIa; level of evidence, B).[10] It has a sensitivity of 85% to 90% and specificity of 65% to 70%, and it is also helpful for prognosis in patients with heart failure and ischemic cardiomyopathy, in which case the myocardial perfusion reserve is a better predictor of cardiac death than LVEF (hazard ratio, 4.11).[72,73]

Cardiac CT New cardiac CT technology allows evaluation of structural abnormalities in the heart that could be the cause for heart failure, as well as evaluation of left ventricular function by

multidetector row CT and of the coronary anatomy by coronary cardiac CT, which has images comparable with those obtained by coronary angiogram. However, there is a lack of studies with CT in heart failure and the radiation exposure is a limitation for this technique. In addition, its use could be limited in patients with renal failure because of the iodine-based contrast used during the angiogram.[69]

Invasive assessment
Endomyocardial biopsy The role of endomyocardial biopsy (EMB) in the diagnosis of patients with heart failure remains controversial. EMB is especially important in the diagnosis of suspected giant cell myocarditis and necrotizing eosinophilic myocarditis, which, although they are associated with a grave prognosis, usually respond well to medical therapy.[74–76] EMB is usually indicated in patients with new-onset heart failure of less than 2 weeks associated with hemodynamic compromise and patients with heart failure of 2 weeks to 3 months associated with new ventricular arrhythmias, second-degree or third-degree heart

block, or failure to response to usual care within 1 to 2 weeks (class I recommendation; level of evidence, B).[77] Other indications for EMB include heart failure associated with dilated cardiomyopathy, suspected allergic reaction with eosinophilic cardiomyopathy anthracycline cardiomyopathy, suspected cardiac tumors or arrhythmogenic right ventricular dysplasia and unexplained hypertrophic cardiomyopathy.[77] EMB is performed under fluoroscopy or echocardiographic guidance. The risk of serious complications associated with EMB has been reported between less than 1% and 3.3% in different series, with risk of death mostly related to cardiac tamponade.[77–79]

Pulmonary artery catheter evaluation Since the Evaluation Study of Congestive Heart Failure and Pulmonary Artery Catheterization Effectiveness (ESCAPE) trial was published, the use of routine hemodynamic monitoring with a pulmonary artery catheter is no longer recommended as part of the routine evaluation of patients with heart failure.[80] In this randomized trial the investigators did not find a significant difference in the end point of days alive out of the hospital between patients with acute heart failure who were treated with pulmonary artery catheter (PAC) catheter–guided therapy compared with those who were not. In addition, more patients in the PAC group experienced adverse events.[80] However, although the AHA/ACC guidelines do not recommend PAC as part of the routine evaluation of patients with heart failure, it is considered reasonable to use PAC-guided therapy in selected patients with refractory end-stage heart failure (level of evidence, C).[10] PAC can also be considered in patients with acute heart failure who fail treatment, when volume status cannot be accurately assessed by clinical evaluation alone, in patients with worsening renal function during treatment, patients with hemodynamic instability, or in patients treated with vasoactive drugs.[81] PAC is also useful in discerning pulmonary and cardiac causes of dyspnea and pulmonary edema, diagnosing pulmonary artery hypertension, and evaluating pulmonary vascular resistance in patients considered for heart transplant or mechanical support.[81]

Left heart catheterization Left heart catheterization and coronary angiography is indicated in the evaluation of patients with heart failure and angina. In addition, it may be useful in identifying causes and aiding decision making in patients with left ventricular dysfunction without angina. Angiography should only be considered in patients who are eligible for revascularization and should be considered in those with heart failure and no prior diagnosis of coronary artery disease.

Prognostication

Scores Prognostication is essential in identifying patients with heart failure at risk for adverse outcomes. Risk factor stratification may guide decision making and identify patients in need of advanced therapies, such as heart transplant or mechanical circulatory support.[10] Several scores have been developed in an attempt to predict mortality in both ambulatory and hospitalized patients with heart failure.[82,83] The Seattle Heart Failure Model, a readily available and well-validated program on the Internet, was developed to predict survival in ambulatory patients based on clinical, laboratory, device, and pharmacologic characteristics of the patients and provides an estimation of 1-year, 2-year, and 3-year survival.[83] The ADHERE (Acute Decompensated Heart Failure National Registry) model estimates in-hospital mortality based on systolic blood pressure, blood urea nitrogen, and serum creatinine on admission.[84] The ESCAPE Risk Model and Discharge Score estimates 6-month mortality in patients with acutely decompensated heart failure based on parameters assessed at discharge. Although these scores are informative, their use may be limited given the advances in heart failure treatment, increased use of mechanical circulatory support, and decrease in number of heart transplants (**Table 4**).

Functional testing The physiologic evaluation of exercise capacity is a key component in the evaluation of patients with chronic heart failure, particularly those being considered for transplant and mechanical circulatory support. Decreased exercise tolerance is one of the most important symptoms of heart failure, and objective evaluation of patients with heart failure is recommended for those that are potential candidates for heart transplant or mechanical support.[10]

- The 6-minute walk test (6MWT) and the cardiopulmonary stress test (CPX) are widely used for risk stratification. 6MWT is inexpensive, reproducible, and distance walked in 6 minutes correlates well with change in symptoms and can be used in several populations.[85–88] The 6MWT is limited by is lack of subjectivity compared with NYHA class, its dependence on patient motivation at the time of the test, and its inability to estimate maximal exercise capacity.[89]
- The CPX provides additional prognostic information. The CPX may be used to determine the severity of the heart failure, to aid in exercise prescription, and to assess the efficacy of the heart failure therapy.[86,89] Maximal

Table 4
Risk scores

Risk Score	Reference/Link
Chronic HF	
All patients with chronic HF	
Seattle Heart Failure Model	Levy WC, Mozaffarian D, Linker DT, et al. The Seattle Heart Failure Model: prediction of survival in heart failure. Circulation 2006;113:1424–33. Available at: http://SeattleHeartFailureModel.org
Heart Failure Survival Score	Aaronson KD, Schwartz JS, Chen TM, et al. Development and prospective validation of a clinical index to predict survival in ambulatory patients referred for cardiac transplant evaluation. Circulation 1997;95:2660–7. Available at: http://handheld.softpedia.com/get/Health/Calculator/HFSS-Calc-37354.shtml
CHARM (Candesartan in Heart Failure: Assessment of Reduction in Mortality and Morbidity) Risk Score	Pocock SJ, Wang D, Pfeffer MA, et al. Predictors of mortality and morbidity in patients with chronic heart failure. Eur Heart J 2006;27:65–75
CORONA Risk Score	Wedel H, McMurray JJ, Lindberg M, et al. Predictors of fatal and non-fatal outcomes in the Controlled Rosuvastatin Multinational Trial in Heart Failure (CORONA): incremental value of apolipoprotein A-1, high sensitivity C-reactive peptide and N-terminal pro B-type natriuretic peptide. Eur J Heart Fail 2009;11:281–91
Specific to chronic Heart Failure with Preserved Ejection Fraction	
I-PRESERVE Score	Komajda M, Carson PE, Hetzel S, et al. Factors associated with outcome in heart failure with preserved ejection fraction: findings from the Irbesartan in Heart Failure with Preserved Ejection Fraction Study (I-PRESERVE). Circ Heart Fail 2011;4:27–35
Acutely Decompensated HF	
ADHERE Classification and Regression Tree Model	Fonarow GC, Adams KF Jr, Abraham WT, et al. Risk stratification for in-hospital mortality in acutely decompensated heart failure: classification and regression tree analysis. JAMA 2005;293:572–80
American Heart Association Get With the Guidelines Score	Peterson PN, Rumsfeld JS, Liang L, et al. A validated risk score for in-hospital mortality in patients with heart failure from the American Heart Association Get With The Guidelines program. Circ Cardiovasc Qual Outcomes 2010;3:25–32. Available at: http://www.heart.org/HEARTORG/HealthcareProfessional/GetWithTheGuidelinesHFStroke/GetWithTheGuidelinesHeartFailureHomePage/Get-With-The-Guidelines-Heart-Failure-Home- %20Page_UCM_306087_SubHomePage.jsp
EFFECT (Enhanced Feedback for Effective Cardiac Treatment) Risk Score	Lee DS, Austin PC, Rouleau JL, et al. Predicting mortality among patients hospitalized for heart failure: derivation and validation of a clinical model. JAMA 2003;290:2581–7. Available at: http://www.ccort.ca/Research/CHFRiskModel.aspx
ESCAPE Risk Model and Discharge Score	O'Connor CM, Hasselblad V, Mehta RH, et al. Triage after hospitalization with advanced heart failure: the ESCAPE (Evaluation Study of Congestive Heart Failure and Pulmonary Artery Catheterization Effectiveness) risk model and discharge score. J Am Coll Cardiol 2010;55:872–8
OPTIMIZE-HF Risk-Prediction Nomogram	Kociol RD, Horton JR, Fonarow GC, et al. Admission, discharge, or change in B-type natriuretic peptide and longterm outcomes: data from Organized Program to Initiate Lifesaving Treatment in Hospitalized Patients with Heart Failure (OPTIMIZE-HF) linked to Medicare claims. Circ Heart Fail 2011;4:628–36

Adapted from Yancy CW, Jessup M, Bozkurt B, et al. 2013 ACC/AHA Guidelines for the Management of Heart Failure: A Report of the American College of Cardiology Foundation/American Heart Association Task Force on Practice Guidelines. Circulation 2013;128(16):e240–319.

oxygen uptake (peak V_{O_2}) and the rate of increase in ventilation per unit increase in carbon dioxide production (VE/V_{CO_2}) are widely used parameters obtained from CPX that are used in the management of heart failure and have prognostic implications. Peak V_{O_2} greater than 14 mL/kg/min is associated with significantly better survival compared with peak V_{O_2} less than 14 mL/kg/min (94% vs 70%).[90–92] Thus, a peak V_{O_2} of 14 mL/kg/min (12 mL/kg/min in patients taking β-blockers) is often used as the cutoff in determining timing of transplant listing. Three-year survival of patients with heart failure with VE/V_{CO_2} slope greater than or equal to 43 is inferior to that of patients with heart transplant, whereas the survival of those with VE/V_{CO_2} slope less than 43 is superior to that of patients with heart transplant.[93]

Although there are widely accepted thresholds for these measurements, both are prognostic across a range of values.[94] VE/V_{CO_2} slope seems to be better in predicting cardiac mortality; correlates with pulmonary capillary wedge pressure; and, unlike peak V_{O_2}, is not dependent on achieving anaerobic threshold.[93,95,96]

Biomarkers BNP and NT-proBNP are useful in evaluating prognosis and disease severity. BNP and NT-proBNP that are persistently increased after aggressive heart failure management are associated with significant risk of death and heart failure admission. Cardiac troponins are similarly associated with increased mortality and progressive left ventricular dysfunction. Cardiac troponins are responsive to treatment and persistent increase is associated with worse prognosis in patients with chronic and acute heart failure.

Emerging Biomarkers and Novel Diagnostic Methods

Biomarkers of renal injury
Cystatin C and neutrophil gelatinase-associated lipocalin (N-GAL) are new biomarkers used to diagnose renal dysfunction earlier than changes in serum creatinine are noted.

Cystatin C is a protease inhibitor produced at a constant rate in nucleated cells. It is not affected by age, sex, race, or muscle mass; it is freely filtered by the glomerular membrane; and it is neither secreted nor reabsorbed in the kidney, which allows estimation of glomerular filtration rate better than with creatinine.[97,98] In patients with heart failure cystatin C is superior to creatinine to detect worsening renal function and it has been associated with worse outcomes.[99–102]

N-GAL is a secretory glycoprotein initially identified in human neutrophil granules that is obtained using genomic microarray technology.[103] Increase in N-GAL levels indicates accumulation of nephrotoxins and renal ischemia that can be identified as early as 48 hours before increase in creatinine levels.[103] In patients with heart failure, N-GAL has a prognostic value, being associated with higher likelihood of worsening renal failure and all causes of death and cardiovascular disease mortality.[104–106]

Biomarkers of myocardial fibrosis
Soluble ST2 and galectin-3 both predict hospitalization and death and add prognostic value to natriuretic peptide levels.[107] The ST2 gene encodes a protein of the interleukin-1 receptor family. The ST2 gene is upregulated in cardiac myocytes and fibroblasts subjected to mechanical strain, and knockout of the ST2 gene leads to severe myocyte hypertrophy and interstitial cardiac fibrosis.[108,109] Galectin-3, a member of the lectin family that binds beta-galactosides, has similarly been implicated in cardiac remodeling.[110]

Noninvasive impedance cardiography
Noninvasive impedance cardiography determines the changes in thoracic fluid content and is based on changes in the conductivity/resistance to propagation of an electrical impulse across the thorax.[111] The original method used several current electrodes placed in the chest wall and neck that produce a constant current measured by voltage electrodes. Based on Ohm's law, which states that voltage is equal to impedance times current, voltage is directly proportional to impedance. Thus, when there is fluid in the body, impedance decreases and conductivity increases.[111]

Impedance cardiography allows calculations of certain hemodynamic parameters including stroke volume, cardiac output, cardiac index, systemic vascular resistance, and left work index. Several studies have shown a good correlation between these measured parameters and invasive hemodynamic evaluation, with correlation indices that range from 0.73 to 0.93.[111]

More recently, intrathoracic impedance has been measured with devices that are added to implanted devices including pacemakers, cardiac resynchronization therapy, and defibrillators. This device has the advantage of continuous monitoring and reduction of variability caused by changes in body position previously seen with the external electrodes.

This technology has shown a strong inverse relationship between intrathoracic impedance and pulmonary capillary wedge pressure,[112] as well as changes in intrathoracic impedance before patients experience symptoms, with a low risk of false-positives, helping to predict risk for heart failure hospitalizations and with a potential benefit in detection of patients with acute decompensated heart failure who are ready for discharge.[98–113]

SUMMARY

Heart failure is one of the most prevalent cardiovascular diseases in the United States, with a steady increase in its incidence in the past several years, and its prompt diagnosis helps to decrease mortality, hospital stay, and costs related to treatment. Identification of risk factors and aggressive treatment are as important as early diagnosis of heart failure. Although a comprehensive history and a complete physical examination are essential parts of the diagnosis of heart failure, it is essential to supplement these with diagnostic tools that provide information regarding the cause of heart failure, related complications, and prognosis in order to prescribe appropriate therapy, monitor response to therapy, and to transition expeditiously to advanced therapies when needed. Emerging technologies and biomarkers may provide better risk stratification and more accurate determination of cause and progression.

REFERENCES

1. Heidenreich PA, Trogdon JG, Khavjou OA, et al, American Heart Association Advocacy Coordinating Committee, Stroke Council. Forecasting the future of cardiovascular disease in the United States: a policy statement from the American Heart Association. Circulation 2011;123(8):933–44.
2. Lloyd-Jones DM, Larson MG, Leip EP, et al, Framingham Heart Study. Lifetime risk for developing congestive heart failure: the Framingham Heart Study. Circulation 2002;106(24):3068–72.
3. Roger VL, Weston SA, Redfield MM, et al. Trends in heart failure incidence and survival in a community-based population. JAMA 2004;292(3):344–50.
4. Matsushita K, Blecker S, Pazin-Filho A, et al. The association of hemoglobin A1c with incident heart failure among people without diabetes: the atherosclerosis risk in communities stud. Diabetes 2010;59(8):2020–6.
5. Bales AC, Sorrentino MJ. Causes of congestive heart failure. Prompt diagnosis may affect prognosis. Postgrad Med 1997;101(1):44–6.
6. Wuerz RC, Meador SA. Effects of prehospital medications on mortality and length of stay in congestive heart failure. Ann Emerg Med 1992;21(6):669–74.
7. McMurray JJ, Adamopoulos S, Anker SD, et al. ESC guidelines for the diagnosis and treatment of acute and chronic heart failure 2012: the Task Force for the Diagnosis and Treatment of Acute and Chronic Heart Failure 2012 of the European Society of Cardiology. Developed in collaboration with the Heart Failure Association (HFA) of the ESC. Eur J Heart Fail 2012;14(8):803–69. http://dx.doi.org/10.1093/eurjhf/hfs105.
8. Cohn JN. Mechanisms in heart failure and the role of angiotensin-converting enzyme inhibition. Am J Cardiol 1990;66(11):2D–6D.
9. Francis GS, McDonald K, Chu C, et al. Pathophysiologic aspects of end-stage heart failure. Am J Cardiol 1995;75(3):11A–6A.
10. Jessup M, Abraham WT, Casey DE, et al. 2009 Focused update: ACCF/AHA guidelines for the diagnosis and management of heart failure in adults: a report of the American College of Cardiology Foundation/American Heart Association Task Force on Practice Guidelines: developed in collaboration with the International Society for Heart and Lung Transplantation. Circulation 2009;119(14):1977–2016. http://dx.doi.org/10.1161/CIRCULATIONAHA.109.192064.
11. Heart Failure Society of America. Conceptualization and working definition of heart failure. J Card Fail 2006;12(1):e10–1. http://dx.doi.org/10.1016/j.cardfail.2005.11.007.
12. Nohria A, Tsang SW, Fang JC, et al. Clinical assessment identifies hemodynamic profiles that predict outcomes in patients admitted with heart failure. J Am Coll Cardiol 2003;41(10):1797–804.
13. Baig MK, Mahon N, McKenna WJ, et al. The pathophysiology of advanced heart failure. Am Heart J 1998;135(6 Pt 2 Su):S216–30.
14. Wang CS, FitzGerald JM, Schulzer M, et al. Does this dyspneic patient in the emergency department have congestive heart failure? JAMA 2005;294(15):1944–56. http://dx.doi.org/10.1001/jama.294.15.1944.
15. Heart Failure Society of America. Evaluation of patients for ventricular dysfunction and heart failure. J Card Fail 2006;12(1):e16–25. http://dx.doi.org/10.1016/j.cardfail.2005.11.009.
16. Stevenson LW, Perloff JK. The limited reliability of physical signs for estimating hemodynamics in chronic heart failure. JAMA 1989;261(6):884–8.
17. Abraham WT, Fonarow GC, Albert NM, et al. Predictors of in-hospital mortality in patients hospitalized for heart failure: insights from the Organized Program to Initiate Lifesaving Treatment in Hospitalized Patients with Heart Failure (OPTIMIZE-HF). J Am Coll Cardiol 2008;52(5):347–56. http://dx.doi.org/10.1016/j.jacc.2008.04.028.
18. Drazner MH, Rame JE, Stevenson LW, et al. Prognostic importance of elevated jugular venous

pressure and a third heart sound in patients with heart failure. N Engl J Med 2001;345(8):574–81.

19. Bettari L, Fiuzat M, Shaw LK, et al. Hyponatremia and long-term outcomes in chronic heart failure–an observational study from the Duke databank for cardiovascular diseases. J Card Fail 2012;18(1):74–81. http://dx.doi.org/10.1016/j.cardfail.2011.09.005.

20. Gheorghiade M, Rossi JS, Cotts W, et al. Characterization and prognostic value of persistent hyponatremia in patients with severe heart failure in the ESCAPE trial. Arch Intern Med 2007;167(18):1998–2005. http://dx.doi.org/10.1001/archinte.167.18.1998.

21. Gheorghiade M, Abraham WT, Albert NM, et al. Relationship between admission serum sodium concentration and clinical outcomes in patients hospitalized for heart failure: an analysis from the OPTIMIZE-HF registry. Eur Heart J 2007;28(8):980–8. http://dx.doi.org/10.1093/eurheartj/ehl542.

22. Konishi M, Haraguchi G, Ohigashi H, et al. Progression of hyponatremia is associated with increased cardiac mortality in patients hospitalized for acute decompensated heart failure. J Card Fail 2012;18(8):620–5. http://dx.doi.org/10.1016/j.cardfail.2012.06.415.

23. Shorr AF, Tabak YP, Johannes RS, et al. Burden of sodium abnormalities in patients hospitalized for heart failure. Congest Heart Fail 2011;17(1):1–7. http://dx.doi.org/10.1111/j.1751-7133.2010.00206.x.

24. Goland S, Naugolny V, Korbut Z, et al. Appropriateness and complications of the use of spironolactone in patients treated in a heart failure clinic. Eur J Intern Med 2011;22(4):424–7. http://dx.doi.org/10.1016/j.ejim.2011.04.008.

25. Kiernan MS, Wentworth D, Francis G, et al. Predicting adverse events during angiotensin receptor blocker treatment in heart failure: results from the HEAAL trial. Eur J Heart Fail 2012;14(12):1401–9. http://dx.doi.org/10.1093/eurjhf/hfs145.

26. Sztramko R, Chau V, Wong R. Adverse drug events and associated factors in heart failure therapy among the very elderly. Can Geriatr J 2011;14(4):79–92. http://dx.doi.org/10.5770/cgj.v14i4.19.

27. De Vecchis R, Ciccarelli A, Ariano C, et al. In chronic heart failure with marked fluid retention, the I.V. high doses of loop diuretic are a predictor of aggravated renal dysfunction, especially in the set of heart failure with normal or only mildly impaired left ventricular systolic function. Minerva Cardioangiol 2011;59(6):543–54.

28. Brisco MA, Coca SG, Chen J, et al. Blood urea nitrogen/creatinine ratio identifies a high-risk but potentially reversible form of renal dysfunction in patients with decompensated heart failure. Circ Heart Fail 2013;6(2):233–9. http://dx.doi.org/10.1161/CIRCHEARTFAILURE.112.968230.

29. Cleland JG, Carubelli V, Castiello T, et al. Renal dysfunction in acute and chronic heart failure: prevalence, incidence and prognosis. Heart Fail Rev 2012;17(2):133–49. http://dx.doi.org/10.1007/s10741-012-9306-2.

30. Filippatos GS, Desai RV, Ahmed MI, et al. Hypoalbuminaemia and incident heart failure in older adults. Eur J Heart Fail 2011;13(10):1078–86. http://dx.doi.org/10.1093/eurjhf/hfr088.

31. Abraham WT, Schrier RW. Edematous disorders: pathophysiology of renal sodium and water retention and treatment with diuretics. Curr Opin Nephrol Hypertens 1993;2(5):798–805.

32. Horwich TB, Kalantar-Zadeh K, MacLellan RW, et al. Albumin levels predict survival in patients with systolic heart failure. Am Heart J 2008;155(5):883–9. http://dx.doi.org/10.1016/j.ahj.2007.11.043.

33. Gencer B, Collet TH, Virgini V, et al. Subclinical thyroid dysfunction and the risk of heart failure events: an individual participant data analysis from 6 prospective cohorts. Circulation 2012;126(9):1040–9. http://dx.doi.org/10.1161/CIRCULATIONAHA.112.096024.

34. Pantos C, Mourouzis I, Cokkinos DV. New insights into the role of thyroid hormone in cardiac remodeling: time to reconsider? Heart Fail Rev 2011;16(1):79–96. http://dx.doi.org/10.1007/s10741-010-9185-3.

35. Pearce EN, Yang Q, Benjamin EJ, et al. Thyroid function and left ventricular structure and function in the Framingham Heart Study. Thyroid 2010;20(4):369–73. http://dx.doi.org/10.1089/thy.2009.0272.

36. Iacoviello M, Guida P, Guastamacchia E, et al. Prognostic role of sub-clinical hypothyroidism in chronic heart failure outpatients. Curr Pharm Des 2008;14(26):2686–92.

37. Galli E, Pingitore A, Iervasi G. The role of thyroid hormone in the pathophysiology of heart failure: clinical evidence. Heart Fail Rev 2010;15(2):155–69. http://dx.doi.org/10.1007/s10741-008-9126-6.

38. Silva-Tinoco R, Castillo-Martinez L, Orea-Tejeda A, et al. Developing thyroid disorders is associated with poor prognosis factors in patient with stable chronic heart failure. Int J Cardiol 2011;147(2):e24–5. http://dx.doi.org/10.1016/j.ijcard.2009.01.012.

39. Kanbay M, Segal M, Afsar B, et al. The role of uric acid in the pathogenesis of human cardiovascular disease. Heart 2013;99(11):759–66.

40. Gotsman I, Keren A, Lotan C, et al. Changes in uric acid levels and allopurinol use in chronic heart failure: association with improved survival. J Card Fail 2012;18(9):694–701.

41. Kim H, Yoon HJ, Park HS, et al. Potentials of cystatin C and uric acid for predicting prognosis of heart failure. Congest Heart Fail 2013;19(3):123–9.

42. Málek F, Ošťádal P, Pařenica J, et al. Uric acid, allo-purinol therapy, and mortality in patients with acute heart failure–results of the acute HEart FAilure data-base registry. J Crit Care 2012;27(6):737.e11–24.

43. Emdin M, Vittorini S, Passino C, et al. Old and new biomarkers of heart failure. Eur J Heart Fail 2009;11(4):331–5. http://dx.doi.org/10.1093/eurjhf/hfp035.

44. Chowdhury P, Choudhary R, Maisel A. The appropriate use of biomarkers in heart failure. Med Clin North Am 2012;96:901.

45. Pandit K, Mukhopadhyay P, Ghosh S, et al. Natriuretic peptides: diagnostic and therapeutic use. Indian J Endocrinol Metab 2011;15(Suppl 4):S345–53. http://dx.doi.org/10.4103/2230-8210.86978.

46. McCullough PA, Nowak RM, McCord J, et al. B-type natriuretic peptide and clinical judgment in emergency diagnosis of heart failure: analysis from Breathing Not Properly (BNP) multinational study. Circulation 2002;106(4):416–22.

47. Maisel AS, McCord J, Nowak RM, et al. Bedside B-type natriuretic peptide in the emergency diagnosis of heart failure with reduced or preserved ejection fraction. Results from the Breathing Not Properly multinational study. J Am Coll Cardiol 2003;41(11):2010–7.

48. Januzzi JL Jr, Camargo CA, Anwaruddin S, et al. The N-terminal pro-BNP investigation of dyspnea in the emergency department (PRIDE) study. Am J Cardiol 2005;95(8):948–54. http://dx.doi.org/10.1016/j.amjcard.2004.12.032.

49. Hall C. Essential biochemistry and physiology of (NT-pro)BNP. Eur J Heart Fail 2004;6(3):257–60.

50. Anand IS, Fisher LD, Chiang YT, et al, Val-HeFT Investigators. Changes in brain natriuretic peptide and norepinephrine over time and mortality and morbidity in the Valsartan Heart Failure Trial (val-HeFT). Circulation 2003;107(9):1278–83.

51. Januzzi JL Jr, Rehman SU, Mohammed AA, et al. Use of amino-terminal pro-B-type natriuretic peptide to guide outpatient therapy of patients with chronic left ventricular systolic dysfunction. J Am Coll Cardiol 2011;58(18):1881–9.

52. Porapakkham P, Porapakkham P, Zimmet H, et al. B-type natriuretic peptide-guided heart failure therapy: a meta-analysis. Arch Intern Med 2010;170(6):507–14.

53. Felker GM, Hasselblad V, Hernandez AF, et al. Biomarker-guided therapy in chronic heart failure: a meta-analysis of randomized controlled trials. Am Heart J 2009;158(3):422–30.

54. Lainchbury JG, Troughton RW, Strangman KM, et al. N-terminal pro-B-type natriuretic peptide-guided treatment for chronic heart failure: results from the BATTLESCARRED (NT-proBNP-assisted treatment to lessen serial cardiac readmissions and death) trial. J Am Coll Cardiol 2009;55(1):53–60.

55. Troughton RW, Frampton CM, Yandle TG, et al. Treatment of heart failure guided by plasma amino-terminal brain natriuretic peptide (N-BNP) concentrations. Lancet 2000;355(9210):1126–30.

56. Pfisterer M, Buser P, Rickli H, et al, TIME-CHF Investigators. BNP-guided vs symptom-guided heart failure therapy: the Trial of Intensified vs Standard Medical Therapy in Elderly Patients with Congestive Heart Failure (TIME-CHF) randomized trial. JAMA 2009;301(4):383–92.

57. Berger R, Moertl D, Peter S, et al. N-terminal pro-B-type natriuretic peptide-guided, intensive patient management in addition to multidisciplinary care in chronic heart failure a 3-arm, prospective, randomized pilot study. J Am Coll Cardiol 2010;55(7):645–53.

58. Maisel AS, Clopton P, Krishnaswamy P, et al. Impact of age, race, and sex on the ability of B-type natriuretic peptide to aid in the emergency diagnosis of heart failure: results from the Breathing Not Properly (BNP) multinational study. Am Heart J 2004;147(6):1078–84. http://dx.doi.org/10.1016/j.ahj.2004.01.013.

59. Redfield MM, Rodeheffer RJ, Jacobsen SJ, et al. Plasma brain natriuretic peptide concentration: impact of age and gender. J Am Coll Cardiol 2002;40(5):976–82.

60. Yancy CW, Jessup M, Bozkurt B, et al. 2013 ACCF/AHA guideline for the management of heart failure: executive summary: a report of the American College of Cardiology Foundation/American Heart Association Task Force on Practice Guidelines. J Am Coll Cardiol 2013. http://dx.doi.org/10.1016/j.jacc.2013.05.020.

61. Metra M, Bettari L, Pagani F, et al. Troponin T levels in patients with acute heart failure: clinical and prognostic significance of their detection and release during hospitalization. Clin Res Cardiol 2012;101(8):663–72.

62. Venge P, Johnston N, Lindahl B, et al. Normal plasma levels of cardiac troponin I measured by the high-sensitivity cardiac troponin I access prototype assay and the impact on the diagnosis of myocardial ischemia. J Am Coll Cardiol 2009;54(13):1165–72.

63. Kusumoto A, Miyata M, Kubozono T, et al. Highly sensitive cardiac troponin T in heart failure: comparison with echocardiographic parameters and natriuretic peptides. J Cardiol 2012;59(2):202–8.

64. Masson S, Anand I, Favero C, et al, Valsartan Heart Failure Trial (Val-HeFT) and Gruppo Italiano per lo Studio della Sopravvivenza nell'Insufficienza Cardiaca–Heart Failure (GISSI-HF) Investigators. Serial measurement of cardiac troponin T using a highly sensitive assay in patients with chronic heart

failure: data from 2 large randomized clinical trials. Circulation 2012;125(2):280–8.

65. Arenja N, Reichlin T, Drexler B, et al. Sensitive cardiac troponin in the diagnosis and risk stratification of acute heart failure. J Intern Med 2012;271(6): 598–607.

66. Nayyar S, Magalski A, Khumri TM, et al. Contrast administration reduces interobserver variability in determination of left ventricular ejection fraction in patients with left ventricular dysfunction and good baseline endocardial border delineation. Am J Cardiol 2006;98(8):1110–4.

67. Liang HY, Cauduro SA, Pellikka PA, et al. Comparison of usefulness of echocardiographic Doppler variables to left ventricular end-diastolic pressure in predicting future heart failure events. Am J Cardiol 2006;97(6):866–71.

68. Meta-analysis Research Group in Echocardiography (MeRGE) Heart Failure Collaborators, Doughty RN, Klein AL, Poppe KK, et al. Independence of restrictive filling pattern and LV ejection fraction with mortality in heart failure: an individual patient meta-analysis. Eur J Heart Fail 2008;10(8): 786–92. http://dx.doi.org/10.1016/j.ejheart.2008. 06.005.

69. Paterson I, Mielniczuk LM, O'Meara E, et al. Imaging heart failure: current and future applications. Can J Cardiol 2013;29(3):317–28.

70. Assomull RG, Shakespeare C, Kalra PR, et al. Role of cardiovascular magnetic resonance as a gatekeeper to invasive coronary angiography in patients presenting with heart failure of unknown etiology. Circulation 2011;124(12):1351–60.

71. Bruder O, Schneider S, Nothnagel D, et al. EuroCMR (European Cardiovascular Magnetic Resonance) registry: results of the German pilot phase. J Am Coll Cardiol 2009;54(15):1457–66.

72. Kim C, Kwok YS, Heagerty P, et al. Pharmacologic stress testing for coronary disease diagnosis: a meta-analysis. Am Heart J 2001;142(6):934–44.

73. Tio RA, Dabeshlim A, Siebelink HM, et al. Comparison between the prognostic value of left ventricular function and myocardial perfusion reserve in patients with ischemic heart disease. J Nucl Med 2009;50(2):214–9.

74. Ardehali H, Qasim A, Cappola T, et al. Endomyocardial biopsy plays a role in diagnosing patients with unexplained cardiomyopathy. Am Heart J 2004;147(5):919–23.

75. Cooper LT Jr, Berry GJ, Shabetai R. Idiopathic giant-cell myocarditis–natural history and treatment. Multicenter giant cell myocarditis study group investigators. N Engl J Med 1997;336(26):1860–6.

76. deMello DE, Liapis H, Jureidini S, et al. Cardiac localization of eosinophil-granule major basic protein in acute necrotizing myocarditis. N Engl J Med 1990;323(22):1542–5.

77. Cooper LT, Baughman KL, Feldman AM, et al, American Heart Association, American College of Cardiology, European Society of Cardiology. The role of endomyocardial biopsy in the management of cardiovascular disease: a scientific statement from the American Heart Association, the American College of Cardiology, and the European Society of Cardiology. Circulation 2007;116(19):2216–33.

78. Deckers JW, Hare JM, Baughman KL. Complications of transvenous right ventricular endomyocardial biopsy in adult patients with cardio-myopathy: a seven-year survey of 546 consecutive diagnostic procedures in a tertiary referral center. J Am Coll Cardiol 1992;19(1):43–7.

79. Fowles RE, Mason JW. Endomyocardial biopsy. Ann Intern Med 1982;97(6):885–94.

80. Binanay C, Califf RM, Hasselblad V, et al, ESCAPE Investigators and ESCAPE Study Coordinators. Evaluation study of congestive heart failure and pulmonary artery effectiveness: the ESCAPE trial. JAMA 2005;594(13):1625–33.

81. Kahwash R, Leier CV, Miller L. Role of the pulmonary artery catheter in diagnosis and management of heart failure. Cardiol Clin 2011;29(2):281–8.

82. Aaronson KD, Schwartz JS, Chen TM, et al. Development and prospective validation of a clinical index to predict survival in ambulatory patients referred for cardiac transplant evaluation. Circulation 1997;95(12):2660–7.

83. Levy WC, Mozaffarian D, Linker DT, et al. The Seattle heart failure model: prediction of survival in heart failure. Circulation 2006;113(11):1424–33.

84. Fonarow GC, Adams KF Jr, Abraham WT, et al, ADHERE Scientific Advisory Committee, Study Group, and Investigators. Risk stratification for in-hospital mortality in acutely decompensated heart failure: classification and regression tree analysis. JAMA 2005;293(5):572–80.

85. Ingle L, Rigby AS, Carroll S, et al. Prognostic value of the 6-min walk test and symptom severity in older patients with left ventricular systolic dysfunction. Eur Heart J 2007;28(5):560–8.

86. Ingle L, Shelton RJ, Rigby AS, et al. The reproducibility and sensitivity of the 6-minute walk test in elderly patients with chronic heart failure. Eur Heart J 2005;26(17):1742–51.

87. Rostagno C, Gensini GF. Six minute walk test: a simple and useful test to evaluate functional capacity in patients with heart failure. Intern Emerg Med 2008;3(3):205–12.

88. Forman DE, Fleg JL, Kitzman DW, et al. 6-min walk test provides prognostic utility comparable to cardiopulmonary exercise testing in ambulatory outpatients with systolic heart failure. J Am Coll Cardiol 2012;60(25):2653–61.

89. Balady GJ, Arena R, Sietsema K, et al, American Heart Association Exercise, Cardiac Rehabilitation,

and Prevention Committee of the Council on Clinical Cardiology, Council on Epidemiology and Prevention, Council on Peripheral Vascular Disease, Interdisciplinary Council on Quality of Care and Outcomes Research. Clinician's guide to cardiopulmonary exercise testing in adults: a scientific statement from the American Heart Association. Circulation 2010;122(2):191–225.

90. Szlachcic J, Massie BM, Kramer BL, et al. Correlates and prognostic implication of exercise capacity in chronic congestive heart failure. Am J Cardiol 1985;55(8):1037–42.

91. Likoff MJ, Chandler SL, Kay HR. Clinical determinants of mortality in chronic congestive heart failure secondary to idiopathic dilated or to ischemic cardiomyopathy. Am J Cardiol 1987; 59(6):634–8.

92. Mancini DM, Eisen H, Kussmaul W, et al. Value of peak exercise consumption for optimal timing of cardiac transplantation in ambulatory patients with heart failure. Circulation 1991;83(3):778–86.

93. Ferreira AM, Tabet JY, Frankenstein L, et al. Ventilatory efficiency and the selection of patients for heart transplantation. Circ Heart Fail 2010;3(3): 378–86.

94. Francis DP, Shamim W, Davies LC, et al. Cardiopulmonary exercise testing for prognosis in chronic heart failure: continuous and independent prognostic value from VE/VCO$_2$ slope and peak VO$_2$. Eur Heart J 2000;21(2):154–61.

95. Arena R, Myers J, Aslam SS, et al. Peak VO$_2$ and VE/VCO$_2$ slope in patients with heart failure: a prognostic comparison. Am Heart J 2004;147(2): 354–60.

96. Nanas SN, Nanas JN, Sakellariou DC, et al. VE/VCO$_2$ slope is associated with abnormal resting haemodynamics and is a predictor of long-term survival in chronic heart failure. Eur J Heart Fail 2006;8(4):420–7.

97. Kostrubiec M, Łabyk A, Pedowska-Włoszek J, et al. Neutrophil gelatinase-associated lipocalin, cystatin C and eGFR indicate acute kidney injury and predict prognosis of patients with acute pulmonary embolism. Heart 2012;98(16):1221–8.

98. Coll E, Botey A, Alvarez L, et al. Serum cystatin C as a new marker for noninvasive estimation of glomerular filtration rate and as a marker for early renal impairment. Am J kidney Dis 2000;36(1):29–34.

99. Damman K, van der Harst P, Smilde TD, et al. Use of cystatin C levels in estimating renal function and prognosis in patients with chronic systolic heart failure. Heart 2012;98(4):319–24.

100. Lassus J, Harjola VP, Sund R, et al, FINN-AKVA Study group. Prognostic value of cystatin C in acute heart failure in relation to other markers of renal function and NT-proBNP. Eur Heart J 2007; 28(15):1841–7.

101. Gao C, Zhong L, Gao Y, et al. Cystatin C levels are associated with the prognosis of systolic heart failure patients. Arch Cardiovasc Dis 2011;104(11): 565–71.

102. Manzano-Fernández S, Boronat-Garcia M, Albaladejo-Otón MD, et al. Complementary prognostic value of cystatin C, N-terminal pro-B-type natriuretic peptide and cardiac troponin T in patients with acute heart failure. Am J Cardiol 2009; 103(12):1753–9.

103. Ronco C. NGAL: an emerging biomarker of acute kidney injury. Int J Artif Organs 2008;31(3):199–200.

104. Aghel A, Shrestha K, Mullens W, et al. Serum neutrophil gelatinase-associated lipocalin (NGAL) in predicting worsening renal function in acute decompensated heart failure. J Card Fail 2010;16(1): 49–54.

105. Alvelos M, Lourenço P, Dias C, et al. Prognostic value of neutrophil gelatinase associated lipocalin in acute heart failure. Int J Cardiol 2013;165(1): 51–5.

106. Daniels LB, Barrett-Connor E, Clopton P, et al. Plasma neutrophil gelatinase associated lipocalin is independently associated with cardiovascular disease and mortality in community-dwelling older adults: the Rancho Bernardo Study. J Am Coll Cardiol 2012;59(12):1101–9.

107. Rehman SU, Mueller T, Januzzi JL Jr. Characteristics of the novel interleukin family biomarker ST2 in patients with acute heart failure. J Am Coll Cardiol 2008;52(18):1458–65.

108. Yanagisawa K, Tsukamoto T, Takagi T, et al. Murine ST2 gene is a member of the primary response gene family induced by growth factors. FEBS Lett 1992;302(1):51–3.

109. Sanada S, Hakuno D, Higgins LJ, et al. IL-33 and ST2 comprise a critical biomechanically induced and cardioprotective signaling system. J Clin Invest 2007;117(6):1538–49.

110. Ho JE, Liu C, Lyass A, et al. Galectin-3, a marker of cardiac fibrosis, predicts incident heart failure in the community. J Am Coll Cardiol 2012;60(14): 1249–56.

111. Bayram M, Yancy CW. Transthoracic impedance cardiography: a noninvasive method of hemodynamic assessment. Heart Fail Clin 2009;5(2):161–8.

112. Yu CM, Wang L, Chau E, et al. Intrathoracic impedance monitoring in patients with heart failure: correlation with fluid status and feasibility of early warning preceding hospitalization. Circulation 2005;112(6): 841–8.

113. Whellan DJ, Droogan CJ, Fitzpatrick J, et al. Change in intrathoracic impedance measures during acute decompensated heart failure admission: results from the diagnostic data for discharge in heart failure patients (3D-HF) pilot study. J Card Fail 2012;18(2):107–12.

Management of ACCF/AHA Stage A and B Patients

Faiz Subzposh, MD, Ashwani Gupta, MBBS,
Shelley R. Hankins, MD,
Howard J. Eisen, MD, FACC, FAHA, FACP*

KEYWORDS

- Stage A heart failure • Stage B heart failure • Screening • Management • Asymptomatic

KEY POINTS

- Patients with Stage A heart failure (HF) are at high risk for development of HF without any evidence of structural heart disease.
- Patients with Stage B HF have structural heart disease without any current or previous symptoms.
- Early detection of patients with Stage A and B with subsequent early intervention can lead to long-term reduction in morbidity and mortality of HF.
- Coronary artery disease, hypertension, and diabetes are the three major risk factors for development of HF.
- Neurohormonal blockade with angiotensin-converting enzyme inhibitors and β-blockers is the foundation of medical treatment in Stage B HF.

INTRODUCTION

Heart failure (HF) remains a major health problem in the United States, affecting 5.8 million Americans.[1] The prevalence of HF continues to rise due to the improved survival of patients. Despite advances in treatment, morbidity and mortality remains very high, with a median survival of about 5 years after the first clinical symptoms.[2] Hence, there has been a paradigm shift toward prevention of HF and identifying patients before the development of the first clinical episode. HF is a progressive disorder that is characterized by cardiac remodeling, typically a change in chamber size and geometry leading to increased hemodynamic stress and ventricular dysfunction. These changes further exacerbate the remodeling process and lead to a vicious cycle culminating in progressive deterioration. In 2001, American College of Cardiology

Foundation/American Heart Association (ACCF/AHA) guidelines identified four stages of progressive development of HF[3]:

1. Stage A: patients at high risk for HF, but without evidence of structural heart disease
2. Stage B: patients with structural heart disease, but without signs or symptoms of HF
3. Stage C: patients with previous or current signs or symptoms of HF
4. Stage D: refractory HF requiring special interventions.

This classification complements the New York Heart Association (NYHA) functional classification, which primarily assesses the severity of clinical symptoms in Stage C or D. It identifies patients at high risk for developing HF and, hence, allows early therapeutic interventions. It is hoped this approach will reduce long-term morbidity and mortality of HF.

The authors have no disclosures.
Division of Cardiology, Drexel University College of Medicine, 245 North 15th Street, Mailstop #1012, Philadelphia, PA 19102, USA
* Corresponding author.
E-mail address: heisen@drexelmed.edu

Cardiol Clin 32 (2014) 63–71
http://dx.doi.org/10.1016/j.ccl.2013.09.003
0733-8651/14/$ – see front matter © 2014 Elsevier Inc. All rights reserved.

cardiology.theclinics.com

STAGE A HF

Stage A patients have high-risk factors for developing HF but do not have any evidence of cardiac structural abnormalities and have normal ventricular function. The prevalence of Stage A HF was 22% in a population-based cross-sectional study of 45-year-old adults.[4] Coronary artery disease (CAD), hypertension, and diabetes are the three major risk factors for development of HF (**Box 1**).[5,6] Early detection and risk reduction are the two most important components of management of Stage A HF. It is important for health care providers to identify patients in Stage A, implement early interventions to delay progression to advanced stages of HF, and reverse the potentially treatable causes. Routine periodic evaluation should be done for signs and symptoms of HF. See later discussion of management strategies for specific risk factors.

CAD

CAD is the most common risk factor for development of HF, especially in male patients.[5] Population-attributable risk (PAR) for CAD was 62% in the National Health and Nutrition Examination Survey (NHANES). In the Framingham Study, combined PAR for angina and myocardial infarction was 39% for men and 18% for women. Secondary prevention of CAD in patients without any

structural heart disease reduces the incidence, as well as delays the development, of HF.[7] Treatment with β-blockers, statins,[8] angiotensin-converting enzyme (ACE) inhibitors,[9] clopidogrel,[10] and revascularization (when appropriate) has reduced the incidence of HF. Most of the benefits are due to the prevention of further coronary syndromes; however, there are other secondary effects leading to reduction of HF. β-blockers can have unfavorable effects on lipid profile and glycemic control; however, benefits outweigh the minor increase in risk. In addition, combined α-blockers and β-blockers do not have these adverse effects.[11] Aggressive primary and secondary prevention of CAD remains the cornerstone of management of Stage A HF.

HYPERTENSION

Hypertension is one of the most important risk factors for development of HF, especially in women and African Americans.[5] Aggressive treatment of systolic, as well as diastolic, hypertension reduces the incidence of HF, with an average risk reduction of 40% to 50%.[12] Diuretics, ACE inhibitors, angiotensin receptor blockers (ARBs), and β-blockers have all decreased the risk of HF with no significant difference among the various agents.[13] However, trials have shown increased incidence of HF with use of doxazosin and nifedipine.[14,15] These medications should be avoided as first-line therapy for treatment of hypertension. Detailed recommendations of blood pressure goals and choice of antihypertensive drugs are provided in guidelines by Joint National Committee on Prevention, Detection, and Treatment of High Blood Pressure.[16]

DIABETES

Diabetes can lead to HF either by development of coronary heart disease or diabetic cardiomyopathy. The risk of developing HF is two times higher in male patients and three to four times higher in female patients with diabetes.[17] Poor glycemic control and duration of diabetes are directly related to the development of HF.[18] Increase in hemoglobin A1c by 1% leads to 8% to 15% increase in risk of developing HF.[19] Tight glycemic control remains the most important goal in management of diabetes and prevention of HF. Blockade of the renin-angiotension system is equally important and provides additional benefit in reduction of microvascular complications, progression of diabetic nephropathy, and the incidence of HF.[11]

Box 1
Risk factors for developing HF

Common Risk Factors	Other Risk Factors
CAD	Sleep apnea
Hypertension	Tachycardia induced
Diabetes	cardiomyopathy
Metabolic	Cardiotoxins (eg,
syndrome	anthracyclines, cocaine,
Smoking	Ephedra, amphetamines,
Dyslipidemia	trastuzumab,
Obesity	cyclophosphamide)
Alcohol use	Right ventricular pacing
Family history	Physical inactivity
Renal disease	Endocrine disorders
	(hypothyroidism or
	hyperthyroidism,
	pheochromocytoma,
	acromegaly)
	HIV
	Mediastinal irradiation
	Connective tissue disorders
	Genetic disorders
	Sarcoidosis

DYSLIPIDEMIA

Dyslipidemia is another important risk factor for development of HF.[20] Low high-density lipoprotein (HDL), elevated non-HDL, high total cholesterol to HDL ratio, and high triglyceride level have all been implicated as risk factors for the development of HF. Despite mixed results from various studies, appropriate management of dyslipidemia is an essential component of reducing risk of HF. Management of dyslipidemia should be done in accordance with guidelines recommended by the National Cholesterol Education Program.[21]

METABOLIC SYNDROME, OBESITY, AND PHYSICAL INACTIVITY

Metabolic syndrome, obesity, and physical inactivity are independent risk factors for the development of HF after adjustment for other established risks factors.[22–24] Multiple mechanisms have been hypothesized in metabolic syndrome, including increased myocardial mass by direct effects of insulin, sympathetic activation, potentiation of effects of angiotension II on myocytes, and increased collagen cross-linking due to increased glycosylation end-products.[22] It is also an inflammatory state, which may be a potential mechanism for increased risk of development of HF. Approximately 11% of HF cases in male patients and 14% in female patients are associated with obesity alone.[23] Physical inactivity leads to increased left ventricular stiffness and decreased compliance with aging.[25] Lifestyle modification, weight loss, and regular exercise are highly recommended for all patients. Although no prospective studies have shown that these interventions lead to reduction in HF, it is a reasonable assumption to make. Further studies are required to prove and quantify the benefits from these interventions.

SLEEP APNEA

Obstructive sleep apnea (OSA) is an independent predictor for development of HF. One study showed an odds ratio of 2.38 for risk of developing HF with OSA.[26] Potential mechanisms include hypoxia, exaggerated negative intrathoracic pressure, sympathetic activation, and systemic hypertension.[27] Effective treatment of sleep apnea by continuous positive airway pressure and weight loss can potentially reduce the risk of developing HF. However, the data for the benefit of these therapies in ameliorating the progression of HF is lacking.

RENAL DISEASE

Prevalence of HF is 10 to 30 times higher in dialysis patients.[28] Myocardial dysfunction is common with renal disease and it worsens with initiation of dialysis.[29] The Kidney Disease Outcomes Quality Initiative (K/DOQI) guidelines recommend that all patients undergo baseline echocardiogram at initiation of dialysis, repeated every 3 years.[30] Echocardiogram should be obtained after the dry weight is obtained. Aggressive blood pressure control, optimizing calcium phosphate homeostasis, and correction of anemia can potentially reduce the risk of developing HF. ACE inhibitors and calcium channel blockers (CCBs) are the antihypertensives of choice in these patients. Some studies have also shown that risk of HF reduces with renal transplantation.[31] Microalbuminuria is also strongly associated with an increased incidence of HF in diabetics as well as nondiabetics.[32] However, treatment with ACE inhibitors has not been shown to reduce risk of HF in these patients.

SMOKING

Smoking is one of the strongest risk factors for developing HF. The effect of smoking is generally mediated through its role in the development of CAD. It is associated with 60% increased risk of HF after adjusting for all the other risk factors.[33] Although smoking cessation has not been shown to reduce risk of developing HF, it has been shown to reduce mortality in patients with established HF.[34] Smoking cessation and abstinence should be advised to all the patients, irrespective of the stage of HF.

ALCOHOL

Mild-to-moderate alcohol use has been associated with reduced risk of HF, probably related to reduced risk of CAD.[35] However, heavy alcohol use is a leading cause of HF, especially in men.[36] Various studies have reported alcohol consumption as the cause for dilated cardiomyopathy in the range of 21% to 50%.[37] Increased apoptosis, direct cardiotoxic effects, activation of the renin-angiotensin system, and nutritional deficiencies have been hypothesized as the potential mechanisms. Avoiding excessive alcohol consumption can be highly successful in reducing the risk of development of HF, apart from other potential health benefits.

CARDIOTOXINS

Cardiotoxic potential of many substances and drugs, such as amphetamines, cocaine, Ephedra, anthracyclines, trastuzumab, cyclophosphamide, has been very well described. Complete abstinence from use of offending illicit drugs and termination of use of therapeutic agents is essential.

Trastuzumab, a monoclonal antibody, is used to treat breast tumors, which overexpress the epidermal growth factor, HER2. It is associated with an increased incidence of HF in all age groups.[38] Cardiac dysfunction from trastuzumab is thought to be due to blocking the ErbB2 signaling pathway and abnormalities in expression of Bcl-2, Bcl-cS, and BAX proteins.[39] The National Comprehensive Cancer Network guidelines recommend assessment of left ventricle (LV) systolic function at baseline, 3, 6, and 9 months after initiation of therapy.[40] Imatinib, a tyrosine kinase inhibitor used to treat Philadelphia chromosome–positive chronic myelogenous leukemia and other malignancies, can rarely be associated with congestive HF.[41]

Cardiac dysfunction from anthracycline therapy occurs because of free radical injury leading to permanent myocyte loss.[42] In patients receiving anthracyclines, evaluation of LV systolic function is recommended at baseline and after administration of cumulative dosage of 300 mg/m[2].[42] Screening is recommended at relatively low cumulative dosage for patients younger than 15 years of age and older than 60 years of age.

Cocaine-induced cardiomyopathy is an underrecognized entity. One small study showed 7% incidence of LV systolic dysfunction 2 weeks after cocaine use in asymptomatic young adults.[43] Sympathomimetic effects of cocaine, increased oxidative stress, and increased risk of thrombosis have been proposed as the potential mechanisms.[44] Complete abstinence from cocaine is essential in the prevention and management of cocaine-induced cardiomyopathy.

RIGHT VENTRICULAR PACING

There has been growing evidence over the last decade that right ventricular pacing leads to increased risk of HF and hospitalization.[45] Patients with chronic right ventricular pacing, such as patients with high-degree AV block, should be regularly examined for the development of HF symptoms. Serial echocardiograms are also recommended to detect asymptomatic left ventricular dysfunction. Some trials have shown the benefit of implantation of biventricular pacemakers, instead of dual chamber pacemakers, in subjects who will require pacing the right ventricle more than 50% of the time.[46]

TACHYCARDIA-INDUCED CARDIOMYOPATHY

Tachycardia-induced cardiomyopathy is also a well-recognized reversible cause of HF. Almost all supraventricular arrhythmias have been associated with tachycardia-induced cardiomyopathy, atrial fibrillation, atrial tachycardia, atrioventricular nodal reentry tachycardia, and atrioventricular reciprocating tachycardia.[47] Frequent ventricular ectopy can also lead to development of left ventricular systolic dysfunction.[48] Restoration of sinus rhythm is the main goal and pharmacologic, electrical cardioversion, or ablative strategies can be used. Rate control can also be effective in refractory arrhythmias using drugs or AV node ablation, if required.

HIV

Left ventricular systolic dysfunction is a well-known complication of HIV, with incidence ranging from 4% to 28% without highly active antiretroviral therapy (HAART).[49,50] There is some evidence that HAART reduces incidence of HF in HIV patients, but this cardioprotective effect decreases over time and, eventually, the incidence of HF becomes similar in patients who are exposed or not exposed to HAART.[51] However, robust data are lacking and further studies are needed. Regardless, HAART therapy should be recommended to all HIV patients and it seems to provide at least some benefit in reduction of incidence of HF. For patients at high risk for cardiovascular disease, some panels have recommended a baseline screening echocardiogram, then every 1 to 2 years or as clinically indicated.[52]

ENDOCRINE DISORDERS

Hyperthyroidism has been associated with development of HF. It was thought to be a high output cardiac failure; however, increased heart rate, atrial fibrillation, systemic hypertension, changes in systemic vascular resistance, and so forth, have been implicated as potential mechanisms.[53] Hypothyroidism, pheochromocytoma, and acromegaly have also been associated with increased risk of HF. Management of underlying endocrine disorder is the mainstay of management and reduction in incidence of HF.

DIAGNOSTIC MODALITIES

Echocardiography is the imaging modality of choice, which can differentiate between Stage A and B HF. The prevalence of systolic and diastolic dysfunction was found to be 8% and 32%, respectively, in patients with Stage A HF and one risk factor. Prevalence increased to 9% and 38%, respectively, with two risk factors and to 15% and 38%, respectively, with three or more risk factors.[54] These numbers may be expected to increase with development of more sensitive techniques of detecting systolic and diastolic dysfunction. Routine echocardiography is strongly recommended for patients with two or more risk factors for development of HF. Brain natriuretic peptide levels in patients older than 60 years of age could provide a cost-effective screening tool.[55]

STAGE B HF

Stage B HF patients are defined as those with evidence of structural heart disease but without current or previous symptoms. Once patients start to manifest symptoms of HF, they advance to stage C HF in the spectrum of this progressive disease. Examples of such patients include those who have recently had a myocardial infarction and have developed LV systolic dysfunction without any symptoms of HF or patients with hypertension and LV remodeling, such as hypertrophy demonstrated by routine echocardiography.

The prevalence of Stage B HF is approximately fourfold greater than patients who have Stage C or D combined.[56] Unless a vigorous screening program is in place, most of these patients go unnoticed until they advance to Stage C. It is also possible that patients minimize their symptoms because of the gradual onset of HF symptoms. In addition, and patients might unconsciously reduce their activity levels to compensate for the decreased exercise tolerance and underreport their symptoms.

MANAGEMENT GOALS

The biggest challenge in managing Stage B patients is identification. Although it is well established that treating these patients early will decrease their morbidity and mortality, a definitive cost-effective screening program has not been developed.[57,58] Screening tools such as echocardiography or plasma brain natriuretic peptide levels are a reasonable approach to these patients.[55,59]

Most of the clinical trials identify CAD as the predominant cause of Stage B HF. The nonischemic causes include, but are not limited to, valvular heart disease, postviral myocarditis, familial dilated cardiomyopathy, and hypertension. It is important to identify the cause of myocardial dysfunction because it guides the therapeutic options (see **Box 1**).

The proportion of patients with Stage B increases when diastolic dysfunction is included. Recent studies have shown that diastolic dysfunction identified by echocardiography has a substantial prognostic significance for those with and without preserved ejection fraction (EF).[60,61] Serial echocardiography for these select individuals is a promising approach for screening and follow-up.[62]

PHARMACOLOGIC TREATMENT
β-Blockers

LV dysfunction activates counteracting mechanisms through the neurohormonal system, including renin-angiotensin and norepinephrine. These mechanisms are initiated much before the development of symptoms.[63]

β-blockers reduce the LV chamber volume and improve EF. The REversal of VEntricular Remodeling with Metoprolol Succinate (REVERT) Trial randomized subjects to receive metoprolol succinate or placebo. Over the course of 12 months, EF, as well as end systolic volumes, significantly decreased compared with baseline or placebo in a dose-dependent fashion. This is the only trial that looked only at Stage B subjects and the effect of β-blockers.[64]

In the Carvedilol Post-Infarct Survival Control in Left Ventricular Dysfunction (CAPRICORN) trial, the long-term effects of carvedilol on ischemic cardiomyopathy were shown to be beneficial. Of the 1959 randomized subjects, 53% were asymptomatic. Over the course of 2 years, carvedilol had a 31% risk reduction in all cause mortality compared with placebo.[65] A further echocardiography substudy showed significant improvements in LV EF and a reduction in LV chamber volumes when compared with placebo.[66]

β-blockers should be introduced early to prevent any further remodeling in an already structurally abnormal LV. The ACCF/AHA guidelines recommend the use of β-blockers in Stage B HF patients, regardless of the cause, as a Class I recommendation.[59]

ACE Inhibitors and ARBs

As previously discussed, the neurohormonal system activation occurs early in the spectrum of this clinical syndrome, which influences the rationale of blocking the renin-angiotensin-aldosterone system (RAAS). The benefit of ACE inhibitors is that they inhibit the formation of angiotensin II, promoting antihypertensive, antifibrotic, and vasodilatory properties to the cardiovascular system.[67] ARBs work in a similar fashion, inhibiting the effects by blocking angiotensin II receptor.

The Studies of Left Ventricular Dysfunction (SOLVD) prevention trial demonstrated the effects of enalapril versus placebo on 4228 Stage B HF subjects with an EF lower than 35%. There were significant reductions in progression of disease, as well as hospitalizations related to HF. There was also a trend toward fewer deaths in the enalapril group, although this difference did not reach statistical significance.[68] ARBs have been shown to have no mortality difference compared with ACE inhibitors in ischemic cardiomyopathy and they are recommended for patients who are intolerant of ACE inhibitors.[69,70]

RAAS blockade is also beneficial in nonischemic causes of HF such as hypertensive heart disease.[67] ACE inhibitors and ARBs have been shown to prevent and reverse hypertrophy and fibrosis. ACCF/AHA guidelines recommend the use of ACE inhibitors in those patients with Stage B HF (Class I) and ARBs can be used in patients intolerant to ACE inhibitors.[59]

CCBs, Digoxin, and Aldosterone Antagonists

The use of CCBs has clinical benefit in the asymptomatic patient with LV systolic dysfunction. Although there have been no studies showing adverse effects, CCBs with negative inotropic effects should not be used in asymptomatic patients with an EF lower than 40%, especially after a myocardial infarction.[71]

Digoxin is also a Class III recommendation in asymptomatic patients with low EF because there is no proven benefit and a high risk of harm.[72]

Most of the data for aldosterone antagonists is available in stage C and D HF. In the Randomized Aldactone Evaluation Study (RALES) and the Eplerenone Post-Acute Myocardial Infarction Heart Failure Efficacy and Survival Study (EPHESUS), there were significant reductions in mortality and morbidity when compared with placebo.[73,74] The effect of aldosterone inhibition on LV remodeling has also been shown to affect patients with HF with preserved EF.[75] Currently, these drugs are not recommended in the ACCF/AHA guidelines for management of asymptomatic patients.[59]

NONPHARMACOLOGICAL TREATMENT

Patients with asymptomatic LV systolic dysfunction are at increased risk for sudden cardiac death. In the Framingham Study population, 43% deaths in subjects with ischemic cardiomyopathy occurred suddenly without overt signs of HF.[58] One trial, which looked at asymptomatic subjects with LV systolic dysfunction and primary prevention of sudden cardiac death, was the Multicenter Automatic Defibrillator Implantation Trial II (MADIT II). In this trial, 1232 subjects with a previous myocardial infarction and an EF less than 30% were randomized to receive an implantable cardioverter-defibrillator (ICD) or conventional medical therapy. One-third of both groups were asymptomatic. Over the follow-up of 20 months, there was a 31% reduction in death in the ICD arm compared with conventional medical therapy.[76] The data for primary prevention in nonischemic patients are derived from the Defibrillators in Non-Ishcemic Cardiomyopathy Treatment Evaluation (DEFINITE) study, which evaluated 458 subjects with EF higher than 36% over a 29-month period (22% were asymptomatic). Overall, there was an insignificant reduction in mortality of 35% and most of the mortality benefit was in the symptomatic subjects.[77] ACCF/AHA guidelines recommend ICD placement in selected, asymptomatic patients with ischemic cardiomyopathy (Class IIa) as well as nonischemic cardiomyopathy (Class IIb).[59]

Some other causes of Stage B HF are valvular heart disease and tachyarrhythmias. Although the patients may not exhibit symptoms, valvular stenosis or regurgitation may be classified as severe by echocardiography. Repair or replacement should be considered for these patients.[78] If tachyarrhythmia has been diagnosed as the primary cause of LV dysfunction, such as supraventricular tachycardia with rapid ventricle response or a high burden of isolated PVCS, efforts should be made to keep the patient in sinus rhythm or control the ventricular response rates as much as possible with either ablation therapy or medications.

SUMMARY

Patients at high risk for developing HF are classified as stage A HF. CAD, diabetes, and hypertension are the three major risk factors. There are various other modifiable, as well as nonmodifiable, risk factors. These patients may advance to stage B HF; however, diagnosis may be difficult because the patients are asymptomatic. Early detection of stage A and B patients with early therapeutic interventions and close monitoring is critically important to slow the progression to advanced stages of HF, and to decrease morbidity and mortality. Left ventricular remodeling and dysfunction are mediated through neurohormonal activation. ACE inhibitors and β-blockers remain the mainstay of medical management of stage B patients. Implantation of ICD may be considered in selected patients to reduce mortality. Routine use of echocardiography in high-risk patients is highly recommended for early detection of stage A and B patients.

REFERENCES

1. American Heart Association. 2010 heart and stroke statistical update. Dallas (TX): American Heart Association; 2010.
2. Levy D, Kenchaiah S, Larson MG, et al. Long-term trends in the incidence of and survival with heart failure. N Engl J Med 2002;347(18):1397–402.
3. Hunt SA, Abraham WT, Chin MH, et al. 2009 Focused update incorporated into the ACC/AHA 2005 guidelines for the diagnosis and management of heart failure in adults: a report of the American College of Cardiology Foundation/American Heart Association task force on practice guidelines: developed in collaboration with the International Society for Heart and Lung Transplantation. Circulation 2009;119:e391–479.
4. Ammar KA, Jacobsen SJ, Mahoney DW, et al. Prevalence and prognostic significance of heart failure stages: application of the American College of Cardiology/American Heart Association heart failure staging criteria in the community. Circulation 2007;115:1563–70.
5. Lloyd-Jones DM, Larson MG, Leip EP, et al. Lifetime risk for developing congestive heart failure: the Framingham Heart Study. Circulation 2002; 106:3068–72.
6. He J, Ogden LG, Bazzano LA, et al. Risk factors for congestive heart failure in US men and women: NHANES I epidemiologic follow-up study. Arch Intern Med 2001;161:996–1002.
7. Kjekshus J, Pedersen TR, Olsson AG, et al. The effects of simvastatin on the incidence of heart failure in patients with coronary heart disease. J Card Fail 1997;3:249–54.
8. LaRosa JC, Grundy SM, Waters DD, et al. Intensive lipid lowering with atorvastatin in patients with stable coronary disease. N Engl J Med 2005;352: 1425–35.
9. Arnold JM, Yusuf S, Young J, et al. Prevention of heart failure in patients in the Heart Outcomes Prevention Evaluation (HOPE) study. Circulation 2003;107:1284–90.
10. Yusuf S, Zhao F, Mehta SR, et al. Effects of clopidogrel in addition to aspirin in patients with acute coronary syndromes without ST-segment elevation. N Engl J Med 2001;345:494–502.
11. Lindholm LH, Ibsen H, Dahlof B, et al. Cardiovascular morbidity and mortality in patients with diabetes in the Losartan Intervention For Endpoint reduction in hypertension study (LIFE): a randomized trial against atenolol. Lancet 2002;359: 1004–10.
12. Psaty BM, Lumley T, Furberg CD, et al. Health outcomes associated with various antihypertensive therapies used as first-line agents: a network meta-analysis. JAMA 2003;289:2534–44.
13. Psaty BM, Smith NL, Siscovick DS, et al. Health outcomes associated with antihypertensive therapies used as first-line agents: a systematic review and meta-analysis. JAMA 1997;277(9):739–45.
14. Major cardiovascular events in hypertensive patients randomized to doxazosin vs chlorthalidone: the Antihypertensive and Lipid-Lowering Treatment to Prevent Heart Attack Trial (ALLHAT). ALLHAT Collaborative Research Group. JAMA 2000;283:1967–75.
15. Brown MJ, Palmer CR, Castaigne A, et al. Morbidity and mortality in patients randomized to double-blind treatment with a long-acting calcium-channel blocker or diuretic in the International Nifedipine GITS study: intervention as a Goal in Hypertension Treatment (INSIGHT). Lancet 2000;356:366–72.
16. Chobanian AV, Bakris GL, Black HR, et al. Seventh report of the Joint National Committee on prevention, detection, evaluation, and treatment of high blood pressure. Hypertension 2003;42:1206–52.
17. Kannel WB, McGee DL. Diabetes and cardiovascular disease: the Framingham Study. JAMA 1979;241(19):2035–8.
18. Whelton PK, Barzilay J, Cushman WC, et al. Clinical outcomes in antihypertensive treatment of type 2 diabetes, impaired fasting glucose concentration, and normoglycemia: Antihypertensive and Lipid-Lowering Treatment to Prevent Heart Attack Trial (ALLHAT). Arch Intern Med 2005; 165:1401–9.
19. Chae CU, Glynn RJ, Manson JE, et al. Diabetes predicts congestive heart failure risk in the elderly. Circulation 1998;98(Suppl I):721.
20. Dhingra R, Sesso HD, Kenchaiah S, et al. Differential effects of lipids on the risk of heart failure and coronary artery disease: the Physicians Health Study. Am Heart J 2008;155:869–75.
21. National Cholesterol Education Program (NCEP) Expert Panel on Detection, Evaluation, and Treatment of High Blood Cholesterol in Adults (Adult Treatment Panel III). Third report of the National Cholesterol Education Program (NCEP) expert panel on detection, evaluation, and treatment of high blood cholesterol in adults (Adult Treatment Panel III) final report. Circulation 2002;106(25): 3143–421.
22. Ingelsson E, Arnlov J, Lind L, et al. Metabolic syndrome and risk for heart failure in middle-aged men. Heart 2006;92:1409–13.
23. Kenchaiah S, Evans JC, Levy D, et al. Obesity and the risk of heart failure. N Engl J Med 2002;347: 305–13.
24. Berry JD, Pandey A, Gao A, et al. Physical fitness and risk for heart failure and coronary artery disease. Circ Heart Fail 2013;6:627–34.
25. Aurigemma GP, Gaasch WH. Diastolic heart failure. N Engl J Med 2004;351:1097–105.

26. Shahar E, Whitney CW, Redline S, et al. Sleep-disordered breathing and cardiovascular disease: cross-sectional results of the Sleep Heart Health Study. Am J Respir Crit Care Med 2001; 163:19–25.

27. Kasai T, Bradley TD. Obstructive sleep apnea and heart failure. J Am Coll Cardiol 2011;57:119–27.

28. Stack AG, Bloembergen WE. A cross-sectional study of the prevalence and clinical correlates of congestive heart failure among incident US dialysis patients. Am J Kidney Dis 2001;38:992–1000.

29. McCullough PA. Cardiovascular disease in chronic kidney disease from a cardiologist's perspective. Curr Opin Nephrol Hypertens 2004;13:591–600.

30. K/DOQI Workgroup. K/DOQI clinical practice guidelines for cardiovascular disease in dialysis patients. Am J Kidney Dis 2005;45:S1–153.

31. DeLima JJ, Vieira ML, Viviani LF, et al. Long-term impact of renal transplantation on carotid artery properties and on ventricular hypertrophy in end-stage renal failure patients. Nephrol Dial Transplant 2002;17:645–51.

32. Vaur L, Gueret P, Lievre M, et al. Development of congestive heart failure in type 2 diabetic patients with microalbuminuria or proteinuria: observations from the DIABHYCAR (type 2 DIABete, Hypertension, Cardiovascular Events and Ramipril) study. Diabetes Care 2003;26:855–60.

33. Eriksson H, Svardsudd K, Larsson B, et al. Risk factors for heart failure in the general population: the study of men born in 1913. Eur Heart J 1989; 10:647–56.

34. Suskin N, Sheth T, Negassa A, et al. Relationship of current and past smoking to mortality and morbidity in patients with left ventricular dysfunction. J Am Coll Cardiol 2001;37:1677–82.

35. Walsh CR, Larson MG, Evans JC, et al. Alcohol consumption and risk for congestive heart failure in the Framingham Heart Study. Ann Intern Med 2002;136:181–91.

36. George A, Figueredo VM. Alcoholic cardiomyopathy: a review. J Card Fail 2011;17(10):844–9.

37. Regan TJ. Alcohol and the cardiovascular system. JAMA 1990;264:377–81.

38. Chen J, Long JB, Hurria A, et al. Incidence of heart failure or cardiomyopathy after adjuvant trastuzumab therapy for breast cancer. J Am Coll Cardiol 2012;60:2504–12.

39. Ewer SM, Ewer MS. Cardiotoxicity profile of trastuzumab. Drug Saf 2008;31:459–67.

40. National Comprehensive Cancer Network. NCCN clinical practice guidelines in oncology. Breast Cancer 2013. Version 3. Available at: http://www.NCCN.com. Accessed November 5, 2013.

41. Kerkela T, Grazette L, Yacoubii R, et al. Cardiotoxicity of the cancer therapeutic agent imatinib mesylate. Nat Med 2006;12:908–16.

42. Wouters KA, Kremer LC, Miller TL, et al. Protecting against anthracycline-induced myocardial damage: a review of the most promising strategies. Br J Haematol 2005;131:561–78.

43. Bertolet B, Freund G, Martin D. Unrecognized left ventricular dysfunction in an apparently healthy cocaine abuse population. Clin Cardiol 1990;13: 323–8.

44. Awtry EH, Philippides GJ. Alcoholic and cocaine-associated cardiomyopathies. Prog Cardiovasc Dis 2010;52(4):289–99.

45. Steinberg JS, Fischer A, Wang P, et al. The clinical implications of cumulative right ventricular pacing in the Multicenter Automatic Defibrillator Trial II. J Cardiovasc Electrophysiol 2005;16:359–65.

46. Yu C, Chan JY, Zhang Q, et al. Biventricular pacing in patients with bradycardia and normal ejection fraction. N Engl J Med 2009;361:2123–34.

47. Khasnis A, Jongnarangsin K, Abela G, et al. Tachycardia-induced cardiomyopathy: a review of literature. Pacing Clin Electrophysiol 2005;28(7): 710–21.

48. Baman TS, Lange DC, Ilg KJ, et al. Relationship between burden of premature ventricular complexes and left ventricular function. Heart Rhythm 2010;7(7):865–9.

49. Lipshultz SE, Easley KA, Orav EJ, et al. Cardiac dysfunction and mortality in HIV-infected children: the prospective P2C2 HIV multicenter study. Pediatric pulmonary and cardiac complications of vertically transmitted HIV infection (P2C2 HIV) study group. Circulation 2000;102:1542–8.

50. Morse CG, Kovacs JA. Metabolic and skeletal complications of HIV infection: the price of success. JAMA 2006;296:844–54.

51. Fisher SD, Easley KA, Orav EJ, et al. Mild dilated cardiomyopathy and increased left ventricular mass predict mortality: the prospective P2C2 HIV multicenter study. Am Heart J 2005;150(3):439–47.

52. Lipshultz SE, Fisher SD, Lai WW, et al. Cardiovascular monitoring and therapy for HIV-infected patients. Ann N Y Acad Sci 2001;946:236–73.

53. Klein I, Danzi S. Thyroid disease and the heart. Circulation 2007;116:1725–35.

54. Carerj S, Carrubba SL, Antonini-Canterin F, et al. The incremental prognostic value of echocardiography in asymptomatic stage A heart failure. J Am Soc Echocardiogr 2010;23:1025–34.

55. Heidenreich PA, Gubens MA, Fonarow GC, et al. Cost-effectiveness of screening with B-type natriuretic peptide to identify patients with reduced left ventricular ejection fraction. J Am Coll Cardiol 2004;43:1019–26.

56. Frigerio M, Oliva F, Turazza FM, et al. Prevention and management of chronic heart failure in management of asymptomatic patients. Am J Cardiol 2003;9:4–9.

57. Goldberg LR, Jessup M. Stage B heart failure management of asymptomatic left ventricular systolic dysfunction. Circulation 2006;24:2851–60.

58. Wang TJ, Evans JC, Benjamin EJ, et al. Natural history of asymptomatic left ventricular systolic dysfunction in the community. Circulation 2003;8: 977–82.

59. Hunt SA, Abraham WT, Chin MH, et al. ACC/AHA 2005 guideline update for the diagnosis and management of chronic heart failure in the adult a report of the American College of Cardiology/ American Heart Association Task Force on Practice Guidelines (Writing Committee to Update the 2001 Guidelines for the Evaluation and Management of Heart Failure): developed in collaboration with the American College of Chest Physicians and the International Society for Heart and Lung Transplantation: endorsed by the Heart Rhythm Society. Circulation 2005;12:e154–235.

60. Redfield MM, Jacobsen SJ, Burnett JC Jr, et al. Burden of systolic and diastolic ventricular dysfunction in the community. JAMA 2003;2:194–202.

61. Aurigemma GP, Gottdiener JS, Shemanski L, et al. Predictive value of systolic and diastolic function for incident congestive heart failure in the elderly: the Cardiovascular Health Study. J Am Coll Cardiol 2001;4:1042–8.

62. Coglianese EE, Wang TJ. Clinical monitoring of stage B heart failure: echocardiography. Heart Fail Clin 2012;2:169–78.

63. Francis GS, Benedict C, Johnstone DE, et al. Comparison of neuroendocrine activation in patients with left ventricular dysfunction with and without congestive heart failure. A substudy of the Studies of Left Ventricular Dysfunction (SOLVD). Circulation 1990;5:1724–9.

64. Colucci WS, Kolias TJ, Adams KF, et al. Metoprolol reverses left ventricular remodeling in patients with asymptomatic systolic dysfunction the REversal of VEntricular Remodeling with Toprol-XL (REVERT) trial. Circulation 2007;1:49–56.

65. Dargie HJ. Effect of carvedilol on outcome after myocardial infarction in patients with left-ventricular dysfunction: the CAPRICORN randomised trial. Lancet 2001;357:1385–90.

66. Doughty RN, Whalley GA, Walsh HA, et al. Effects of carvedilol on left ventricular remodelling in patients following acute myocardial infarction: the CAPRICORN echo substudy. Circulation 2004;2: 201–6.

67. Collier P, McDonald KM. The role of renin angiotensin system intervention in stage B heart failure. Heart Fail Clin 2012;2:225–36.

68. Nicklas JM, Pitt B, Timmis G, et al. Effect of enalapril on mortality and the development of heart-failure in asymptomatic patients with reduced left-ventricular ejection fractions. N Engl J Med 1992; 10:685–91.

69. Dickstein K, Kjekshus J. Effects of losartan and captopril on mortality and morbidity in high-risk patients after acute myocardial infarction: the OPTIMAAL randomised trial. Lancet 2002;360:752–60.

70. Pfeffer MA, McMurray JJ, Velazquez EJ, et al. Valsartan, captopril, or both in myocardial infarction complicated by heart failure, left ventricular dysfunction, or both. N Engl J Med 2003;20:1893–906.

71. The effect of diltiazem on mortality and reinfarction after myocardial infarction. Multicenter Diltiazem Postinfarction Trial Research Group. N Engl J Med 1988;7:385–92.

72. Trial M. The effect of digoxin on mortality and morbidity in patients with heart failure. N Engl J Med 1997;336:525–33.

73. Pitt B, Zannad F, Remme WJ, et al. The effect of spironolactone on morbidity and mortality in patients with severe heart failure. N Engl J Med 1999;10:709–17.

74. Pitt B, Remme W, Zannad F, et al. Eplerenone, a selective aldosterone blocker, in patients with left ventricular dysfunction after myocardial infarction. N Engl J Med 2003;14:1309–21.

75. Mak GJ, Ledwidge MT, Watson CJ, et al. Natural history of markers of collagen turnover in patients with early diastolic dysfunction and impact of eplerenone. J Am Coll Cardiol 2009;18:1674–82.

76. Moss AJ, Zareba W, Wall WJ, et al, Multicenter Automatic Defibrillator Implantation Trial II Investigators. Prophylactic implantation of a defibrillator in patients with myocardial infarction and reduced ejection fraction. N Engl J Med 2002;12:877–83.

77. Kadish A, Dyer A, Daubert JP, et al. Prophylactic defibrillator implantation in patients with nonischemic dilated cardiomyopathy. N Engl J Med 2004; 21:2151–8.

78. Bonow RO, Carabello BA, Chatterjee K, et al. ACC/AHA 2006 guidelines for the management of patients with valvular heart disease a report of the American College of Cardiology/American Heart Association Task Force on Practice Guidelines (writing committee to revise the 1998 guidelines for the management of patients with valvular heart disease) developed in Collaboration With the Society of Cardiovascular Anesthesiologists Endorsed by the Society for Cardiovascular Angiography and Interventions and the Society of Thoracic Surgeons. J Am Coll Cardiol 2006;3:e1–148.

Management of ACCF/AHA Stage C Heart Failure

Sasikanth Adigopula, MD, Rey P. Vivo, MD,
Eugene C. DePasquale, MD, Ali Nsair, MD,
Mario C. Deng, MD, FESC*

KEYWORDS

- Heart failure • Stage C • Drug therapy • Surgical treatment

KEY POINTS

- American College of Cardiology Stage C heart failure (HF) includes those patients with prior or current symptoms of heart failure in the context of an underlying structural heart problem who are primarily managed with medical therapy.
- Although there is guideline-based medical therapy for those who have HF with reduced ejection fraction (HFrEF), therapies in heart failure with preserved ejection fraction (HFpEF) have thus far proven elusive.
- Emerging therapies, such as serelaxin, are currently under investigation and may prove beneficial.
- The role of advanced surgical therapies, such as mechanical circulatory support, in this population is not well defined; further investigation is warranted for these therapies in patients with Stage C HF.

STAGE C HEART FAILURE

Heart failure (HF) terminology is varied and at times imprecise. Stage C HF, as described by the American College of Cardiology Foundation (ACCF)/American Heart Association (AHA) classification system, includes patients with structural heart disease with prior or current symptoms of HF. The 2 most widely used HF classification schemes are the previously mentioned ACCF/AHA system and the New York Heart Association (NYHA) functional classification. The ACCF/AHA staging system, however, emphasizes the development and progression of disease, whereas the NYHA classes focus on exercise capacity and the symptomatic status of the disease. Both these classifications are complementary, but increasingly the ACCF/AHA staging system is being used more commonly. The ACCF/AHA staging system includes asymptomatic stages (risk factors, structural heart disease), thereby underscoring the importance of preventive medicine, and reflecting the progressive nature of the HF syndrome. The stages are progressive, as a patient may progress from stage A to stage D, but cannot return to stage A. This is in contrast to the NYHA classification in which response or lack thereof to treatment can alter the functional status of a patient and therefore the NYHA class.

EDUCATION AND EXERCISE

One of the most important and challenging parts of HF management is educating the patient regarding adherence and compliance with medications, salt restriction, appropriate physical activity, lifestyle modifications, and weight loss. It is critical to educate patients on understanding their disease process, symptoms, fluid changes, and weight fluctuations. Readmission rates were significantly

The authors have nothing to disclose.
Mechanical Circulatory Support & Heart Transplantation Program, Ahmanson-UCLA Cardiomyopathy Center, David Geffen School of Medicine, University of California, Los Angeles, 100 UCLA Medical Plaza, Suite 630 East, Los Angeles, CA 90095, USA
* Corresponding author. Ronald Reagan UCLA Medical Center, David Geffen School of Medicine, University of California, Los Angeles, 100 UCLA Medical Plaza, Suite 630 East, Los Angeles, CA 90095.
E-mail address: mdeng@mednet.ucla.edu

Cardiol Clin 32 (2014) 73–93
http://dx.doi.org/10.1016/j.ccl.2013.09.012
0733-8651/14/$ – see front matter © 2014 Elsevier Inc. All rights reserved.

lower in patients who were educated in all 6 categories of the HF core measures from the Joint Commission on Accreditation of Healthcare Organizations.[1] Discharge education led to fewer days of hospitalization, lower cost, and lower mortality rates within a 6-month follow-up.[2]

Physical activity must be encouraged in patients with HF, similar to other cardiovascular (CV) diseases (**Table 1**). In those able to participate, regular physical activity and exercise is safe and effective and helps in improving functional status.[3–7] Exercise and rehabilitation improves endothelial function, increases peripheral oxygen extraction, and reduces hospital readmissions. Cardiac rehabilitation can be useful in clinically stable patients with HF to improve functional capacity, exercise duration, health-related quality of life, and mortality.[8,9]

SODIUM RESTRICTION

Sodium intake is related to hypertension, left ventricular (LV) hypertrophy, and CV disease. Physicians have therefore traditionally recommended dietary sodium restriction in patients with HF for decades. Reduction in dietary sodium reduces fluid retention and risk for hospitalizations.[10,11] The 2013 ACCF/AHA guidelines recommend restricting sodium to 1500 mg/d for patients with stage A and B HF and less than 3000 mg/d for patients with stage C and D HF (see **Table 1**). Some studies have signaled a worsening neurohormonal profile with sodium restriction in HF[12,13]; however, these patients did not receive optimal medical therapy at that time. Further studies are required to evaluate the effects of sodium restriction on neurohormonal activation and outcomes in optimally treated patients with HF.

OBESITY AND OBSTRUCTIVE SLEEP APNEA

People with body mass index (BMI) of 30 kg/m^2 or higher are considered obese. The "obesity paradox" is well known in HF, as patients with BMI between 30 and 35 kg/m^2 have lower mortality and hospitalization rates than those with a BMI in the normal range.[14] However, this is not maintained in morbidly obese patients whose BMI is more than 35 kg/m^2. Advanced HF can lead to higher total energy expenditure that may lead to weight loss, contributing to cardiac cachexia, which has been demonstrated to predict a worse prognosis.[15]

Obesity is a major risk factor for obstructive sleep apnea (OSA). The prevalence of OSA progressively increases as BMI and associated markers (eg, neck circumference, waist-to-hip ratio) increase. Patients with HF and OSA do not routinely present with excessive daytime sleepiness. Hence, clinical judgment is imperative in identifying these patients. Continuous positive airway pressure (CPAP) can be beneficial to increase left ventricular ejection fraction (LVEF) and improve functional status in patients with HF and sleep apnea.[3,16–18] CPAP has been demonstrated to decrease the apnea-hypopnea index, improve nocturnal oxygenation, increase LVEF, lower norepinephrine levels, and increase the distance walked in the 6-minute walk test in those with OSA. These benefits were sustained for up to 2 years.[17]

Table 1
2013 ACCF/AHA recommendations for nonpharmacologic treatment in stage C HF

Non-Pharmacologic Intervention	Class of Recommendation	Level of Evidence
Patients with HF should receive specific education to facilitate HF self-care	I	B
Sodium restriction in patients with symptomatic HF to reduce congestive symptoms	IIa	C
CPAP can be beneficial to increase LVEF and improve functional status in patients with HF and sleep apnea	IIa	B
Exercise training (or regular physical activity) is recommended as safe and effective for patients with HF who are able to participate to improve functional status	I	A
Cardiac rehabilitation can be useful in clinically stable patients with HF to improve functional capacity, exercise duration, HRQOL, and mortality	IIa	B

Abbreviations: ACCF, American College of Cardiology Foundation; AHA, American Heart Association; CPAP, continuous positive airway pressure; HF, heart failure; HRQOL, health-related quality of life; LVEF, left ventricular ejection fraction.

PHARMACOLOGIC THERAPY

Recommendations for stage A and B HF hold true for stage C as well. These include evaluation and treatment of hypertension, lipid disorders, advocating cessation of substance abuse, including smoking, alcohol, and illicit drug usage, obtaining detailed family history to assess for a familial component, assessing sudden cardiac death (SCD) risk and assessment for structural heart disease, left ventricular hypertrophy (LVH), ischemia, and valvular heart disease as clinically indicated.

ANGIOTENSIN-CONVERTING ENZYME INHIBITORS

Angiotensin-converting enzyme inhibitors (ACE-I) decrease the conversion of angiotensin I to angiotensin II, thereby reducing the maladaptive effects of angiotensin II. Furthermore, there is a decrease in the breakdown of bradykinin, which promotes vasodilatation in the vascular endothelium and promotes natriuresis. Unless contraindicated, ACE inhibitors are recommended in all patients with HF with reduced ejection fraction (HFrEF).[19–21] ACE-Is reduce the risk of death and hospitalization in HFrEF patients (**Table 2**). ACE-Is are frequently used in conjunction with beta blockers (BB). ACE-Is are beneficial in ischemic and nonischemic cardiomyopathies, as well as in patients with HF with mild, moderate, or severe symptoms.

Table 2
Recommendations for the use of ACE-I

Treatment – Use of ACE-I	Class of Recommendation	Level of Evidence
ACE-I in patients with a history of MI and reduced EF to prevent HF	I	A
ACE-Is should be used in all patients with a reduced EF to prevent HF	I	A
ACE-I in HFrEF with current or prior symptoms	I	A

Recommendations summarized from current literature and data referenced in this article; see reference list.

Abbreviations: ACE-I, angiotensin-converting enzyme inhibitor; EF, ejection fraction; HF, heart failure; HFrEF, HF with reduced ejection fraction; MI, myocardial infarction.

Data supporting use of ACE inhibitors in HF dates back to more than 25 years ago when the Cooperative North Scandinavian Enalapril Survival Study (CONSENSUS-I) was reported in 1987 (**Table 3**).[22] In this trial, 253 patients in NYHA class IV HF were randomized to enalapril or placebo with

Table 3
ACE-I trials supporting current guideline recommendations

Study	Aim of Study	Baseline Therapy	Results
CONSENSUS,[22] 1987	Study the effect of enalapril on prognosis of NYHA class IV HF	Diuretics (spironolactone 53%), digitalis (93%), other; Vasodilators except ACE-I (nitrates 46%)	40% reduction in mortality at 6 mo ($P = .002$) 31% reduction in mortality at 1 y ($P = .001$)
SOLVD,[20] 1991	Study the effect of enalapril on mortality and hospitalization in patients with chronic HF and LVEF <35%	Diuretics and digoxin	16% reduction in mortality ($P = .0036$)
ATLAS,[23] 1999	To compare the efficacy and safety of low and high doses of ACE-I on the risk of death and hospitalization in chronic HF	Diuretics, digoxin, and vasodilators	High-dose ACE-I group: • 8% lower risk of all-cause mortality ($P = .128$) • 12% lower risk of death or hospitalization ($P = .002$) • 24% fewer hospitalizations for HF ($P = .002$)

Abbreviations: ACE-I, angiotensin-converting enzyme inhibitor; HF, heart failure; LVEF, left ventricular ejection fraction; NYHA, New York Heart Association.

a 40% reduction in mortality demonstrated in the enalapril cohort. A 10-year follow-up to this study revealed a sustained 30% risk reduction in the enalapril group and a higher mortality among patients not receiving open ACE-I therapy.[24]

The SOLVD (Studies Of Left Ventricular Dysfunction) study randomized 2569 patients with symptomatic NYHA class II to III HF and ejection fraction of 35% or less to either placebo or enalapril. The predominant etiology was ischemic cardiomyopathy (72%). There was a 16% reduction in mortality demonstrated in the enalapril cohort.[20] In addition, the 12-year follow-up to the SOLVD study showed that enalapril extended median survival by 9.4 months in the combined SOLVD prevention and treatment trial.[25]

There are no significant differences among available ACE inhibitors in their effects on symptoms or survival.[21] Initial treatment usually begins with a low-dose ACE-I that is gradually uptitrated to goal doses used in clinical trials (**Table 4**).[20] If the target dose cannot be tolerated, then the maximum tolerable dose should be used for treatment. Serum potassium and creatinine should be assessed within 1 to 2 weeks of initiation of therapy and periodically thereafter.

Overall, ACE-Is are well tolerated. Adverse effects of ACE-Is are related to angiotensin suppression and kinin potentiation. ACE inhibitors are contraindicated in those who have experienced life-threatening adverse reactions (ie, angioedema) during previous medication exposure or if they are pregnant or plan to become pregnant. ACE inhibitors must also be avoided or used with extreme caution in patients with markedly increased serum creatinine (>3 mg/dL), bilateral renal artery stenosis, elevated levels of serum potassium (>5.0 mEq/L), and hypotension (systolic blood pressure <80 mm Hg). Other adverse effects include cough in up to 20% of the patients, rash and taste disturbances.

ANGIOTENSIN RECEPTOR BLOCKERS

Angiotensin II production continues in the presence of ACE inhibition, driven through alternative enzyme pathways. Angiotensin receptor blockers (ARBs) act by blocking the binding of angiotensin II to the AT1 receptor. ARBs are now considered an alternative to ACE-I as first-line drugs in patients with HFrEF. These agents are especially useful in patients who are ACE-I intolerant, as it does not lead to kinin production. Although the incidence of cough and angioedema are much lower compared with ACE-I, they have to be used cautiously, as these can be life-threatening as well.[26] As with ACE-I therapy, ARBs must be started at a low dose and uptitrated toward doses used in clinical trials (**Table 5**). The side effects of ARBs are from suppression of angiotensin stimulation. It is prudent to check renal function and potassium every week for the first 2 weeks and monthly thereafter.

ARBs have also been demonstrated to reduce mortality and morbidity in those who are already on an ACE inhibitor and a BB and do not have an indication for or are intolerant of an aldosterone antagonist in those who are persistently symptomatic (**Table 6**).[27] When used in such a combination it is especially important to closely monitor for renal function, potassium, and hypotension. It should be emphasized that this combination is not recommended routinely and only in those who remain symptomatic despite the approaches discussed. It is not recommended to combine ACE-I, ARB, and aldosterone antagonist therapy.

The ARBs studied in clinical trials (Candesartan [CHARM], Valsartan [Val-HeFT, VALIANT], and Losartan [HEAAL]) have all shown significant reduction in mortality and readmissions in patients with HF. The first major trial evaluating the use of ARBs in HF was the Val-HeFT study. Valsartan was added to ACE-I, BB, digoxin, and diuretic therapies to evaluate the long-term effects of adding ARBs to standard HF therapy. In this trial, valsartan significantly reduced the combined end point of mortality and morbidity as well as improved clinical signs and symptoms in patients with HF compared with placebo. This difference was predominantly driven by a 24% reduction in the rate of HF hospitalizations, without a clear benefit for mortality

Table 4
Recommendations for appropriate doses of ACEIs

Drug	Initial Dose	Maximum Dose	Clinical Trials	Mean Dose Achieved
Lisinopril	2.5–5.0 mg qD	20–40 mg qD	ATLAS	32.5–35 mg/d
Captopril	6.25 mg TID	50 mg TID	ELITE	122.7 mg/d
Enalapril	2.5 mg BID	10–20 mg BID	SOLVD	16.6 mg/d

Recommendations summarized from current literature and data referenced in this article; see reference list.
Abbreviations: ACE-I, angiotensin-converting enzyme inhibitor; BID, twice a day; qD, every day; TID, 3 times a day.

Table 5
Recommendations for appropriate doses of ARBs

Drug	Initial Dose	Maximum Dose	Clinical Trial	Mean Dose Achieved
Losartan	25–50 mg qD	50–150 mg qD	HEAAL	129 mg/d
Valsartan	20–40 mg BID	160 mg BID	Val-HeFT	254 mg/d
Candesartan	4–8 mg qD	32 mg qD	CHARM	24 mg/d

Recommendations summarized from current literature and data referenced in this article; see reference list.
   Abbreviations: ARB, angiotensin receptor blocker; BID, twice a day; qD, every day.

alone (**Table 7**). However, the post hoc observation of adverse effects on mortality and morbidity in the subgroup receiving combined valsartan, an ACE inhibitor, and a β-blocker raised concern about the potential safety of this specific combination.[25] Hence, regular use of an ACE inhibitor, ARB, and aldosterone antagonist combination is not recommended and is potentially harmful for patients with HFrEF.[3]

The CHARM trial (Candesartan in Heart Failure Assessment of Reduction in Mortality and morbidity) was a complementary parallel trial with CHARM-Alternative (2028 patients) investigating use of ARBs in patients who were ACE-I intolerant, and CHARM-Added (2548 patients) investigating use of ARBs in patients who were already on ACE-I.[28] NYHA II-IV patients with HF with LVEF of 40% or lower were randomized to candesartan or placebo. The primary end point was a composite of CV death or hospital admission for HF. The study revealed an absolute reduction of 7 major events per 100 patients treated in CHARM-Alternative and an absolute reduction of 4.4 major events per 100 patients treated in CHARM-Added.[29] However, the investigators concluded that because of

adverse effects, especially with concomitant use of ACE-I therapy, routine monitoring of blood pressure, serum creatinine, and serum potassium is warranted.[32]

Other trials, including Evaluation of Losartan in the Elderly (ELITE II),[33] Optimal Trial in Myocardial Infarction with the Angiotensin II Antagonist Losartan (OPTIMAAL),[34] and Valsartan in Acute Myocardial Infarction (VALIANT),[30] which have assessed ARBs in comparison with ACE-Is for treatment of HF have shown no clear benefit of one pharmacologic agent over the other for mortality in patients with HFrEF.

ALDOSTERONE ANTAGONISTS

Despite the inhibition of the ACE with ACE-I therapy, there is evidence of increased plasma levels of aldosterone. Aldosterone has pleiotropic effects, resulting in increased sodium retention, constriction of systemic arterioles, stimulation of cytokine production, inflammatory-cell adhesion, activation of macrophages, and stimulation of growth of fibroblasts and the synthesis of type I and III fibrillar collagens involved in scar formation.[35]

Table 6
Current recommendations for the use of ARBs

Treatment – Use of ARB	Class of Recommendation	Level of Evidence
ARB in patients with a history of MI and reduced EF to prevent HF	I	A
ARBs are recommended in patients with HFrEF with current or prior symptoms who are ACE-I intolerant	I	A
ARBs are reasonable to reduce morbidity and mortality as alternatives to ACE-Is as first-line therapy for patients with HFrEF, especially for patients already taking ARBs for other indications	IIa	A
Addition of an ARB may be considered in persistently symptomatic patients with HFrEF who are already being treated with an ACE-I and a BB in whom an aldosterone antagonist is not indicated or tolerated	IIa	B

Recommendations summarized from current literature and data referenced in this article; see reference list.
   Abbreviations: ACE-I, angiotensin-converting enzyme inhibitor; ARB, angiotensin receptor blocker; BB, beta blocker; EF, ejection fraction; HF, heart failure; HFrEF, HF with reduced ejection fraction; MI, myocardial infarction.

Table 7
ARB trials supporting current guideline recommendations

Study	Aim of Study	Baseline Therapy	Results
CHARM Alternative,[28] 2003	To study the effect of ARBs in symptomatic HF with LVEF <40% and not taking an ACE-I (intolerant)	Diuretics BB 55% Spironolactone 24% Digoxin 46%	Absolute reduction of 7 major events per 100 patients treated NNT 14 patients to prevent 1 CV death or hospitalization HR: 0.77 (95% CI: 0.67–0.89); $P = .0004$
CHARM ADDED,[29] 2003	To investigate if ARB + ACE-I in patients with CHF and LVEF <40% improve clinical outcomes	BB 55% Digoxin 59% Spironolactone 17%	Absolute reduction of 4.4 major events per 100 patients treated NNT of 23 to prevent first event of CV death or CHF hospitalization RR: 0.85 (95% CI: 0.75–0.96); $P = .011$
VALIANT,[30] 2003	Compare the effect of an ARB, ACE-I, and the combination of the 2 on mortality in patients with LV systolic dysfunction (LVEF <35%)	BBs ASA	1-y mortality in the 3 groups: Valsartan 12.5% Captopril 13.2% Combination 12.3%
Val-HeFT,[25] 2001	Evaluate long-term effects of adding ARB to standard therapy for HF (NYHA II–IV with LVEF <40%)	Diuretics Digoxin 67% BB 35% ACE-I 93%	Mortality similar for the 2 treatment groups. For the combined end point of mortality and morbidity: RR: 0.87, 97.5% (CI, 0.77–0.97) $P = .009$
HEAAL,[31] 2009	To study the effects of high-dose vs low-dose losartan on clinical outcomes in patients with HF (NYHA class II–IV, LVEF <40%)	Diuretics (77%), BBs (72%), ARBs (38%)	635 patients in high-dose (150 mg) group vs 665 in 50-mg group died (HR: 0.94, 95% CI: 0.84–1.04, $P = .24$) 450 patients in high-dose vs 503 patients in low-dose group admitted for HF (0.87, 0.76–0.98, $P = .025$)

Abbreviations: ACE-I, angiotensin-converting enzyme inhibitor; ARB, angiotensin receptor blocker; ASA, aspirin; BB, beta blocker; CHF, chronic heart failure; CI, confidence interval; CV, cardiovascular; HF, heart failure; HFrEF, HF with reduced ejection fraction; HR, hazard ratio; LVEF, left ventricular ejection fraction; MI, myocardial infarction; NNT, number needed to treat; NYHA, New York Heart Association; RR, relative risk.

Aldosterone receptor antagonists are recommended in patients with NYHA class II–IV and who have an LVEF of 35% or less, unless contraindicated, to reduce morbidity and mortality (**Table 8**).[3] In the landmark RALES (Randomized Aldactone Evaluation Study) trial, 1663 NYHA class III–IV patients with severe HF and LVEF of 35% or less who were being treated with an ACE-I, a loop diuretic, and in most cases digoxin, were randomly assigned to receive spironolactone daily (25 mg) or placebo. After a mean follow-up period of 24 months, there was a 46% mortality rate in the placebo group compared with a reduced mortality rate of 35% in the spironolactone group.[36] Reduced risk of SCD and HF hospitalizations were also demonstrated.

Eplerenone has been shown to reduce all-cause deaths, CV deaths, or HF hospitalizations in a wider range of patients with HFrEF.[37] The Eplerenone Post-Acute Myocardial Infarction Heart

Table 8
Current recommendations for the use of aldosterone antagonists

Treatment – Use of MRAs	Class of Recommendation	Level of Evidence
MRAs are recommended in patients with NYHA class II–IV and who have LVEF ≤35%	I	A
MRA in post-MI patients who have LVEF ≤40% who develop symptoms of HF or who have a history of diabetes mellitus	I	B

Recommendations summarized from current literature and data referenced in this article; see reference list.
Abbreviations: HF, heart failure; LVEF, left ventricular ejection fraction; MI, myocardial infarction; MRA, mineralocorticoid receptor antagonists; NYHA, New York Heart Association.

Failure Efficacy and Survival Study (EPHESUS) trial demonstrated that eplerenone significantly reduced mortality in patients with HF or diabetes mellitus with LVEF of 40% or less after myocardial infarction (MI).[38] More recently, the Eplerenone in Mild Patients Hospitalization and Survival Study in Heart Failure (EMPHASIS-HF) trial studied eplerenone in patients with HF with LVEF of 30% or less (or 30%–35% if QRS duration ≥130 ms) with milder NYHA class II symptoms. In this population, aldosterone antagonism was also associated with improved survival (**Table 9**).[37]

Mineralocorticoid receptor antagonists (MRAs) cannot be used in patients with serum creatinine more than 2.5 mg/dL in men or more than 2.0 mg/dL in women (or estimated glomerular filtration rate <30 mL/min/1.73 m²), and/or potassium more than 5.0 mEq/L.[39,40] Careful monitoring of potassium, renal function, and diuretic dosing should be performed at initiation and closely followed thereafter to minimize risk of hyperkalemia and renal insufficiency.[36,37] In RALES, there was increased incidence (10%) of gynecomastia or breast pain with use of spironolactone (nonselective antagonist). The incidence of these adverse events was less than 1% in EPHESUS (Eplerenone Post-Acute Myocardial Infarction Heart Failure Efficacy and Survival Study) and EMPHASIS-HF without any difference in adverse events between eplerenone and placebo.[39,40]

The initial dose for spironolactone is 12.5 to 25.0 mg daily, and for eplerenone is 25.0 mg/d,

increasing to 50.0 mg daily. Every-other-day dosing can be used if there is any concern about hyperkalemia and renal insufficiency. Potassium levels and renal function should be checked within 2 to 3 days and again at 7 days after initiation of an aldosterone receptor antagonist.[3] Serial labs to monitor renal function and potassium must be performed at least monthly for the first 3 months and every 3 months thereafter.

β-ADRENERGIC BLOCKADE

BBs are recommended in all patients with HFrEF (**Table 10**). Unlike ACE-Is, there is no class effect with BBs.[3] The 3 BBs that have been demonstrated to be effective in clinical trials are metoprolol succinate, carvedilol, and bisoprolol (**Table 11**). The current ACC guidelines recommend prompt initiation of BBs as well as initiation during ACE-I optimization in hemodynamically stable patients. BBs can be safely started in patients hospitalized for HF who are not on intravenous inotropes.[41] The addition of a BB produces greater symptom improvement and mortality risk reduction than ACE inhibition even when reaching target doses demonstrated in clinical trials.[23,42] The Carvedilol and ACE-inhibitor Remodeling Mild Heart Failure Evaluation (CARMEN) study revealed that combination of BB and ACE-I therapy is superior to ACE-I alone for left ventricular (LV) remodeling as assessed by LV end-systolic volume index on transthoracic echo.[43]

Table 9
Recommendations for appropriate doses of aldosterone antagonists

Drug	Initial Dose	Maximum Dose	Clinical Trial	Mean Dose Achieved
Spironolactone	12.5–25 mg qD	25 mg qD-BID	RALES	26 mg/d
Eplerenone	25 mg qD	50 mg qD	EPHESUS	42.6 mg/d

Recommendations summarized from current literature and data referenced in this article; see reference list.
Abbreviations: BID, twice a day; qD, every day.

Table 10
Current recommendations for the use of BBs

Treatment – Use of BBs	Class of Recommendation	Level of Evidence
BB in patients with a history of MI and reduced EF to prevent HF	I	B
BBs should be used in all patients with a reduced EF to prevent HF	I	C
Use of 1 of the 3 BBs (Bisoprolol, Carvedilol, and Sustained-release metoprolol succinate) is recommended for all patients with current or prior symptoms of HFrEF	I	A

Recommendations summarized from current literature and data referenced in this article; see reference list.
Abbreviations: BB, beta blocker; EF, ejection fraction; HF, heart failure; HFrEF, HF with reduced ejection fraction; HR, hazard ratio; MI, myocardial infarction.

The Metoprolol CR/XL Randomized Intervention Trial in Congestive Heart Failure (MERIT-HF) study group investigated whether metoprolol succinate, which selectively blocks beta-1 receptors, in addition to standard therapy (ACEI and diuretics) would lower mortality in patients with decreased LVEF and HF symptoms. The study randomized approximately 2000 NYHA class II–IV patients with chronic HF and with LVEF of 40% or less to either metoprolol succinate or placebo. All-cause mortality, sudden death, and death from worsening HF were lower in the metoprolol group.[44]

The CIBIS (Cardiac Insufficiency Bisoprolol Study) study group investigated the efficacy of bisoprolol, a beta-1 selective adrenergic receptor blocker, in decreasing all-cause mortality in chronic HF in a multicenter trial in Europe. In this trial, 2647 NYHA III–IV patients with LVEF of 35% or less receiving standard therapy (diuretics and ACE-Is) were randomized to bisoprolol or placebo. CIBIS-II was stopped early because bisoprolol showed a significant mortality benefit. Treatment effects were independent of the severity or cause of HF. The investigators concluded that BB therapy had survival benefit in stable patients with HF.[45]

The Carvedilol Prospective Randomized Cumulative Survival (COPERNICUS) trial demonstrated the beneficial effects of carvedilol, which blocks alpha-1, beta-1, and beta-2 receptors, on mortality in NYHA class IV patients with chronic HF. All subgroups including those with the most advanced HF showed the same beneficial effect on mortality.[46]

The Carvedilol or Metoprolol European Trial (COMET) demonstrated a significant survival benefit for carvedilol over metoprolol tartrate in patients with mild-to-severe chronic HF.[47] However, target dosing of metoprolol tartrate (50 mg twice daily) and carvedilol (25 mg twice daily) is not equivalent, with the carvedilol dose reached being substantially higher.[48] Further, shorter-acting metoprolol tartrate was used in this trial rather than longer-acting metoprolol succinate (**Table 12**).

In the US Carvedilol Heart Failure Study, 1094 patients with chronic HF were randomly assigned to receive either placebo or the BB carvedilol; background therapy with digoxin, diuretics, and an ACE-I remained constant.[49] At the end of 6 months, the overall mortality rate was 7.8% in the placebo group and 3.2% in the carvedilol group; the reduction in risk attributable to carvedilol was 65% (95% confidence interval; $P<.001$). This finding led the Data and Safety Monitoring Board to recommend termination of the study before its scheduled completion. In addition, as compared with placebo, carvedilol therapy was accompanied by a 27% reduction in the risk of hospitalization for CV causes (19.6% vs 14.1%, $P<.036$).

Table 11
Recommendations for appropriate doses of BBs

Drug	Initial Dose	Maximum Dose	Clinical Trial	Mean Dose Achieved
Metoprolol succinate	12.25 mg qD	200 mg qD	MERIT-HF	159 mg/d
Carvedilol	3.125 mg BID	50 mg BID	CAPRICORN	37 mg/d
Bisoprolol	1.25 mg qD	10 mg qD	CIBIS-II	8.6 mg/d

Recommendations summarized from current literature and data referenced in this article; see reference list.
Abbreviations: BB, beta blocker; BID, twice a day; qD, every day.

Table 12
BB trials supporting current guideline recommendations

Study	Aim of Study	Baseline Therapy	Results
MERIT HF,[44] 1999	To investigate whether Metoprolol XL lowered mortality in patients with NYHA II–IV and LVEF <40%	Diuretics + ACE-I [Amiodarone NOT allowed]	All-cause mortality was 11.0% in the placebo group vs 7.2% in the Metoprolol Group ($P = .00009$)
CIBIS II,[45] 1999	To assess the efficacy of bisoprolol in decreasing all-cause mortality in chronic HF (NYHA class III or IV with EF <35%)	Diuretics + ACE-I (amiodarone allowed 16%)	Annualized mortality was 13.2% in the placebo group vs 8.8% in the Bisoprolol group HR: 0.66 (95% CI 0.54–0.81) $P<.0001$
COPERNICUS,[46] 2002	To study if Carvedilol is beneficial in patients with NYHA class IV and LVEF <25%	Diuretics + ACE-I (or ARB) (Amiodarone allowed 18%)	All-cause mortality was 18.5% in placebo group and 11.4% in Carvedilol group ($P = .0014$)
CAPRICORN,[49] 2001	To investigate the long-term efficacy of carvedilol on patients with LV dysfunction post-acute MI already treated with ACE-I	ACE-I 98% Aspirin 86%	All-cause mortality was 15.0% in the placebo group vs 12% in the Carvedilol Group ($P = .03$)
US CARVEDILOL,[50] 1996	To investigate the effect of BB on survival of patients with chronic heart failure	Digoxin + Loop Diuretic + ACE-I 90%	All-cause mortality was 7.8% in the placebo group vs 3.2% in the Carvedilol Group ($P<.001$)

Abbreviations: ACE-I, angiotensin-converting enzyme inhibitor; ARB, angiotensin receptor blocker; BB, beta blocker; CI, confidence interval; EF, ejection fraction; HF, heart failure; HR, hazard ratio; LVEF, left ventricular ejection fraction; MI, myocardial infarction; NYHA, New York Heart Association.

The Carvedilol Post-Infarct Survival Control in LV Dysfunction (CAPRICORN) study enrolled 1959 patients with a proven acute MI and a LVEF of 40% or less that were randomly assigned 6.25 mg carvedilol or placebo[50]; 98% of these patients were receiving an ACE-I and 86% were receiving aspirin. Carvedilol was progressively increased to a maximum of 25 mg twice daily during the next 6 weeks, and patients were followed until the requisite number of primary end points had occurred. The primary end point was all-cause mortality or hospital admission for CV problems. Analysis was by intention to treat. All-cause mortality was lower in the carvedilol group than in the placebo group (12% vs 15%, $P = .03$). CV mortality, nonfatal MIs, and all-cause mortality or nonfatal MI were also lower on carvedilol than on placebo. The reduction in all-cause mortality was additional to the effects of ACE inhibitors, which was prescribed in 98% of patients.

BBs should be initiated at low doses and titrated up as tolerated by the patient to target doses used in clinical trials.[42] While uptitrating the dose, patients must be monitored for adverse effects that can include bradycardia, heart block, hypotension, fluid retention and worsening HF, fatigue and worsening of depression, and reactive airway disease. If there is evidence of fluid overload, BB must be used in conjunction with diuretics.[51,52] BBs have been demonstrated to reduce mortality and risk of hospitalization in HF,[23,42–45] as well as reduce the risks of disease progression, clinical deterioration, and sudden death.[53–55] Withdrawing BBs abruptly should be avoided, as it could lead to worsening of HF.[56] For these reasons, we recommend that adverse effects be closely monitored and dose reduction be pursued first before permanently and abruptly withdrawing BB therapy.

DIURETICS

Diuretics inhibit the reabsorption of sodium or chloride at specific sites in the renal tubules. Loop diuretics act in the thick ascending limb of the loop of Henle, whereas thiazide-type diuretics act in the distal tubule and connecting segments. Potassium-sparing diuretics act in the aldosterone-sensitive principal cells in the cortical collecting tubule.

Fluid retention may be present in patients who have dyspnea, an increase in weight from baseline of more than 2 kg in fewer than 3 days, raised jugular venous pressure, crepitations on chest auscultation, hepatomegaly, or signs of peripheral edema. Diuretics are used to increase urinary sodium excretion and decrease physical signs of fluid retention in patients with HF (**Table 13**).[57,58] Although diuretics have not been shown to change mortality or morbidity, they have been shown to improve symptoms and exercise tolerance in patients with HF.[59,60]

Most patients with HF are initially treated with loop diuretics because of their potency. However, in hypertensive HF with mild congestion, thiazide diuretics are preferred, as they present a more persistent effect on blood pressure. Potassium-sparing diuretics may be helpful in people with hypokalemia and in conjunction with loop diuretics (**Table 14**).

Diuretic therapy is commonly initiated with low doses, and the dose is increased until urine output increases and weight decreases, generally by 1 to 2 lb daily. Lower doses may result in fluid retention, whereas higher doses can lead to volume contraction, which may lead to hypotension, renal insufficiency, and electrolyte abnormalities. Electrolyte abnormalities need to be monitored closely, as hypokalemia and hypomagnesemia can predispose patients to serious cardiac arrhythmias.[61] Other rare side effects are loop diuretic–induced ototoxicity and hypersensitivity reactions, as they are sulfonamides.

Furosemide has a bioavailability of only about 50% with substantial interpatient and intrapatient variability (10%–100%).[62,63] As a result, there may be a greater response to oral torsemide or

Table 14
Recommendations for appropriate doses of diuretics

Drug	Initial Dose	Maximum Dose
Loop diuretics		
Furosemide	20–40 mg qD/BID	600 mg
Bumetanide	0.5–1 mg qD/BID	10 mg
Torsemide	10–20 mg qD	200 mg
Thiazide diuretics		
Chlorthiazide	250–500 mg BID	1000 mg
Chlorthalidone	12.5–25 mg qD	100 mg
Hydrochlorothiazide	25 mg qD/BID	200 mg
Indapamide	2.5 mg qD	5 mg
Metolazone	2.5 mg qD	20 mg
Potassium-sparing diuretics		
Amiloride	5 mg qD	20 mg
Spironolactone	12.5–25 mg qD	50 mg
Triamterene	50–75 mg BID	200 mg
Eplerenone	25 qD	50 qD

Recommendations summarized from current literature and data referenced in this article; see reference list.
Abbreviations: BID, twice a day; qD, every day.

bumetanide, which are more predictably absorbed.[53,54,64] In advanced stages, bowel edema and hypoperfusion may further delay absorption and delivery,[63] and, therefore, increasing doses may be required to achieve an appropriate effect. Diuretic resistance can usually be overcome by parenteral administration,[55] the use of 2 or more diuretics in combination (eg, furosemide and metolazone),[65] or the addition of drugs that increase renal blood flow (eg, positive inotropic agents).

ORAL VASODILATORS

Hydralazine produces arterial vasodilation and systemic vascular resistance reduction by increasing intracellular cyclic guanosine monophosphate and promoting smooth muscle relaxation. Nitrates are transformed in smooth muscle cells into nitric oxide and subsequently vasodilation. The Vasodilator-Heart Failure Trial (V-HeFT) study randomized

Table 13
Current recommendations for the use of diuretics

Treatment – Use of Diuretics	Class of Recommendation	Level of Evidence
Diuretics for fluid retention in HFrEF	I	C

Recommendations summarized from current literature and data referenced in this article; see reference list.
Abbreviation: HFrEF, heart failure with reduced ejection fraction.

HFrEF patients who were on digoxin and diuretic to receive additional therapy with placebo, prazosin, or combination of isosorbide dinitrate-hydralazine (ISDN-HYD). It showed reduced mortality in the ISDN-HYD cohort compared with placebo at 2 years.[66] In a subsequent study, the V-HeFT II trial randomized 804 patients to either ISDN-HYD or enalapril on background therapy of digoxin and diuretics. This study showed that enalapril resulted in significantly improved survival compared with ISDN-HYD in patients with HF.

In addition, the Hy-C trial demonstrated that captopril produced more favorable effects on survival in comparison with vasodilators.[67] A post hoc retrospective analysis of these vasodilator trials demonstrated particular efficacy of isosorbide dinitrate and hydralazine in the African American population.[68] This was subsequently validated in the A-Heft trial. This trial randomized African Americans with advanced HF, who were receiving standard therapy (including BBs and ACEIs), to ISDN-HYD or placebo. This study demonstrated that the addition of fixed-dose isosorbide dinitrate and hydralazine enhanced survival and decreased hospitalizations.[69]

Combination therapy with hydralazine and nitrates is recommended for patients with contra-indications to ACE-Is or ARBs (angioedema, persistent hyperkalemia, acute kidney injury), as well as in African American patients with HF who remain symptomatic (NYHA functional class III–IV) despite optimal medical therapy (**Table 15**).[3]

Adverse effects of these vasodilators may include headache, dizziness, and gastrointestinal complaints.[66] Hypotension can be a major limitation to the use of vasodilator therapy in the elderly. However, nitrates are useful when a reduction of preload is necessary when diuretic use can be limited, such as in renal failure.[70]

DIGOXIN

Digoxin is a positive inotropic agent. Digoxin also attenuates carotid sinus baroreceptors and has sympatho-inhibitory effects that lead to a decrease in norepinephrine, renin, and possibly aldosterone levels.[71,72] In the only randomized controlled trial of digoxin therapy (DIG trial), patients with HF (LVEF<45%) were randomized to receive digoxin or placebo and were followed for 37 months; approximately 30% of these patients were older than 70 years. There was no difference in the primary end point of mortality from any cause with digoxin compared with placebo, but fewer patients were hospitalized for worsening HF when treated with digoxin as compared with placebo (relative risk [RR] 0.72; 95% confidence interval [CI] 0.66–0.79, P<.001).[73]

A Cochrane systematic review of 13 studies showed that digoxin reduced the combined end point of death and hospital admission in those with both HF with reduced ejection fraction and HF with preserved ejection fraction. However, most of these studies were conducted in patients who were not taking a BB.[74,75] Other placebo-controlled trials have shown that treatment with digoxin for 1 to 3 months can improve symptoms, health-related quality of life, and exercise tolerance in patients with mild to moderate HF (**Table 16**).[76–79] In HFrEF patients who are symptomatic despite optimal therapy with neurohormonal antagonists, digoxin may be added for symptomatic relief. In patients with atrial fibrillation, BBs are usually more effective when added to digoxin in controlling the ventricular response, particularly during exercise.[80,81]

The dosage of digoxin should be adjusted to obtain serum levels between 0.6 and 1.2 ng/mL. A post hoc analysis found that patients with HF with LVEF less than 45% with serum digoxin

Table 15 Current recommendations for the use of oral vasodilators		
Treatment: Use of Oral Vasodilators	Class of Recommendation	Level of Evidence
The combination of hydralazine and isosorbide dinitrate in African Americans with NYHA class III–IV HFrEF receiving optimal therapy with ACE-I and BB	I	A
The combination of hydralazine and isosorbide dinitrate in patients with current or prior symptomatic HFrEF who cannot be given an ACE-I or ARB because of drug intolerance, hypotension, or renal insufficiency	IIa	B

Recommendations summarized from current literature and data referenced in this article; see reference list.

Abbreviations: ACE-I, angiotensin-converting enzyme inhibitor; ARB, angiotensin receptor blocker; BB, beta blocker; HFrEF, HF with reduced ejection fraction; NYHA, New York Heart Association.

Table 16
Current recommendations for the use of digoxin

Treatment: Use of Digoxin	Class of Recommendation	Level of Evidence
Digoxin can be beneficial in patients with HFrEF, unless contraindicated, to decrease hospitalizations for HF	IIa	B

Recommendations summarized from current literature and data referenced in this article; see reference list.

Abbreviations: HF, heart failure; HFrEF, HF with reduced ejection fraction.

concentrations of 0.5 to 0.8 ng/mL had a 6% reduced mortality compared with those who had concentrations of 0.8 to 1.1 ng/mL. Thus, serum digoxin concentrations and targeting lower concentrations seem to be the critical point of digoxin therapy, especially in elderly and lean patients in whom adverse effects, such as increased volume of distribution, renal insufficiency, and hypokalemia, are frequent. Other common side effects include cardiac arrhythmias (heart block, ectopic and re-entrant cardiac rhythms), gastrointestinal symptoms (eg, anorexia, nausea, and vomiting), and neurologic complaints (eg, visual disturbances, disorientation, and confusion). Although toxicity is commonly associated with high serum digoxin levels (>2 ng/mL), it may occur with lower levels, especially if there is concomitant hypokalemia, hypomagnesemia, or hypothyroidism.[82,83]

HF WITH PRESERVED EJECTION FRACTION

HF with preserved ejection fraction (HFpEF) is a clinical syndrome encompassing symptoms and signs of HF together with a normal LVEF. The prevalence of HFpEF increases with age (15%, 33%, and 50% at ages 50, 50–70, and 70 years, respectively).[84] Despite improved understanding of the pathophysiology of HFpEF, specific pharmacologic treatment has thus far proven disappointing. Management for HFpEF is currently directed at symptoms, especially comorbidities, and risk factors that may worsen CV disease (such as treatment of hypertension, ventricular rate in atrial fibrillation) as trials for HFpEF have generally been disappointing with various therapies.[85] For example, atrial fibrillation with rapid ventricular rate may worsen HF symptoms in this population by leading to shortened diastolic filling time and the loss of atrial contribution to LV diastolic filling.

In those patients with HFpEF and hypertension, the major therapeutic goal is the improvement of diastolic function by controlling blood pressure and regression of left ventricular hypertrophy. Improved blood pressure control reduces hospitalization for HF.[86] It also leads to decreased CV events and mortality.[87] In the hypertensive population, ACE inhibitors and/or ARBs may be used. Coronary artery disease (CAD) is also common in patients with HFpEF[88]; however, there are no studies examining the impact of revascularization on symptoms or outcomes in this population. It is reasonable to consider revascularization in symptomatic HFpEF patients for whom ischemia appears to contributing to HF symptoms (**Table 17**).

The CHARM-Preserved trial,[89] which enrolled 3023 patients with NYHA class II to IV HF and

Table 17
Current recommendations for treatment of stage C HF with preserved EF

Heart Failure with Preserved Ejection Fraction	Class of Recommendation	Level of Evidence
Systolic and diastolic blood pressure to be controlled	I	B
Diuretics for symptomatic relief from volume overload	I	C
Use BB, ACE-I, ARBs in patients with HTN	IIa	C
Coronary revascularization is reasonable in patients with CAD in whom symptoms (angina) or demonstrable myocardial ischemia is judged to be having an adverse effect on symptomatic HFpEF despite optimized medical therapy	IIa	C
Consider use of ARBs to decrease hospitalizations	IIb	B

Recommendations summarized from current literature and data referenced in this article; see reference list.

Abbreviations: ACE-I, angiotensin-converting enzyme inhibitor; ARB, angiotensin receptor blocker; BB, beta blocker; CAD, coronary artery disease; HFpEF, HF with preserved ejection fraction; HTN, hypertension.

LVEF greater than 40%, demonstrated that candesartan was not significantly associated with mortality or morbidity reduction in patients with HFpEF (CV-related death or hospitalization for HF: hazard ratio [HR] = 0.86; 95% CI, 0.74–1.00). In this trial, diastolic function was not strictly defined and patients with ejection fraction greater than 40% were included. This could have allowed inclusion of patients who had systolic HF but had improved their ejection fraction by use of ACE inhibitors and BBs.

The I-PRESERVE study examined the effects of irbesartan in patients with HFpEF. This study had a more specific definition of HFpEF than CHARM-Preserved. Patients were included if LVEF was greater than 45% and a there was corroborative objective evidence of HF or a cardiac substrate for diastolic dysfunction. After a mean follow-up duration of 49.5 months, the primary event rates of death from any cause or hospitalization for a CV cause in the irbesartan and placebo groups were similar (HR = 0.95; 95% CI 0.86–1.05).[90] The PEP-CHF (Perindopril in Elderly People with Chronic Heart failure) trial evaluated the effects of perindopril in 850 elderly patients with HFpEF. Unfortunately, perindopril was not associated with improved primary outcomes in a subgroup of patients with HFpEF.[91] See **Box 1** for the ABC strategy to achieve success with drug therapy in patients with stage C HF.

DEVICE THERAPY
Implantable Cardioverter-Defibrillator

Despite optimal medical therapy, patients with HF with reduced ejection fraction (HFrEF) carry a residual increased risk for SCD due to tachyarrhythmias. Evidence supporting the current guideline recommendations for implantable cardioverter-defibrillator (ICD) therapy is summarized in **Table 18**. Additionally, separate topics on arrhythmias and heart failure, and sudden cardiac death and heart failure are discussed in this series.

Primary prevention
According to the 2013 ACCF/AHA guidelines for the management of HF, there are 2 Class I indications for ICD therapy in the context of primary prevention[3]:

1. In patients with nonischemic or ischemic heart cardiomyopathy 40 or more days post-MI with LVEF of 35% or less and NYHA class II or III symptoms on optimal medical therapy, who have expected survival for more than 1 year (Level of Evidence: A)
2. In patients 40 or more days post-MI with LVEF of 30% or less and NYHA class I symptoms on

Box 1
The ABC strategy to achieve success with drug therapy in patients with Stage C HF

A: ACE-I/ARB: in all patients with HF unless contraindicated.

B: BB: use as early as possible in patients withHFrEF.

C: Compliance with medications, sodium restriction, and follow-up visits must be reinforced.

D: Dosage: Start low; go slow, try to achieve target doses used in clinical trials.

E: Education: Educate patient, family, and caretakers.

F: Fluid status to be carefully assessed at every visit.

G: Guidelines-based therapy to be followed.

H: Hydralazine and…

I: Isosorbide dinitrate as combination in African Americans with HF.

J: Judicious use while combining any of the following: ACE-I, ARB, MRA, diuretics.

K: K1 Mg1 BUN, Cr to be closely monitored.

L: Loop diuretics (first line) and other diuretics in appropriate doses to maintain euvolemia.

M: MRAs can also be used in NYHA Class II.

N: Nonsteroidal anti-inflammatory drugs to be avoided in HF.

Abbreviations: ACE-I, angiotensin-converting enzyme inhibitor; ARB, angiotensin receptor blocker; BB, beta blocker; BUN, blood urea nitrogen; Cr, creatinine; HF, heart failure; HFrEF, HF with reduced ejection fraction; MRA, mineralocorticoid receptor antagonists; NYHA, New York Heart Association.

optimal medical therapy, who have expected survival for more than 1 year (Level of Evidence: B)

Secondary prevention
There are several Class I indications for ICD therapy in the setting of secondary prevention for survivors of SCD and individuals with previously documented ventricular arrhythmias, based on the 2008 ACC/AHA/Heart Rhythm Society device-based therapy guidelines[100]:

1. In patients who are survivors of cardiac arrest due to ventricular fibrillation (VF) or hemodynamically unstable sustained ventricular tachycardia (VT) after exclusion of any completely reversible cause (Level of Evidence: A)
2. In patients with structural heart disease and spontaneous sustained VT (Level of Evidence: B)

Table 18
ICD trials supporting current guideline recommendations

Study (Year, Reference)	Patient Population	Primary End Point/Findings
Primary prevention		
MADIT,[92] 1996	196 pxs, prior MI, NSVT, or inducible VT/VF EF ≤35% ICD vs medical therapy	All-cause mortality: ICD associated with a 54% risk reduction during mean follow up of 27 mo (P = .009)
MUSTT,[93] 1999	704 pxs, CAD/MI, NSVT, or inducible VT EF ≤40% EP-guided therapy (ICD or anti-arrhythmic drugs) vs none	Cardiac arrest or arrhythmic death: EP-guided therapy (largely due to ICDs) associated with 27% risk reduction during median follow-up of 39 mo (P = .04)
MADIT-II,[94] 2002	1232 pxs, prior MI EF ≤30% ICD vs medical therapy	All-cause mortality: ICD associated with a 31% risk reduction during mean follow-up of 2 y (P = .016)
DINAMIT,[95] 2004	674 pxs, 6–40 d post-MI EF ≤35%, impaired cardiac autonomic function ICD vs medical therapy	All-cause mortality: HR for ICD: 1.08 (P = .66)
SCD-HeFT,[96] 2005	2521 pxs, CAD and DCM EF ≤35%, NYHA II–III ICD vs amiodarone vs medical therapy	All-cause mortality: ICD associated with a 23% risk reduction during median follow-up of 46 mo (P = .007)
Secondary prevention		
AVID,[97] 1997	1016 pxs, survivors of VF or sustained VT, EF ≤40% CAD 81%; mean EF 32% ± 13% ICD vs anti-arrhythmic drugs	Overall survival: 89.3% vs 82.3% (1 y) 81.6% vs 74.7% (2 y) 75.4% vs 64.1% (3 y) (P<.02)
CIDS,[98] 2000	659 pxs, resuscitated VF or VT or with unmonitored syncope 77% prior MI, mean EF = 34% ± 14% ICD vs amiodarone	All-cause mortality: ICD reduced risk from 10.2%/y to 8.3%/y (19.7% RRR) (P = .142)
CASH,[99] 2000	288 pxs, survivors of SCD 73% CAD, mean EF = 46% ± 18% ICD vs amiodarone vs metoprolol	All-cause mortality: ICD associated with a 23% risk reduction during 9 y of follow-up (P = .081)

Abbreviations: CAD, coronary artery disease; DCM, dilated cardiomyopathy; EF, ejection fraction; EP, electrophysiology; HR, hazard ratio; ICD, implantable cardioverter-defibrillator; MI, myocardial infarction; NSVT, non-sustained ventricular tachycardia; NYHA, New York Heart Association; pxs, provexis; RRR, relative risk reduction; SCD, sudden cardiac death; VF, ventricular fibrillation; VT, ventricular tachycardia.

3. In patients with syncope of undetermined origin with hemodynamically significant sustained VT or VF during electrophysiological study (EPS) (Level of Evidence: B)
4. In patients with nonsustained VT due to prior MI, LVEF of 40% or less, and inducible VF or sustained VT at EPS (Level of Evidence: B).

Cardiac Resynchronization Therapy

Progressive LV dysfunction may result in ventricular electromechanical discoordination or LV dyssynchrony, which constitutes the rationale for cardiac resynchronization therapy (CRT). In addition to improving systolic function, functional mitral regurgitation, exercise capacity, and hospitalization rates, CRT has been shown to prolong survival. Current guidelines support Class I recommendations for CRT in patients with LVEF of 35% or less, sinus rhythm, left bundle-branch block (LBBB), QRS duration of 150 ms or more, and NYHA class II, III, or ambulatory IV symptoms on optimal medical therapy (Level of Evidence: A for NYHA class III/IV; Level of Evidence: B for NYHA class II). Class IIa recommendations are applicable in similar patients with non-LBBB pattern with QRS duration of 150 ms or more, LBBB and QRS 120–149 ms, or atrial fibrillation requiring near 100% ventricular pacing. Trial data supporting these guidelines for CRT are summarized in **Table 19**.

SURGICAL INTERVENTIONS
Coronary Artery Bypass Graft Surgery

The goals of coronary artery bypass graft (CABG) surgery in ischemic cardiomyopathy are to increase survival and improve symptoms. In addition to the severity of LV systolic dysfunction and

CAD, the presence of angina and myocardial viability need to be considered before revascularization. Contemporary guidelines designate a Class I recommendation for CABG for patients with HF with angina and left main stenosis (>50%) or left main equivalent (LMEQ) disease (ie, ≥70% stenosis in the proximal left anterior descending [LAD] and proximal left circumflex coronary arteries) and who are on optimal medical therapy (Level of Evidence: C).[3,108] Data from the Coronary Artery Surgery Study (CASS) Registry

Table 19
CRT trials supporting current guideline recommendations

Study (Year, Reference)	Patient Population	Primary End Point/Findings
NYHA Class III-IV		
MUSTIC,[101] 2001	58 pxs, EF ≤35%, QRS >150 ms, SR, NYHA III CRT-P vs no pacing	6-min walk distance: 22% improved during 6 mo of follow-up (P<.001)
MIRACLE,[102] 2002	453 pxs, EF <35%, QRS >130 ms, SR, NYHA III–IV CRT vs medical therapy	6-min walk distance improved: +39 vs +10 m (P = .005); functional class improved (P<.001); quality of life improved: −18.0 vs −9.0 points (P = .001)
COMPANION,[103] 2004	1520 pxs, EF <35%, QRS >120 ms, SR, NYHA III–IV CRT-P vs CRT-D vs medical therapy	Time to death from or hospitalization for any cause: decreased in the CRT-P group (HR 0.81, P = .014) and in the CRT-D (HR 0.80, P = .01) compared with medical therapy alone over 15 mo
CARE-HF,[104] 2005	814 pxs, EF <35%, QRS >120 ms, SR, NYHA III-IV CRT-P vs medical therapy	Time to death from any cause or an unplanned hospitalization for a major CV event: reached by 39% in the CRT group vs 55% in the control group (HR, 0.63; P<.001) for a mean follow-up of 29 mo
NYHA Class I-II		
REVERSE,[105] 2008	610 pxs, EF ≤40%, QRS ≥120 ms, NYHA I–II CRT-D vs no CRT	HF clinical composite response: 16% worsened in the CRT vs 21% in the no CRT group over 12 mo; P = .10
MADIT-CRT II,[106] 2009	1820 pxs, EF ≤30%, QRS ≥130 ms, NYHA I–II CRT-D vs ICD	HF event or death: 17.2% in CRT-D vs 25.3% in ICD only; 34% risk reduction (HR in the CRT-D group: 0.66) in 28 mo; P = .001
RAFT,[107] 2010	1798 pxs, EF ≤30%, QRS ≥120 ms/≥200 ms paced, NYHA II–III CRT-D vs ICD	HF hospitalization or death: 33.2% in CRT-D vs 40.3% in ICD only; 25% risk reduction (HR in CRT-D: 0.75) over 40 mo; P<.001; when confined to NYHA II patients only, there was 27% reduction in the primary end point; P = .001

Abbreviations: CRT, cardiac resynchronization therapy; CRT-D, CRT-defibrillator; CRT-P, CRT-pacing; CV, cardiovascular; EF, ejection fraction; HF, heart failure; HR, hazard ratio; ICD, implantable cardioverter-defibrillator; NYHA, New York Heart Association; SR, sinus rhythm.

revealed that among patients with LMEQ disease, the median survival was 13.1 years and 6.2 years in the CABG surgery and medical therapy groups, respectively (P<.0001).[109] However, CABG surgery did not prolong median survival in the subset of patients with normal LVEF.

Class IIa indications are endorsed for CABG in 2 groups: (1) to improve survival in patients with LVEF of 35% to 50% and significant (≥70% diameter stenosis) multivessel CAD or proximal LAD stenosis when viability is present (Level of Evidence: B), and (2) to improve morbidity and CV mortality for patients with LVEF less than 35%, HF, and significant CAD (Level of Evidence: B). (3) Although older studies have shown lower mortality in patients with mild to moderate LV systolic dysfunction who are treated surgically than medically,[110,111] survival benefit from CABG is less compelling in those with much lower LVEF. The Surgical Treatment for Ischemic Heart Failure (STICH) trial randomized patients with LVEF of 35% or less and surgically amenable CAD to medical therapy plus CABG or medical therapy alone.[112] Over a follow-up of 56 months, there was no significant difference in the primary outcome of all-cause death in the comparison groups (HR with CABG, 0.86; 95% CI 0.72–1.04; P = .12). CABG was superior to medical therapy for the secondary outcomes of CV death, and of death from any cause or CV hospitalization. A substudy of the STICH trial evaluated whether myocardial viability, assessed by single-photon-emission computed tomography, dobutamine echocardiography, or both, could identify patients with greater survival benefit from CABG.[113] The presence of viable myocardium was associated with a greater likelihood of survival in this population (HR for death in patients with viability, 0.64; 95% CI 0.48–0.86; P = .003), but this association was not significant after adjustment for other baseline variables (P = .21).

Mitral Valve Repair

In patients with HF with severe LV systolic dysfunction and significant functional mitral regurgitation (MR), mitral valve repair (MVR), either surgically or percutaneously, has been associated with improved ventricular mechanics and patient morbidity but has not shown any survival benefit superior to medical therapy. Among 73 patients with LVEF higher than 30% and moderate MR who were randomized to receive CABG plus MVR or CABG alone, 1-year mortality was similar in both groups (9% vs 5%, respectively; P = .66).[114] Combined MVR and CABG resulted in better LV reverse remodeling, B-type natriuretic peptide

levels, and functional capacity compared with CABG alone. In reference to the impact of a percutaneously implanted MV clip on patient outcomes, the Endovascular Valve Edge-to-Edge Repair Study (EVEREST) II trial investigated 279 patients with at least moderately severe MR (mean LVEF 61%) who were randomized to undergo either percutaneous or conventional MVR.[115,116] The primary efficacy end point (freedom from death and from surgery for MV dysfunction at 12 months) was reached in 55% in the percutaneous group and 73% in the surgery group (P = .007). Major adverse events at 30 days occurred in 15% and 48% in the percutaneous and surgery groups, respectively (P<.001). An observational study on patients with end-stage HF and severe LV systolic dysfunction reported that at 6 months, percutaneous MVR significantly improved B-type natriuretic peptide levels, LVEF and volumes, NYHA functional class, and 6-minute walk test.[117]

Ventricular Reconstruction

Surgical reverse remodeling or LV reconstruction is a Class IIb indication for carefully selected patients with LV systolic dysfunction and specific conditions, including intractable HF and ventricular arrhythmias (Level of Evidence: B).[3] In post-anterior MI patients with HF with LVEF of 35% or lower, data have shown that surgical ventricular restoration is associated with improved LV systolic function and geometry, and NYHA functional class but is not associated with a significant reduction in death and CV hospitalizations.[117,118]

SUMMARY

ACC Stage C HF includes those patients with prior or current symptoms of HF in the context of an underlying structural heart problem who are primarily managed with medical therapy. Although there is guideline-based medical therapy for those with HFrEF, therapies in HFpEF have thus far proven elusive. Emerging therapies, such as serelaxin, are currently under investigation and may prove beneficial. The role of advanced surgical therapies, such as mechanical circulatory support, in this population is not well defined. Further investigation is warranted for these therapies in patients with stage C HF.

REFERENCES

1. VanSuch M, Naessens JM, Stroebel RJ, et al. Effect of discharge instructions on readmission of hospitalised patients with heart failure: do all of the Joint Commission on Accreditation of Healthcare

Organizations heart failure core measures reflect better care? Qual Saf Health Care 2006;15:414–7.

2. Koelling TM, Johnson ML, Cody RJ, et al. Discharge education improves clinical outcomes in patients with chronic heart failure. Circulation 2005;111:179–85.

3. Yancy CW, Jessup M, Bozkurt B, et al. 2013 ACCF/AHA guideline for the management of heart failure: a report of the American College of Cardiology Foundation/American Heart Association task force on practice guidelines. J Am Coll Cardiol 2013; 62(16):e147–239.

4. Davies EJ, Moxham TT, Rees KK, et al. Exercise training for systolic heart failure: Cochrane systematic review and meta-analysis. Eur J Heart Fail 2010;12:706–15.

5. McKelvie RS. Exercise training in patients with heart failure: clinical outcomes, safety, and indications. Heart Fail Rev 2008;13:3–11.

6. O'Connor CM, Whellan DJ, Lee KL, et al. Efficacy and safety of exercise training in patients with chronic heart failure: HF-ACTION randomized controlled trial. JAMA 2009;301:1439–50.

7. Piña IL, Apstein CS, Balady GJ, et al. Exercise and heart failure: a statement from the American Heart Association Committee on exercise, rehabilitation, and prevention. Circulation 2003;107: 1210–25.

8. Smart NN, Marwick TH. Exercise training for patients with heart failure: a systematic review of factors that improve mortality and morbidity. Am J Med 2004;116:14.

9. Piepoli MF, Davos CC, Francis DP, et al. Exercise training meta-analysis of trials in patients with chronic heart failure (ExTraMATCH). BMJ 2004; 328:189.

10. Arcand JJ, Ivanov JJ, Sasson AA, et al. A high-sodium diet is associated with acute decompensated heart failure in ambulatory heart failure patients: a prospective follow-up study. Audio, Transactions of the IRE Professional Group on. Am J Clin Nutr 2011;93:332–7.

11. Damgaard MM, Norsk PP, Gustafsson FF, et al. Hemodynamic and neuroendocrine responses to changes in sodium intake in compensated heart failure. Am J Physiol Regul Integr Comp Physiol 2006;290:R1294–301.

12. Volpe MM, Tritto CC, DeLuca NN, et al. Abnormalities of sodium handling and of cardiovascular adaptations during high salt diet in patients with mild heart failure. Circulation 1993;88:1620–7.

13. He FJ, MacGregor GA. Effect of longer-term modest salt reduction on blood pressure. Cochrane Database Syst Rev 2004;(3):CD004937.

14. Kenchaiah S, Evans JC, Levy D, et al. Obesity and the risk of heart failure. N Engl J Med 2002;347: 305–13.

15. Anker SD, Ponikowski P, Varney S, et al. Wasting as independent risk factor for mortality in chronic heart failure. Lancet 1997;349:4.

16. Arzt M, Floras JS, Logan AG, et al. Suppression of central sleep apnea by continuous positive airway pressure and transplant-free survival in heart failure: a post hoc analysis of the Canadian continuous positive airway pressure for patients with central sleep apnea and heart failure trial (CANPAP). Circulation 2007;115:3173–80.

17. Bradley TD, Logan AG, Kimoff RJ, et al. Continuous positive airway pressure for central sleep apnea and heart failure. N Engl J Med 2005;353:2025–33.

18. Kaneko Y, Floras JS, Usui K, et al. Cardiovascular effects of continuous positive airway pressure in patients with heart failure and obstructive sleep apnea. N Engl J Med 2003;348:1233–41.

19. Effects of enalapril on mortality in severe congestive heart failure. Results of the Cooperative North Scandinavian Enalapril Survival Study (CONSENSUS). The CONSENSUS Trial Study Group. N Engl J Med 1987;316:1429–35.

20. Effect of enalapril on survival in patients with reduced left ventricular ejection fractions and congestive heart failure. The SOLVD Investigators. N Engl J Med 1991;325:293–302.

21. Garg RR, Yusuf SS. Overview of randomized trials of angiotensin-converting enzyme inhibitors on mortality and morbidity in patients with heart failure. Collaborative Group on ACE Inhibitor Trials. JAMA 1995;273:1450–6.

22. Swedberg KK, Kjekshus JJ. Effects of enalapril on mortality in severe congestive heart failure: results of the Cooperative North Scandinavian Enalapril Survival Study (CONSENSUS). Am J Cardiol 1988;62:60A–6A.

23. Packer M, Poole-Wilson PA, Armstrong PW, et al. Comparative effects of low and high doses of the angiotensin-converting enzyme inhibitor, lisinopril, on morbidity and mortality in chronic heart failure. ATLAS Study Group. Circulation 1999;100:2312–8.

24. Swedberg KK, Kjekshus JJ, Snapinn SS. Long-term survival in severe heart failure in patients treated with enalapril; ten year follow-up of CONSENSUS I. Eur Heart J 1999;20:4.

25. Cohn JN, Tognoni GG. A randomized trial of the angiotensin-receptor blocker valsartan in chronic heart failure. N Engl J Med 2001;345:1667–75.

26. Cicardi MM, Zingale LC, Bergamaschini LL, et al. Angioedema associated with angiotensin-converting enzyme inhibitor use: outcome after switching to a different treatment. Arch Intern Med 2004;164:910–3.

27. Velazquez EJ, Pfeffer MA, McMurray JV, et al. VALsartan In Acute myocardial iNfarcTion (VALIANT) trial: baseline characteristics in context. Eur J Heart Fail 2003;5:537–44.

28. Granger CB, McMurray JJ, Yusuf S, et al, CHARM Investigators and Committees. Effects of candesartan in patients with chronic heart failure and reduced left-ventricular systolic function intolerant to angiotensin-converting-enzyme inhibitors: the CHARM-Alternative trial. Lancet 2003;362(9386): 772–6.

29. McMurray JJ, Ostergren J, Swedberg K, et al, CHARM Investigators and Committees. Effects of candesartan in patients with chronic heart failure and reduced left-ventricular systolic function taking angiotensin-converting-enzyme inhibitors: the CHARM-Added trial. Lancet 2003;362(9386): 767–71.

30. Pfeffer MA, McMurray JJ, Velazquez EJ, et al. Valsartan, captopril, or both in myocardial infarction complicated by heart failure, left ventricular dysfunction, or both. N Engl J Med 2003;349: 1893–906.

31. Konstam MA, Neaton JD, Dickstein K, et al, HEAAL Investigators. Effects of high-dose versus low-dose losartan on clinical outcomes in patients with heart failure (HEAAL study): a randomised, double-blind trial. Lancet 2009;374(9704):1840–8. http://dx.doi.org/10.1016/S0140-6736(09)61913-9.

32. Young JB, Dunlap ME, Pfeffer MA, et al. Mortality and morbidity reduction with Candesartan in patients with chronic heart failure and left ventricular systolic dysfunction: results of the CHARM low-left ventricular ejection fraction trials. Circulation 2004;110:2618–26.

33. Pitt BB, Poole-Wilson PA, Segal RR, et al. Effect of losartan compared with captopril on mortality in patients with symptomatic heart failure: randomised trial–the Losartan Heart Failure Survival Study ELITE II. Lancet 2000;355:1582–7.

34. Dickstein K, Kjekshus J, Group OSCOTOS. Effects of losartan and captopril on mortality and morbidity in high-risk patients after acute myocardial infarction: the OPTIMAAL randomised trial. Lancet 2002;360:9.

35. Weber KT. Aldosterone in congestive heart failure. N Engl J Med 2001;345:1689–97.

36. Pitt BB, Zannad FF, Remme WJ, et al. The effect of spironolactone on morbidity and mortality in patients with severe heart failure. Randomized Aldactone Evaluation Study Investigators. N Engl J Med 1999;341:709–17.

37. Zannad FF, McMurray JJ, Krum HH, et al. Eplerenone in patients with systolic heart failure and mild symptoms. N Engl J Med 2011;364:11–21.

38. Pitt B, Remme W, Zannad F, et al. Eplerenone, a selective aldosterone blocker, in patients with left ventricular dysfunction after myocardial infarction. N Engl J Med 2003;348:1309–21.

39. Juurlink DN, Mamdani MM, Lee DS, et al. Rates of hyperkalemia after publication of the randomized aldactone evaluation study. N Engl J Med 2004; 351:543–51.

40. Bozkurt BB, Agoston II, Knowlton AA. Complications of inappropriate use of spironolactone in heart failure: when an old medicine spirals out of new guidelines. J Am Coll Cardiol 2003;41: 211–4.

41. Gattis WA, O'Connor CM, Gallup DS, et al. Predischarge initiation of carvedilol in patients hospitalized for decompensated heart failure—results of the initiation management predischarge: process for assessment of carvedilol therapy in heart failure (IMPACT-HF) trial. J Am Coll Cardiol 2004;43:8.

42. Clinical outcome with enalapril in symptomatic chronic heart failure; a dose comparison. The NETWORK Investigators. Eur Heart J 1998;19: 481–9.

43. Remme WJ, Riegger GG, Hildebrandt PP, et al. The benefits of early combination treatment of carvedilol and an ACE-inhibitor in mild heart failure and left ventricular systolic dysfunction. The carvedilol and ACE-inhibitor remodelling mild heart failure evaluation trial (CARMEN). Cardiovasc Drugs Ther 2004; 18:57–66.

44. Effect of metoprolol CR/XL in chronic heart failure: Metoprolol CR/XL Randomised Intervention Trial in Congestive Heart Failure (MERIT-HF). Lancet 1999;353:7.

45. The cardiac insufficiency bisoprolol study II (CIBIS-II): a randomised trial. Lancet 1999;353:9–13.

46. Packer M, Coats AJ, Fowler MB, et al. Effect of carvedilol on survival in severe chronic heart failure. N Engl J Med 2001;344:1651–8.

47. Poole-Wilson PA, Swedberg K, Cleland JG, et al. Comparison of carvedilol and metoprolol on clinical outcomes in patients with chronic heart failure in the Carvedilol or Metoprolol European Trial (COMET): randomised controlled trial. Lancet 2003;362:7–13.

48. Hjalmarson A, Waagstein F. COMET: a proposed mechanism of action to explain the results and concerns about dose. Lancet 2003;362:1077–8.

49. Dargie HJ. Effect of carvedilol on outcome after myocardial infarction in patients with left-ventricular dysfunction: the CAPRICORN randomised trial; the CAPRICORN Investigators. Lancet 2001;357(9266):1385–90.

50. Packer M, Bristow MR, Cohn JN, et al. The effect of carvedilol on morbidity and mortality in patients with chronic heart failure. US Carvedilol Heart Failure Study Group. N Engl J Med 1996;334(21): 1349–55.

51. Epstein SE, Braunwald E. The effect of beta adrenergic blockade on patterns of urinary sodium excretion. Studies in normal subjects and in patients with heart disease. Ann Intern Med 1966; 65:20–7.

52. Weil JV, Chidsey CA. Plasma volume expansion resulting from interference with adrenergic function in normal man. Circulation 1968;37:54–61.

53. Müller KK, Gamba GG, Jaquet FF, et al. Torasemide vs. furosemide in primary care patients with chronic heart failure NYHA II to IV—efficacy and quality of life. Eur J Heart Fail 2003;5:793–801.

54. Wargo KA, Banta WM. A comprehensive review of the loop diuretics: should furosemide be first line? Ann Pharmacother 2009;43:1836–47.

55. Dormans TP, van Meyel JJ, Gerlag PG, et al. Diuretic efficacy of high dose furosemide in severe heart failure: bolus injection versus continuous infusion. J Am Coll Cardiol 1996;28:376–82.

56. Waagstein FF, Caidahl KK, Wallentin II, et al. Long-term beta-blockade in dilated cardiomyopathy. Effects of short- and long-term metoprolol treatment followed by withdrawal and readministration of metoprolol. Circulation 1989;80:551–63.

57. Patterson JH, Adams KF, Applefeld MM, et al. Oral torsemide in patients with chronic congestive heart failure: effects on body weight, edema, and electrolyte excretion. Torsemide Investigators Group. Pharmacotherapy 1994;14:514–21.

58. Sherman LG, Liang CS, Baumgardner SS, et al. Piretanide, a potent diuretic with potassium-sparing properties, for the treatment of congestive heart failure. Clin Pharmacol Ther 1986;40:587–94.

59. Wilson JR, Reichek NN, Dunkman WB, et al. Effect of diuresis on the performance of the failing left ventricle in man. Am J Med 1981;70:234–9.

60. Richardson A, Bayliss J, Scriven AJ, et al. Double-blind comparison of captopril alone against frusemide plus amiloride in mild heart failure. Lancet 1987;2:709–11.

61. Steiness EE, Olesen KH. Cardiac arrhythmias induced by hypokalaemia and potassium loss during maintenance digoxin therapy. Heart 1976;38:167–72.

62. Brater DC. Diuretic therapy. N Engl J Med 1998;339:387–95.

63. Vargo DL, Kramer WG, Black PK, et al. Bioavailability, pharmacokinetics, and pharmacodynamics of torsemide and furosemide in patients with congestive heart failure. Clin Pharmacol Ther 1995;57:601–9.

64. Murray MD, Deer MM, Ferguson JA, et al. Open-label randomized trial of torsemide compared with furosemide therapy for patients with heart failure. Am J Med 2001;111:513–20.

65. Sica DA, Gehr TW. Diuretic combinations in refractory oedema states: pharmacokinetic-pharmacodynamic relationships. Clin Pharmacokinet 1996;30:229–49.

66. Cohn JN, Archibald DG, Ziesche SS, et al. Effect of vasodilator therapy on mortality in chronic congestive heart failure. Results of a Veterans Administration Cooperative Study. N Engl J Med 1986;314:1547–52.

67. Fonarow GC, Chelimsky-Fallick CC, Stevenson LW, et al. Effect of direct vasodilation with hydralazine versus angiotensin-converting enzyme inhibition with captopril on mortality in advanced heart failure: the Hy-C trial. J Am Coll Cardiol 1992;19:842–50.

68. Carson PP, Ziesche SS, Johnson GG, et al. Racial differences in response to therapy for heart failure: analysis of the vasodilator-heart failure trials. Vasodilator-Heart Failure Trial Study Group. J Card Fail 1999;5:178–87.

69. Taylor AL, Ziesche SS, Yancy CC, et al. Combination of isosorbide dinitrate and hydralazine in blacks with heart failure. N Engl J Med 2004;351:2049–57.

70. McMurray JJ, Adamopoulos SS, Anker SD, et al. ESC guidelines for the diagnosis and treatment of acute and chronic heart failure 2012: the task force for the diagnosis and treatment of acute and chronic heart failure 2012 of the European Society of Cardiology. Developed in collaboration with the Heart Failure Association (HFA) of the ESC. Eur J Heart Fail 2012;14:803–69.

71. Gheorghiade MM, Ferguson DD. Digoxin. A neurohormonal modulator in heart failure? Circulation 1991;84:2181–6.

72. Gheorghiade M, Adams KF, Colucci WS. Digoxin in the management of cardiovascular disorders. Circulation 2004;109:2959–64.

73. The effect of digoxin on mortality and morbidity in patients with heart failure. The Digitalis Investigation Group. N Engl J Med 1997;336:525–33.

74. Meyer P, White M, Mujib M, et al. Digoxin and reduction of heart failure hospitalization in chronic systolic and diastolic heart failure. Am J Cardiol 2008;102:6.

75. Hood WB, Dans AL, Guyatt GH, et al. Digitalis for treatment of congestive heart failure in patients in sinus rhythm. Cochrane Database Syst Rev 2004;(2):CD002901.

76. Comparative effects of therapy with captopril and digoxin in patients with mild to moderate heart failure. The Captopril-Digoxin Multicenter Research Group. JAMA 1988;259:539–44.

77. Lee DC, Johnson RA, Bingham JB, et al. Heart failure in outpatients: a randomized trial of digoxin versus placebo. CORD Conference Proceedings. N Engl J Med 1982;306:699–705.

78. Guyatt GH, Sullivan MJ, Fallen EL, et al. A controlled trial of digoxin in congestive heart failure. Am J Cardiol 1988;61:371–5.

79. DiBianco R, Shabetai R, Kostuk W, et al. A comparison of oral milrinone, digoxin, and their combination in the treatment of patients with chronic heart failure. CORD Conference Proceedings. N Engl J Med 1989;320:677–83.

80. Matsuda MM, Matsuda YY, Yamagishi TT, et al. Effects of digoxin, propranolol, and verapamil on exercise in patients with chronic isolated atrial fibrillation. Cardiovasc Res 1991;25:453–7.

81. David DD, Segni ED, Klein HO, et al. Inefficacy of digitalis in the control of heart rate in patients with chronic atrial fibrillation: beneficial effect of an added beta adrenergic blocking agent. Am J Cardiol 1979;44:1378–82.

82. Fogelman AM, La Mont JT, Finkelstein S, et al. Fallibility of plasma-digoxin in differentiating toxic from non-toxic patients. Lancet 1971;2:727–9.

83. Ingelfinger JA, Goldman P. The serum digitalis concentration—does it diagnose digitalis toxicity? N Engl J Med 1976;294:867–70.

84. McDonald K. Diastolic heart failure in the elderly: underlying mechanisms and clinical relevance. Int J Cardiol 2008;125:6.

85. Edelmann FF, Wachter RR, Schmidt AG, et al. Effect of spironolactone on diastolic function and exercise capacity in patients with heart failure with preserved ejection fraction: the Aldo-DHF randomized controlled trial. JAMA 2013;309:781–91.

86. Piller LB, Baraniuk SS, Simpson LM, et al. Long-term follow-up of participants with heart failure in the antihypertensive and lipid-lowering treatment to prevent heart attack trial (ALLHAT). Circulation 2011;124:1811–8.

87. Beckett NS, Peters R, Fletcher AE, et al. Treatment of hypertension in patients 80 years of age or older. N Engl J Med 2008;358:1887–98.

88. Abraham WT, Adams KF, Fonarow GC, et al. In-hospital mortality in patients with acute decompensated heart failure requiring intravenous vasoactive medications: an analysis from the Acute Decompensated Heart Failure National Registry (ADHERE). J Am Coll Cardiol 2005;46:57–64.

89. Yusuf S, Pfeffer MA, Swedberg K, et al. Effects of candesartan in patients with chronic heart failure and preserved left-ventricular ejection fraction: the CHARM-Preserved Trial. Lancet 2003;362:777–81.

90. Massie BM, Carson PE, McMurray JJ, et al. Irbesartan in patients with heart failure and preserved ejection fraction. N Engl J Med 2008; 359:2456–67.

91. Cleland JG, Tendera MM, Adamus JJ, et al. The perindopril in elderly people with chronic heart failure (PEP-CHF) study. Eur Heart J 2006;27: 2338–45.

92. Moss AJ, Hall WJ, Cannom DS, et al. Improved survival with an implanted defibrillator in patients with coronary disease at high risk for ventricular arrhythmia. Multicenter Automatic Defibrillator Implantation Trial Investigators. N Engl J Med 1996; 335:1933–40, 2013;1–8.

93. Buxton AE, Lee KL, Fisher JD, et al. A randomized study of the prevention of sudden death in patients with coronary artery disease. Multicenter Unsustained Tachycardia Trial Investigators. N Engl J Med 1999;341:1882–90.

94. Moss AJ, Zareba W, Hall WJ, et al, Multicenter Automatic Defibrillator Implantation Trial II Investigators. Prophylactic implantation of a defibrillator in patients with myocardial infarction and reduced ejection fraction. N Engl J Med 2002; 346:877–83.

95. Hohnloser SH, Kuck KH, Dorian P, et al. Prophylactic use of an implantable cardioverter-defibrillator after acute myocardial infarction. N Engl J Med 2004;351:2481–8.

96. Bardy GH, Lee KL, Mark DB, et al, Sudden Cardiac Death in Heart Failure Trial (SCD-HeFT) Investigators. Amiodarone or an implantable cardioverter-defibrillator for congestive heart failure. N Engl J Med 2005;352:225–37.

97. Investigators TAVID. The Antiarrhythmics Versus Implantable Defibrillators (AVID) Investigators. A comparison of antiarrhythmic-drug therapy with implantable defibrillators in patients resuscitated from near-fatal ventricular arrhythmias. N Engl J Med 1997;337:1576–83.

98. Connolly SJ, Gent M, Roberts RS, et al. Canadian implantable defibrillator study (CIDS): a randomized trial of the implantable cardioverter defibrillator against amiodarone. Circulation 2000;101:1297–302.

99. Kuck KH, Cappato R, Siebels J, et al. Randomized comparison of antiarrhythmic drug therapy with implantable defibrillators in patients resuscitated from cardiac arrest: the Cardiac Arrest Study Hamburg (CASH). Circulation 2000;102:748–54.

100. Epstein AE, DiMarco JP, Ellenbogen KA, et al. ACC/AHA/HRS 2008 guidelines for device-based therapy of cardiac rhythm abnormalities. J Am Coll Cardiol 2008;51:e1–62.

101. Cazeau SS, Leclercq CC, Lavergne TT, et al. Effects of multisite biventricular pacing in patients with heart failure and intraventricular conduction delay. N Engl J Med 2001;344:873–80.

102. Abraham WT, Fisher WG, Smith AL, et al, MIRACLE Study Group. Multicenter insync randomized clinical evaluation. Cardiac Resynchronization in Chronic Heart Failure. N Engl J Med 2002;346: 1845–53.

103. Bristow MR, Saxon LA, Boehmer J, et al. Cardiac-resynchronization therapy with or without an implantable defibrillator in advanced chronic heart failure. N Engl J Med 2004;350:2140–50. ACC Current Journal Review 2004;13:1.

104. Cleland JG, Daubert JC, Erdmann EE, et al. The effect of cardiac resynchronization on morbidity and mortality in heart failure. N Engl J Med 2005;352: 1539–49.

105. Linde C, Abraham WT, Gold MR, et al. Randomized trial of cardiac resynchronization in mildly

symptomatic heart failure patients and in asymptomatic patients with left ventricular dysfunction and previous heart failure symptoms. J Am Coll Cardiol 2008;52:1834–43.

106. Moss AJ, Hall WJ, Cannom DS, et al. Cardiac-resynchronization therapy for the prevention of heart-failure events. N Engl J Med 2009;361:1329–38.

107. Tang AS, Wells GA, Talajic M, et al. Cardiac-resynchronization therapy for mild-to-moderate heart failure. N Engl J Med 2010;363:2385–95.

108. Hillis LD, Smith PK, Anderson JL, et al. 2011 ACCF/AHA guideline for coronary artery bypass graft surgery: a report of the American College of Cardiology Foundation/American heart association task force on practice guidelines. Circulation 2013;11:1–178. http://dx.doi.org/10.1161/CIR.0b013e31823c074e.

109. Caracciolo EA, Davis KB, Sopko GG, et al. Comparison of surgical and medical group survival in patients with left main equivalent coronary artery disease. Long-term CASS experience. Circulation 1995;91:2335–44.

110. Eighteen-year follow-up in the Veterans Affairs Cooperative Study of coronary artery bypass surgery for stable angina. The VA Coronary Artery Bypass Surgery Cooperative Study Group. Circulation 1992;86:121–30.

111. Phillips HR, O'Connor CM, Rogers JJ, et al. Revascularization for heart failure. Am Heart J 2007;153:65–73. Audio, Transactions of the IRE Professional Group on 2007;153:65–73.

112. Velazquez EJ, Lee KL, Deja MA, et al. Coronary-artery bypass surgery in patients with left ventricular dysfunction. N Engl J Med 2011;364:1607–16.

113. Bonow RO, Maurer G, Lee KL, et al. Myocardial viability and survival in ischemic left ventricular dysfunction. N Engl J Med 2011;364:1617–25.

114. Chan KM, Punjabi PP, Flather M, et al, for the RIME Investigators. Coronary artery bypass surgery with or without mitral valve annuloplasty in moderate functional ischemic mitral regurgitation: final results of the randomized ischemic mitral evaluation (RIME) trial. Circulation 2012;126:2502–10.

115. Feldman T, Foster E, Glower DD, et al. Percutaneous repair or surgery for mitral regurgitation. N Engl J Med 2011;364:1395–406.

116. Franzen O, van der Heyden J, Baldus S, et al. MitraClip(R) therapy in patients with end-stage systolic heart failure. Eur J Heart Fail 2011;13:569–76.

117. Jones RH, Velazquez EJ, Michler RE, et al. Coronary bypass surgery with or without surgical ventricular reconstruction. N Engl J Med 2009;360:1705–17.

118. Athanasuleas CL, Buckberg GD, Stanley AW, et al. Surgical ventricular restoration in the treatment of congestive heart failure due to post-infarction ventricular dilation. J Am Coll Cardiol 2004;44:1439–45.

Management of the ACC/AHA Stage D Patient
Cardiac Transplantation

Michelle M. Kittleson, MD, PhD, Jon A. Kobashigawa, MD*

KEYWORDS

- Cardiac transplantation • End-stage heart failure • Rejection • Immunosuppression

KEY POINTS

- Heart transplantation is indicated in patients with heart failure despite optimal medical and device therapy, manifesting as intractable angina, refractory heart failure, or intractable ventricular arrhythmias.
- The evaluation for heart transplantation focuses on assessment of the presence of optimal medical management, the stability of extracardiac function, and adequate compliance and caregiver support.
- Standard immunosuppression after transplantation consists of triple-drug therapy with corticosteroids, calcineurin inhibitors (most commonly tacrolimus), and antiproliferative agents (most commonly mycophenolate mofetil).
- Treatment of rejection is progressively more aggressive as the patient's clinical status worsens, and ranges from an oral corticosteroid bolus and taper to intravenous pulse corticosteroids, cytolytic therapy with antithymocyte globulin, intravenous immune globulin, plasmapheresis, and circulatory support with inotropic therapy, intra-aortic balloon counterpulsation, and extracorporeal membrane oxygenation.
- The major long-term complications of heart transplantation are cardiac allograft vasculopathy, infections, and malignancy.

INTRODUCTION

Despite advances in pharmacologic and device treatment of chronic heart failure, long-term morbidity and mortality remain unacceptably high, with many patients progressing to end-stage heart failure. The 5-year mortality for patients with symptomatic heart failure approaches 50%, and may be as high as 80% at 1 year for the end-stage patients.[1] Over the last 4 decades, cardiac transplantation has become the preferred therapy for select patients with end-stage heart disease. Approximately 2400 heart transplants are performed annually in the United States. According to the registry of the International Society of Heart and Lung Transplantation, the median survival of patients after transplantation is currently 10 years, and up to14 years for those surviving the first year (**Fig. 1**), a significant improvement over that of medical therapy for heart failure.[2]

The purpose of this article is to provide an overview of heart transplantation in the current era, focusing on the evaluation process for heart transplantation, the physiology of the transplanted heart, immunosuppressive regimens, and early and long-term complications.

There are no relevant financial relationships to disclose.
Division of Cardiology, Cedars-Sinai Heart Institute, Los Angeles, CA, USA
* Corresponding author. 8536 Wilshire Boulevard, Suite 301, Beverly Hills, Los Angeles, CA 90211.
E-mail address: jon.kobashigawa@cshs.org

cardiology.theclinics.com

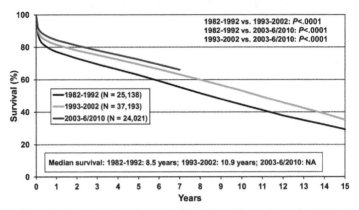

Fig. 1. Survival by era from the International Society of Heart and Lung Transplantation Registry. The median survival for the cohort of 96,273 adult and pediatric heart recipients who completed at least 1 year of follow-up is 10 years. For patients who survive the first year, the half-life is 14 years. When survival is stratified by the era of transplant, there has been a continued improvement in survival over the past 3 decades. (*From* Stehlik J, Edwards LB, Kucheryavaya AY, et al. The Registry of the International Society for Heart and Lung Transplantation: 29th official adult heart transplant report—2012. J Heart Lung Transplant 2012;31(10):1056; with permission.)

EVALUATION FOR HEART TRANSPLANTATION
Indications

The 3 major indications for heart transplantation are heart failure, angina, and ventricular arrhythmias refractory to maximal medical therapy. The most common indication for heart transplantation is refractory heart failure. Angina alone is often not considered an indication for transplantation in the absence of heart failure, as it is not clear if the survival of such patients is improved with heart transplantation. Intractable ventricular arrhythmias, commonly referred to as "VT storm," may merit heart transplant evaluation, and often urgent listing, given the association with hemodynamic compromise. The relative scarcity of donor organs makes it essential to determine whether patients are truly refractory to maximal medical therapy and require heart transplantation (**Fig. 2**).

Objective measurements that may help stratify the severity of illness include cardiopulmonary exercise stress testing and right heart catheterization. The cardiopulmonary exercise stress test measures maximal oxygen consumption (Vo_2max), which is proportional to cardiac output. A compensated patient with a Vo_2max of 12 to 14 mL/kg/min with adequate effort indicates poor survival over the next year and is an indication to proceed with evaluation.[3] Adequate effort is defined as the patient's achievement of anaerobic threshold, at which point CO_2 production exceeds O_2 consumption (indicated by respiratory exchange ratio [RER] >1).

Performing right heart catheterization once the patient is euvolemic is helpful in assessing the degree of fixed postcapillary pulmonary hypertension and cardiac output at rest. A cardiac index value of less than 2.5 L/min/m^2 suggests poor reserve and the need for transplant evaluation.[4]

Contraindications

The 2 major contraindications for heart transplantation are medical and social/psychological. The standard testing for the heart transplant evaluation is outlined in **Box 1**, and the potential contraindications are described in detail in **Table 1**. Many of these factors are not absolute, and need to be considered in the context of the severity of the patient's heart disease and associated comorbidities.

PHYSIOLOGY OF THE TRANSPLANTED HEART
Lack of Innervation to the Transplantation Heart

When the donor heart is placed into the recipient, both afferent (from the heart to the central nervous system) and efferent (from the central nervous system to the heart) nerve supply is lost. The loss of afferent nerve supply means that the recipient will not experience angina. Therefore, chest discomfort in a heart transplant recipient, especially early after transplant, is likely not caused by coronary ischemia, and coronary ischemia will likely not present with chest discomfort. The standard practice of annual angiograms for surveillance of transplant coronary artery disease is a direct consequence of the lack of afferent nerves supplying the transplanted heart.

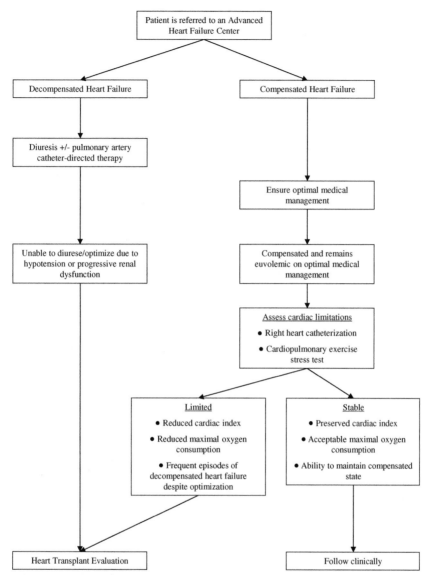

Fig. 2. Clinical algorithm to determine whether patients with advanced heart failure are limited enough to merit heart transplant evaluation. (*From* Kittleson MM, Kobashigawa JA. Management of advanced heart failure: the role of heart transplantation. Circulation 2011;123(14):1570; with permission.)

The consequences of the loss of efferent nerves are related to the loss of vagal tone and the postganglionic direct release of norepinephrine stores in response to exercise. With the loss of vagal tone, heart transplant recipients have a higher than normal resting heart rate of around 90 to 110 beats per minute. The lack of efferent nerves also means that the transplant recipient must rely on circulating catecholamines to respond to exercise, so there is a blunting of the heart rate's response to exercise. Similarly, after exercise, the heart rate returns to baseline more slowly because of the gradual decline of circulating catecholamine concentrations to baseline.

Heart transplant recipients lack the baroreceptor reflex, which relies on intact baroreceptors and sympathetic and parasympathetic innervation. Thus, heart transplant recipients are more susceptible to orthostasis, and carotid sinus massage will not break a reentrant tachycardia in these patients.

Nevertheless, some heart transplant recipients often experience reinnervation of the heart, with return of angina, an improvement in exercise tolerance, and a decrease in resting heart rate. This

---

Box 1
Recommended tests for baseline evaluation for heart transplantation

Weight/body mass index

Immunocompatibility

  ABO typing

  Human leukocyte antigen tissue typing

  Panel reactive antibodies and flow cytometry

Assessment of severity of heart failure

  Cardiopulmonary exercise test

  Echocardiogram

  Right heart catheterization

Evaluation of multiorgan function

  Routine laboratory work (basic metabolic profile, complete blood count, liver function tests)

  Urinalysis

  24-hour urine collection for protein and creatinine

  Pulmonary function tests

  Chest radiograph

  Abdominal ultrasonography

  Carotid Doppler (if >50 years or with ischemic heart disease)

  Ankle-brachial indices (if >50 years or with ischemic heart disease)

  Dental examination

  Ophthalmologic examination (if diabetic)

Infectious serology and vaccination

  Hepatitis B surface Ag, Ab, core Ab

  Hepatitis C Ab

  Human immunodeficiency virus

  Rapid plasma reagin

  Immunoglobulin G for herpes simplex virus, cytomegalovirus, toxoplasmosis, Epstein-Barr virus, varicella

  Purified protein derivative

  Immunizations: influenza, pneumovax, hepatitis B

Preventive and malignancy

  Stool for occult blood × 3

  Colonoscopy (if indicated or if >50 years)

  Mammography (if indicated or if >40 years)

  Papanicolaou smear

  Prostate-specific antigen and digital rectal examination (men >50 years)

General consultations

  Social work

  Psychiatry

  Financial

  As indicated: pulmonology, nephrology, infectious disease, endocrinology

Adapted from Mehra MR, Kobashigawa J, Starling R, et al. Listing criteria for heart transplantation: International Society for Heart and Lung Transplantation guidelines for the care of cardiac transplant candidates—2006. J Heart Lung Transplant 2006;25(9):1036; with permission.

---

process is inconsistent among patients, although it tends to increase over time.

Response to Medications

Some cardiac drugs are not effective in the denervated heart. Because of the lack of vagal tone, digoxin will have little effect on sinoatrial and atrioventricular conduction velocity, and will not achieve rate control if the transplanted heart develops atrial fibrillation. However, the inotropic effects of digoxin persist after transplantation. Similarly, the parasympatholytic effect of atropine will not increase the heart rate in transplanted hearts. Owing to the lack of baroreceptor reflexes, vasodilators such as nifedipine and hydralazine will not cause reflex tachycardia.

The lack of postganglionic sympathetic nerves in the transplanted heart results in increased receptor density, and thus more sensitivity to sympathetic agonists and antagonists. Clinically this is most often seen with β-blockers; heart transplant recipients will often have exaggerated fatigue and, occasionally, bradycardia in response to administration of β-blockers, especially with exercise.

IMMUNOSUPPRESSION
Induction Therapy

Purpose
The purpose of induction therapy was originally to induce tolerance in the graft. Although this goal has not been realized, the benefits of induction therapy include a marked reduction in rejection in the first 4 to 6 weeks after transplantation, and the ability to delay the introduction of calcineurin inhibitors to prevent worsening renal dysfunction.[5,6] The disadvantages of induction therapy include increased risk of infection, risk of malignancy, and rates of late rejection after therapy is completed.[7] At 1 year, the rejection rates of

Table 1
Contraindications to heart transplantation

Age	>70 y is a relative contraindication depending on associated comorbidities
Obesity	Body mass index (BMI) <30 kg/m² is recommended; most centers will tolerate BMI <35 kg/m²
Malignancy	Active neoplasm, except nonmelanoma skin cancer, is an absolute contraindication; cancers that are low grade (such as prostate) or in remission may be acceptable in consultation with an oncologist
Pulmonary hypertension	The inability to achieve pulmonary vascular resistance <2.5 with vasodilator or inotropic therapy is a contraindication; such patients may benefit from long-term unloading with a ventricular assist device
Diabetes	Uncontrolled diabetes or that associated with significant end-organ damage is an absolute contraindication
Renal dysfunction	If due to diabetes, may be an absolute contraindication
Peripheral vascular disease	Severe disease not amenable to revascularization is an absolute contraindication
Infection	Human immunodeficiency virus and hepatitis C are absolute contraindications at most centers
Substance use	6 mo of abstinence from smoking, alcohol, and illicit drugs is required; in critically ill patients, consultation with psychiatry and social work is essential
Psychosocial issues	Noncompliance, lack of caregiver support, and dementia are absolute contraindications; mental retardation may be a relative contraindication

Adapted from Kittleson MM, Kobashigawa JA. Management of advanced heart failure: the role of heart transplantation. Circulation 2011;123(14):1572; with permission.

patients receiving induction are usually similar to those not receiving induction.

Regimens

Regimens for induction therapy include the cytolytic agent antithymocyte globulin and the interleukin-2 receptor (IL-2R) antagonist dacluzimab (**Fig. 3**). However, despite widespread use, no randomized trials of cytolytic agents as induction therapy have been performed in heart transplant recipients. Retrospective evaluations from a large, multi-institutional database have suggested that cytolytic therapy reduces the risk of early rejection but increases the risk of infection. In a randomized trial of induction therapy with dacluzimab in heart transplant recipients, such recipients had less rejection but an increased risk of death from infection; because of the blinded nature of the study, some patients received both the IL-2R antagonist and cytolytic induction therapy.[7]

Based on these results, induction therapy is not standard practice at many centers. Instead such therapy, most often with antithymocyte globulin, may be reserved for those patients at the highest risk for rejection, including patients who are highly sensitized with donor-specific antibodies, or those

with significant renal dysfunction in whom delay of calcineurin inhibition is advisable.

Maintenance Therapy

The purpose of maintenance immunosuppressive therapy is to prevent long-term rejection in transplant recipients. Triple-drug therapy most commonly consists of steroids, a calcineurin inhibitor such as cyclosporine or tacrolimus, and an antiproliferative agent such as azathioprine or mycophenolate mofetil (MMF) (**Table 2**). In special situations a proliferation signal inhibitor (PSI), such as sirolimus or everolimus, may replace the calcineurin inhibitor or antiproliferative agent. Although the optimal maintenance immunosuppressive regimen has yet to be identified, there is evidence that regimens may be tailored to the individual patient, as detailed here.

Steroid therapy
Mechanism of action Corticosteroids are potent immunosuppressive and anti-inflammatory agents (see **Fig. 3**). Corticosteroids diffuse freely across cell membranes and ultimately alter the expression of genes involved in the immune and inflammatory

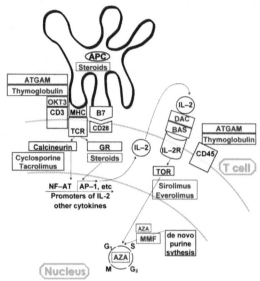

Fig. 3. Immunologic mechanisms leading to graft rejection and sites of action of immunosuppressive drugs. Immunologic mechanisms are shown in blue; immunosuppressive drugs and their site of action are shown in red. Acute rejection begins with recognition of donor antigens that differ from those of recipient by recipient antigen-presenting cells (APCs) (indirect allorecognition). Donor APCs (carried passively in graft) may also be recognized by recipient T cells (direct allorecognition). Alloantigens carried by APCs are recognized by the TCR-CD3 complex on the surface of the T cell. When accompanied by costimulatory signals between APC and T cells such as B7-CD28, T-cell activation occurs, resulting in activation of calcineurin. Calcineurin dephosphorylates transcription factor NF-AT, allowing it to enter the nucleus and bind to promoters of interleukin (IL)-2 and other cytokines. IL-2 activates cell surface receptors (IL-2R), stimulating clonal expansion of T cells (T-helper cells). IL-2, along with other cytokines produced by T-helper cells, stimulates expansion of other cells of the immune system. Activation of IL-2R stimulates target of rapamycin (TOR), which regulates translation of mRNAs to proteins that regulate the cell cycle. Sites of action of individual drugs (highlighted in red) demonstrate multiple sites of action of these drugs, underscoring the rationale for combination therapy. AZA, azathioprine; BAS, basiliximab; DAC, daclizumab; GR, glucocorticoid receptor; MMF, mycophenolate mofetil. (*From* Lindenfeld J, Miller GG, Shakar SF, et al. Drug therapy in the heart transplant recipient: part II: immunosuppressive drugs. Circulation 2004;110(25):3862; with permission.)

response, affecting the number, distribution, and function of all leukocytes.

Administration Corticosteroids are first given as an intravenous bolus of methylprednisolone during the transplant surgery. Oral prednisone is then given in a standard taper, which can differ at various institutions. At the authors' center, patients receive prednisone 40 mg twice daily, decreasing by 5 mg increments until the patient is on 10 mg twice daily. At 1 month after transplantation, the patient will start a prednisone taper so that by 3 months, the prednisone is reduced to 10 mg once daily and by 6 months, decreased to 5 mg once daily. In this program, patients with no rejection in the first 6 months are candidates to be weaned off prednisone completely by 1 year after transplantation.

Side effects Steroid therapy has significant short-term and long-term side effects.[8] Short-term side effects include tremors, emotional lability, easy bruisability, poor wound healing, weight gain, fluid retention, and hyperglycemia. Long-term adverse effects include hypertension, cataracts, ulcer disease, risk of infection, and osteoporosis. Long-term administration of steroids may result in chronic adrenal suppression, and adrenal insufficiency can follow a steroid taper or stress, such as infection or surgery.

Calcineurin inhibitor therapy

Mechanism of action Calcineurin inhibitors have become a cornerstone of maintenance therapy. The 2 calcineurin inhibitors used in clinical practice are cyclosporine and tacrolimus, both of which act by blocking calcium-activated calcineurin (see **Fig. 3**). Cyclosporine binds to cyclophilin and tacrolimus binds to FK-binding protein. The complex then binds to calcineurin, which dephosphorylates nuclear factor of activated T cells (NF-AT). Dephosphorylated NF-AT then binds to specific DNA sites and ultimately inhibits transcription of interleukin-2 and other cytokines.

Clinical trials Tacrolimus has been compared with cyclosporine in several randomized clinical trials. Both tacrolimus and cyclosporine have demonstrated comparable survival in heart transplantation, but tacrolimus may be associated with less treated rejection.[9,10] Tacrolimus is currently the calcineurin inhibitor of choice for maintenance immunosuppression therapy.

Administration Either cyclosporine or tacrolimus is given orally immediately following surgery. For cyclosporine, the dose is titrated to achieve target therapeutic trough levels of 250 to 350 ng/mL. Over the long term, cyclosporine doses are reduced to achieve target trough levels between 100 and 200 ng/mL. Tacrolimus is titrated to achieve target therapeutic levels of 10 to 15 ng/mL initially postoperatively and, over the longer term, doses are reduced to achieve target levels between 5 and 10 ng/mL. At some centers, higher levels of

Table 2
Maintenance immunosuppression

Class	Mechanism	Drugs	Usage
Corticosteroids	Alter expression of genes involved in the immune and inflammatory response, affecting the number, distribution, and function of all leukocytes	Methylprednisolone Prednisone	For all patients in the first year posttransplant Some patients weaned off after the first 6–12 mo
Calcineurin inhibitors	Cyclosporine binds to cyclophilin and tacrolimus binds to FK-binding protein. The complex then binds to calcineurin, which dephosphorylates NF-AT (nuclear factor of activated T cells). Dephosphorylated NF-AT then binds to specific DNA sites and ultimately inhibits transcription of interleukin-2 and other cytokines	Cyclosporine Tacrolimus	For all patients after transplantation May be stopped because of renal insufficiency and replaced with a proliferation signal inhibitor Tacrolimus is associated with less rejection in clinical trials
Antimetabolites	Azathioprine is converted in cells to a purine analogue incorporated into DNA, thus inhibiting its synthesis and the proliferation of both T and B lymphocytes. Mycophenolate mofetil (MMF) is an inhibitor of a key enzyme in the de novo synthesis of guanine nucleotides. Because proliferating lymphocytes are dependent on this pathway for DNA replication, MMF is a selective inhibitor of lymphocyte proliferation	Azathioprine Mycophenolate mofetil	Azathioprine cannot be given with allopurinol MMF is associated with less rejection in clinical trials
Proliferation signal inhibitors	Sirolimus and everolimus inhibit a kinase, target of rapamycin, ultimately inhibiting proliferation of T and B lymphocytes, smooth muscle cells, and endothelial cells	Sirolimus Everolimus	Only sirolimus is approved by the Food and Drug Administration for use in heart transplant recipients Not recommended for de novo use posttransplant

tacrolimus are targeted in an attempt to reduce the need for corticosteroids and antiproliferative agents.[11]

Side effects Cyclosporine causes nephrotoxicity, hypertension, dyslipidemia, neurologic toxicity, hypertrichosis, and gingival hyperplasia.[8] Tacrolimus has a similar side-effect profile, but does not cause hypertrichosis or gingival hyperplasia; in fact, alopecia may occur. Hyperglycemia and neurologic toxicity are more common with tacrolimus.

Antiproliferative therapy
Mechanism of action Azathioprine and MMF are the antiproliferative agents used most commonly after heart transplantation (see **Fig. 3**). Azathioprine is ultimately converted in cells to a purine analogue incorporated into DNA, thus inhibiting its synthesis and the proliferation of both T and B lymphocytes. MMF is an inhibitor of a key enzyme in the de novo synthesis of guanine nucleotides. Because proliferating lymphocytes depend on

this pathway for DNA replication (other cells use both de novo and salvage pathways), MMF is a selective inhibitor of lymphocyte proliferation.

Clinical trials A multicenter, randomized clinical trial compared azathioprine and MMF in combination with cyclosporine and steroids, and demonstrated that MMF-treated patients had improved survival, less rejection, and less cardiac allograft vasculopathy over time.[12] MMF is thus the antimetabolite of choice for standard maintenance therapy in heart transplant recipients.

Administration Either azathioprine or MMF is given orally immediately after transplantation. Azathioprine doses range from 50 to 150 mg daily. MMF is usually prescribed at 1500 mg twice daily, although dose reductions may be necessary because of gastrointestinal upset or leukopenia. Though not standardized, trough levels of mycophenolic acid are often checked with a goal level of greater than 1.5 μg/mL.

Side effects The major side effect of azathioprine is myelosuppression. Furthermore, azathioprine should not be prescribed with allopurinol because allopurinol inhibits xanthine oxidase, leading to increased accumulation of 6-mercaptopurine, a metabolite of azathioprine, and a greater chance of myelosuppression. Major side effects of MMF include nausea, vomiting, and diarrhea, which usually respond to a decrease in dosage[8] or a switch to a sustained-release preparation.[13]

Proliferation signal inhibitors

Mechanism of action There are 2 PSIs, sirolimus and everolimus, although only sirolimus has been approved by the US Food and Drug Administration for use in heart transplant recipients, and everolimus is approved for patients after kidney and liver transplantation. These agents inhibit a kinase, target of rapamycin (see **Fig. 3**), ultimately inhibiting proliferation of T and B lymphocytes, smooth muscle cells, and endothelial cells.

Clinical trials In de novo transplant recipients, compared with azathioprine, sirolimus demonstrated less rejection and less cardiac allograft vasculopathy as measured by intravascular ultrasonography in the first 2 years.[14] However, de novo patients receiving sirolimus were more likely to develop renal dysfunction, pneumonia, and impaired wound healing, and were less likely to develop cytomegalovirus (CMV) infection. Similarly, when everolimus was compared with azathioprine and mycophenolate in de novo heart transplant recipients, there was less rejection, cardiac allograft vasculopathy, and viral infections, but

worsening renal function and a higher incidence of bacterial infections.[15,16] Furthermore, high-dose everolimus (3.0 mg daily) was associated with increased mortality, and this arm was prematurely terminated. Low-dose everolimus (1.5 mg daily) was not associated with higher mortality.[16]

Administration Based on the results of the aforementioned trials, sirolimus and everolimus are rarely started de novo after heart transplantation. In the authors' institution, sirolimus or everolimus is substituted for MMF in patients with rejection, cardiac allograft vasculopathy, neoplasm, and viral infections such as CMV. PSIs may also be used in place of a calcineurin inhibitor to ameliorate renal dysfunction.[5,17]

Side effects The major side effects of PSIs include hypertriglyceridemia, myelosuppression, fluid retention, diarrhea, fatigue, and oral ulcers. Some of these side effects respond to a reduction in dose, although many patients do not tolerate PSIs because of their adverse effects.

LONG-TERM COMPLICATIONS
Rejection

Diagnosis
Transplant rejection remains one of the major causes of death after heart transplantation.[18] Rejection is most frequent during the first month after heart transplantation and declines thereafter. Because clinical symptoms of rejection are often vague, routine testing for rejection in the absence of symptoms is standard practice. Unlike renal or liver transplantation, there are no laboratory markers for rejection in heart transplantation and, thus, the endomyocardial biopsy is the standard approach for the routine surveillance of rejection. Endomyocardial biopsy is most commonly performed in an outpatient setting via a right internal jugular venous approach under fluoroscopic guidance. The most serious complications (which occur in 0.5% of cases) include tricuspid valve injury and cardiac perforation, which can result in tamponade.[19,20] Although the timing of biopsies varies from center to center, in general biopsies are performed frequently early after transplantation and less frequently as time goes on. At the authors' center, after year 1, biopsies are performed only if the heart transplant recipient develops symptoms or signs of rejection.

The purpose of the endomyocardial biopsy is to assess for myocardial damage in the form of cellular or antibody-mediated rejection. The diagnosis of cellular rejection is made in accordance with the revised International Society for Heart and Lung Transplantation (ISHLT) grading scale, published in 2005, which simplifies the prior 1990 classification.[21,22] Biopsies are classified as: Grade 0 R, no rejection (no change from 1990); Grade 1 R, mild rejection (1990 Grades 1A, 1B, and 2); Grade 2 R, moderate rejection (1990 Grade 3A); and Grade 3 R, severe rejection (1990 Grades 3B and 4). Grade 2 R or higher rejection on biopsy is considered significant and meriting of treatment, as discussed in further detail in the next section.

The diagnosis of antibody-mediated rejection is less straightforward, but has achieved greater standardization after a consensus conference in 2010.[23] By the proposed classification, endomyocardial biopsies are graded based on the presence of histologic and immunologic findings consistent with antibody-mediated rejection (**Fig. 4**). Histologic findings include endothelial activation with intravascular macrophages and capillary destruction. Immunologic findings encompass complement and human leukocyte antigen (HLA) deposition.

Though not required for the diagnosis of antibody-mediated rejection, the authors also perform screening for anti-HLA antibodies posttransplantation. Antibodies are checked at months 1, 3, 6, and 12 after transplantation and then annually. The presence of high levels of donor-specific anti-HLA antibodies (usually median fluorescent intensity >10,000 or standard fluorescent intensity >200,000) is considered potentially cytotoxic and may merit a change in treatment, depending on the clinical situation.

Immunopathology

		−	+
Histology	−	pAMR0 _Negative_	pAMR1i _Suspicious_
	+	pAMR1h _Suspicious_	pAMR2 _Positive_ pAMR3 _Severe_

Fig. 4. Histologic findings include endothelial activation with intravascular macrophages and capillary destruction. Immunologic findings encompass complement and human leukocyte antigen deposition. The grading scheme stratifies biopsies based on: no histologic or immunologic evidence of antibody-mediated rejection (negative, pAMR0); either histologic or immunologic evidence of antibody-mediated rejection (suspicious, pAMR1h or pARM1i, respectively); both histologic and immunologic evidence of antibody-mediated rejection (positive, pAMR2); and a final category for severe findings of myocardial destruction, pAMR3. (_From_ Kittleson MM, Kobashigawa JA. Antibody-mediated rejection. Curr Opin Organ Transplant 2012;17(5):554; with permission.)

Although performing an endomyocardial biopsy is straightforward, the morbidity associated with this invasive procedure has led to attempts to identify other means of diagnosing rejection. The Allomap, an 11-gene expression signature derived from peripheral blood mononuclear cells, may predict cellular rejection.[24] In a clinical trial in patients more than 6 months posttransplant, the Allomap gene-expression profile was noninferior to biopsy in the diagnosis of cellular rejection.[25] However, the Allomap has not yet been widely incorporated into clinical practice, mainly because of concerns with the randomized trial protocol, the low event rate in the clinical trial, and limitations of its generalized use.[26,27] A recent randomized controlled trial of the Allomap in the first 6 months after transplantation has also demonstrated noninferiority to the biopsy.[28] However, problems with the Allomap test include the inability to detect antibody-mediated rejection, and the fact that this test cannot be used within the first 55 days after transplant and cannot be used in patients who have received blood transfusions or hematopoietic growth factors affecting leukocytes (such as granulocyte-colony stimulating factor) within the past 30 days.[24] Thus, the widespread use of Allomap instead of endomyocardial biopsy will likely require further clinical use and experience before adoption by most transplant centers.

Treatment

The management of rejection proceeds in a stepwise fashion, based on the severity of rejection detected on biopsy and the patient's presentation (**Fig. 5**). Rejection most often occurs early after transplantation, and treatment is similar regardless of the timing of presentation. Grade 1 R cellular rejection or findings suspicious for antibody-mediated rejection (AMR1) in the absence of clinical or hemodynamic compromise generally merits no intervention. The management of AMR1 is controversial at present, and at some centers treatment may proceed as for higher levels of rejection, as described next.

More serious findings on the biopsy, including Grade 2 R or higher cellular rejection, or higher antibody-mediated rejection (AMR2), require treatment. The intensity of treatment depends on the patient's presentation. If the patient has no symptoms of heart failure and normal left ventricular ejection fraction, treatment options include oral or intravenous pulse steroids, targeting higher levels of immunosuppressive medications, switching from cyclosporine to tacrolimus,[9,10] or switching from MMF to a PSI.[14,15,29] Given the equivalent success of intravenous and oral corticosteroid therapy for the treatment of

		Asymptomatic	Reduced EF	Heart Failure/Shock
Cellular		• Target higher CNI levels • Oral steroid bolus + taper • MMF → PSI	• Oral steroid bolus/taper *or* • IV pulse steroids	• IV pulse steroids • Cytolytic therapy (ATG) • Plasmapheresis (before ATG dose)
Antibody-Mediated	No/↓ DSA	Observe	• Oral steroid bolus/taper *or* IV pulse steroids +/- • IV immune globulin	• IV immune globulin • Inotropic therapy • IV heparin • IABP or ECMO support
	↑DSA	Oral steroid bolus/taper	• IV pulse steroids • IV immune globulin • *consider* ATG	

Fig. 5. Treatment of rejection. Treatment proceeds in a stepwise fashion based on the severity of rejection detected on biopsy and the patient's presentation. ATG, antithymocyte globulin; CNI, calcineurin inhibitor; DSA, donor-specific antibodies; ECMO, extracorporeal membrane oxygenation; IABP, intra-aortic balloon counterpulsation; IV, intravenous; MMF, mycophenolate mofetil; PSI, proliferation signal inhibitor.

asymptomatic cellular rejection,[30] an outpatient course of oral corticosteroids is often the first-line treatment for asymptomatic cellular rejection. Asymptomatic antibody-mediated rejection is more challenging. Recent studies indicate that it may be associated with poor outcomes,[31–33] but it is unclear whether treatment affects outcomes. At the authors' institution such patients will receive an oral corticosteroid bolus, consideration of intravenous immune globulin, and close monitoring of donor-specific HLA antibodies.

For patients with a reduced ejection fraction on echocardiogram, treatment is more aggressive. A reduction in ejection fraction in the absence of biopsy evidence for rejection may be treated with intravenous corticosteroids and cytolytic therapy with antithymocyte globulin in addition to the adjustments in immunosuppressive medications outlined earlier. If there is evidence of AMR2 or higher, such patients will also receive intravenous immune globulin. If donor-specific anti-HLA antibodies are present in the setting of antibody-mediated rejection or a decrease in ejection fraction, patients may receive a steroid bolus and taper, or more intensive therapy with intravenous immune globulin, rituximab, or bortezomib.

Finally, in patients presenting with cardiogenic shock the results of the biopsy are less important, and aggressive empiric treatment includes intravenous corticosteroids, cytolytic therapy, plasmapheresis, intravenous immune globulin, intravenous heparin (as patients often have thrombotic occlusion of the cardiac microvasculature on postmortem examination[34,35]), and hemodynamic support with intra-aortic balloon counterpulsation or even extracorporeal membrane oxygenation.[36]

The protocols for the treatment of rejection will vary between transplant centers, as there are no randomized trials comparing strategies. However, given the relatively small number of heart transplants performed internationally and the relative rarity of rejection, such trials would be difficult to conduct or power to assess differences between treatment strategies. Thus, as a clinician, one must rely on experience and judgment to formulate the treatment plan that maximizes benefit and minimizes toxicity of these therapies.

Long-term management

Whereas cellular rejection is often successfully treated with corticosteroids and cytolytic therapy, resulting in a resolution of heart failure and normalization of the ejection fraction,[37] management of antibody-mediated rejection is often more complicated. Patients often have a persistent reduction in ejection fraction, restrictive physiology leading to recurrent symptoms of heart failure, and accelerated progression of transplant coronary artery disease.[37]

The management of such patients with a persistent drop in ejection fraction after treatment of symptomatic rejection is not well established (**Fig. 6**). The authors often rely on therapies to reduce the levels of donor-specific anti-HLA antibodies, including rituximab and bortezomib, as well as photopheresis to alter the function of T cells. In small case series, such therapies have

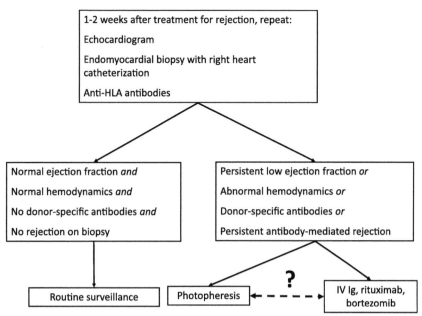

Fig. 6. Long-term management of antibody-mediated rejection. After treatment of antibody-mediated rejection, patients may have a persistent reduction in ejection fraction, restrictive physiology leading to recurrent symptoms of heart failure, and accelerated progression of transplant coronary artery disease. The management of such patients with a persistent drop in ejection fraction after treatment of symptomatic rejection is not well established. The authors often rely on rituximab, bortezomib, or photopheresis. The choice between rituximab, bortezomib, and photopheresis is not well established, and is often decided on a case-by-case basis. Ig, immunoglobulin. (*From* Kittleson MM, Kobashigawa JA. Antibody-mediated rejection. Curr Opin Organ Transplant 2012;17(5):556; with permission.)

shown benefit,[38,39] although often such patients go on to require redo transplantation.

Cardiac Allograft Vasculopathy

Incidence and prognosis
The incidence of cardiac allograft vasculopathy (CAV) varies widely, owing to differences in the definition of disease and patient populations. In one of the largest cohorts studied, of more than 6000 angiograms performed in more than 2600 patients from 39 institutions, angiographically significant CAV was noted in 42% of the patients at 5 years.[40] In a more recent study, although only 10% of heart transplant recipients developed CAV at 5 years there was a substantial increase in incidence thereafter, with 50% having developed disease by 10 years.[41] CAV can occur as soon as 1 year after transplantation, and this early disease is more aggressive and is associated with a worse prognosis.[42] In one study, those with angiographic disease had a 3.4-fold increased risk of major cardiac events and a 4.6-fold increase risk of death over a 3.5-year follow-up.[43] In patients without apparent angiographic epicardial disease, microvascular abnormalities may be present, and are associated with adverse outcomes.[44]

Clinical presentation
Given the denervation of the transplanted heart, patients do not experience typical angina, and the presentation of CAV differs from that of nontransplant CAV, as outlined in **Table 3**.[45] However,

Table 3 Features distinguishing cardiac allograft vasculopathy from nontransplant atherosclerosis	
Nontransplant Atherosclerosis	**Cardiac Allograft Vasculopathy**
Most epicardial disease	Panvascular disease (including microvasculature)
Slow progression	Rapid progression
Eccentric lesions	Concentric lesions (generally)
Lipid rich	Generally lipid poor
Early calcification	Late calcification
Compensatory remodeling with early dilation (Glagov phenomenon)	Arterial constriction

over time patients may develop cardiac reinnervation, and chest pain caused by ischemia and infarction in transplant patients has been documented.[46–48] Electrocardiographic changes with myocardial infarction may be atypical, owing to baseline abnormalities or heterogeneous disease resulting from diffuse vasculopathy.[49] In general, the atypical presentation often leads to lower utilization of revascularization therapies and, consequently, worse outcomes,[43,49] including heart failure, arrhythmia, or sudden death. For this reason, routine surveillance angiography is performed in cardiac transplant recipients, usually at 1-year intervals.

Detecting cardiac allograft vasculopathy

CAV is usually beyond therapeutic intervention by the time symptoms develop, so surveillance is essential to monitoring the development of CAV. Coronary angiography remains the mainstay of CAV detection, although it has limitations. Coronary angiography relies on the ability to compare normal segments of the vessel with diseased segments. The diffuse nature of CAV often results in underestimation of disease because there is no reference segment whereby the normal diameter of the vessel can be assessed. Comparison with prior studies may help, but requires the use of the same angiographic protocol at each study to avoid confounding by technical factors such as angiographic projections and magnification.

Intravascular ultrasonography (IVUS) is currently the only technique offering cross-sectional images of the coronary vessel wall comparable with histologic sections (**Fig. 7**). Intimal area can be quantitatively assessed to detect even early plaque burden. Sequential images are usually obtained as the catheter is pulled back to determine the extent of the disease along a vessel wall. In several studies, IVUS is more sensitive than angiography in detecting CAV.[50–53] IVUS also has prognostic value: progression of intimal thickening greater than 0.5 mm in the first year after heart transplantation is associated with an increased risk of death and development of angiographic CAV up to 5 years after transplantation.[42] Nevertheless, IVUS has several limitations: it is highly invasive, requires anticoagulation and the use of expensive single-use catheters, and its evaluation is mainly limited to the major epicardial vessels.

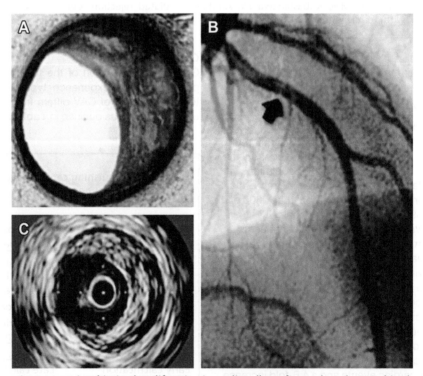

Fig. 7. Concentric or eccentric subintimal proliferation in cardiac allograft vasculopathy seen histologically (*A*) are underestimated in lesion severity angiographically (*B, arrow*), but are better appreciated by intravascular ultrasonography (*C*). (*From* Patel JK, Kobashigawa JA. Cardiac allograft vasculopathy. In: Ahsan N, editor. Chronic allograft failure: natural history, pathogenesis, diagnosis and management. Austin (TX): Landes Bioscience; 2008; with permission.)

Treatment of cardiac allograft vasculopathy

Clinically apparent CAV is associated with a poor prognosis, so prevention is an important strategy (**Box 2**). Agents used in the treatment and prevention of conventional atherosclerosis are used for CAV. Aspirin is given, because of its established role in nontransplant coronary disease. Control of hypertension and hyperlipidemia is paramount. 3-Hydoxy-3-methyl-glutaryl coenzyme A reductase inhibitors are particularly important, as they also prevent allograft rejection.[54] The PSIs also show significant promise in reducing the progression of intimal thickening by IVUS.[14–16]

Once clinically significant CAV is apparent, percutaneous coronary intervention (PCI) is successful for focal disease, although restenosis is common in the transplant setting.[55] Drug-eluting stents may help, but restenosis rates continue to be higher than for similar interventions in the nontransplant population.[56,57] There is no evidence to date that PCI alters the prognosis of CAV and, because many patients with significant disease are asymptomatic, intervention often presents a dilemma. Patients with multivessel focal disease with adequate distal target vessels may be candidates for surgical revascularization with coronary artery bypass grafting (CABG). Efficacy is difficult to determine as relatively small numbers have been reported, reflecting the many patients who do not have adequate targets and the preferential use of PCI.

Retransplantation may be a consideration for many patients with advanced CAV who are not amenable to PCI or CABG. After retransplantation, patients have survival comparable with that of patients undergoing a first transplant, with no increased incidence of CAV in the second donor heart.[58] The scarcity of donor hearts, however, creates an ethical dilemma. Some argue that it is better to maximally distribute organs rather than to allocate 2 organs to the same individual. Others contend that patients needing a second transplant should be considered on the same basis as those being evaluated for a first transplant.

Infection

Because of immunosuppressive therapy, cardiac transplant recipients are at risk for infection in a generally predictable pattern based on time after transplantation.[59] A summary of the infection risk is provided in **Fig. 8**, and antimicrobial prophylaxis is summarized in **Table 4**.

As with acute rejection, monitoring for immune status and infection risk remains problematic. This problem has led to several attempts to investigate monitoring assays, none of which are well validated at present, and there is currently no standard approach to accurately assess the risk for infection in a transplant recipient. However, an immune-monitoring assay (ImmuKnow; Cylex, Columbia, MD) performed on peripheral blood, which measures adenosine triphosphate (ATP) release from activated lymphocytes, may offer some guidance in profoundly immunosuppressed patients.[60,61] In the largest study to date in heart transplant recipients, the average T-cell immune function (TCIF) score was significantly lower in patients who developed an episode of infection within 1 month after the measurement, compared with steady-state patients.[62] A TCIF score of less than 200 ng ATP/mL was associated with future infection. The authors have used this information to tailor immunosuppression. In a patient with infection, if the TCIF score is less than 200 ng ATP/mL, immunosuppression will be reduced either by decreasing the dose of MMF or by targeting lower drug levels of the calcineurin inhibitor or PSI. If the TCIF score is 200 to 500 ng ATP/mL, the patient has an adequate level of immunosuppression. If the TCIF score is greater than 500 ng ATP/mL, the patient may be under-immunosuppressed and the MMF dose may be increased, or high drug levels of the calcineurin inhibitor or PSI may be targeted.

Malignancy

Malignancy is one of the most common causes of mortality in heart transplant recipients.[18] The

---

Box 2
Treatment options for cardiac allograft vasculopathy

Prevention

  Aspirin

  Control of hypertension (calcium-channel blockers, angiotensin-converting enzyme inhibitors)

  Hydroxymethylglutaryl coenzyme A reductase inhibitors

  Control of diabetes

  Mycophenolate mofetil

  Proliferation signal inhibitors (sirolimus, everolimus)

Treatment

  Drug-eluting stents

  Proliferation signal inhibitors

  Surgical revascularization

  Retransplantation

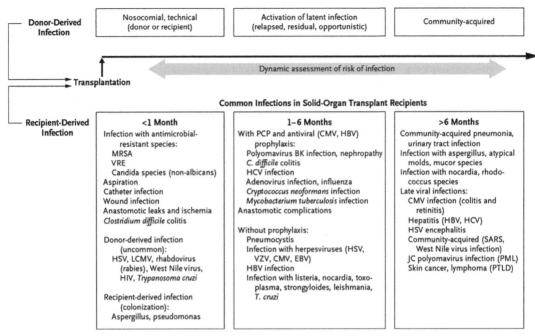

Fig. 8. Changing timeline of infection after organ transplantation. Infections occur in a generally predictable pattern after solid-organ transplantation. The development of infection is delayed by prophylaxis and is accelerated by intensified immunosuppression, toxic drug effects that may cause leukopenia, or immunomodulatory viral infections such as infection with cytomegalovirus (CMV), hepatitis C virus (HCV), or Epstein-Barr virus (EBV). At the time of transplantation, a patient's short-term and long-term risk of infection can be stratified according to donor and recipient screening, the technical outcome of surgery, and the intensity of immunosuppression required to prevent graft rejection. Subsequently, an ongoing assessment of the risk of infection is used to adjust both prophylaxis and immunosuppressive therapy. HBV, hepatitis B virus; HIV, human immunodeficiency virus; HSV, herpes simplex virus; LCMV, lymphocytic choriomeningitis virus; MRSA, methicillin-resistant *Staphylococcus aureus*; PCP, *Pneumocystis carinii* pneumonia; PML, progressive multifocal leukoencephalopathy; PTLD, posttransplantation lymphoproliferative disorder; SARS, severe acute respiratory syndrome; VRE, vancomycin-resistant *Enterococcus faecalis*; VZV, varicella zoster virus. (*Reproduced from* Fishman JA. Infection in solid-organ transplant recipients. N Engl J Med 2007;357(25):2606; with permission.)

ISHLT registry demonstrates that cumulative risk of malignancy is 26% by 8 years, mostly (18%) attributable to skin cancer.[18] A detailed discussion of posttransplant malignancy is beyond the scope of this review. However, the most critical point of treatment of malignancies is prevention. The authors encourage all heart transplant recipients at their institution to undergo routine health

Table 4
Recommended antimicrobial prophylaxis after heart transplantation

Infection	Antimicrobial	Duration
Toxoplasmosis *Pneumocystis* pneumonia	Trimethoprim/sulfamethoxazole Atovaquone or Dapsone if allergic to sulfa drugs	1 y
Cytomegalovirus	Valganciclovir	CMV IgG donor (D)/CMV IgG recipient (R) status: D−/R−: 3 mo (consider acyclovir, a less expensive alternative, for such low-risk patients) D−/R+: 6 mo D+/R+: 6 mo D+/R−: 12 mo
Oral candidiasis	Clotrimoxazole	3 mo

Abbreviations: CMV, cytomegalovirus; IgG, immunoglobulin G.

Table 5
Drug-drug interactions

Drugs that Increase Cyclosporine/ Tacrolimus Levels	Drugs that Decrease Cyclosporine/Tacrolimus Levels	Drugs that Enhance Nephrotoxicity
Cyclosporine		
Calcium-channel blockers: diltiazem, verapamil, nifedipine, nicardipine	Antibiotics: nafcillin and rifampin	Antibiotics: gentamicin, tobramycin, vancomycin, trimethoprim/ sulfamethoxazole
Antibiotics: erythromycin, clarithromycin, doxycycline	Anticonvulsants: phenytoin, phenobarbital, and carbamazepine	
Antifungal: ketoconazole, voriconazole	Miscellaneous: hypericum perforatum, ticlopidine, cholestyramine	Nonsteroidal anti-inflammatory drugs: all formulations, colchicine
Gastrointestinal (GI) agents: Metoclopramide		Antivirals: acyclovir
Miscellaneous: amiodarone, allopurinol, grapefruit, grapefruit juice		GI agents: cimetidine, ranitidine
Tacrolimus		
Calcium-channel blockers: diltiazem, verapamil, nifedipine, nicardipine	Antibiotics: rifampin	Antibiotics: aminoglycosides
Antibiotics: erythromycin, clarithromycin	Anticonvulsants: phenytoin, phenobarbital, carbamazepine	Antifungals: amphotericin B
Antifungal: ketoconazole, voriconazole, fluconazole	Miscellaneous: hypericum perforatum, cholestyramine	Antineoplastics: cisplatin
GI agents: metoclopramide, cimetidine, omeprazole		Cyclosporine
HIV protease inhibitors		
Miscellaneous: methylprednisolone, grapefruit, grapefruit juice		

Adapted from Kansara P, Kobashigawa JA. Management of heart transplant recipients: reference for primary care physicians. Postgrad Med 2012;124:219. Copyright © 2012, with permission from JTE Multimedia.

maintenance screenings with their primary care physicians. In addition, patients are instructed to use sun protection and to establish care with a dermatologist for routine skin examinations. The initial approach to malignancy is reduction of immunosuppression, and switching patients with newly diagnosed malignancy to a PSI such as sirolimus or everolimus instead of a calcineurin inhibitor or MMF, because of the possible protective effect of PSIs in malignancies.[63–65]

General Medical Management

It is essential that all heart transplant recipients receive regular care from an internist for routine health maintenance. Such patients require the same general medical surveillance as nontransplant patients, including age-appropriate cancer screening for malignancies of the cervix, breast, colon, and prostate. Internists may also manage the long-term complications of heart transplant recipients, including renal dysfunction, hypertension, dyslipidemia, diabetes, osteoporosis, and gout. However, it is essential to instruct transplant recipients to inform the transplant center of any new medication recommended by the internist,

as there may be unforeseen interactions that should be monitored (**Table 5**).

SUMMARY

Over the last 4 decades, cardiac transplantation has become the preferred therapy for select patients with end-stage heart disease. Improvements in immunosuppression and posttransplant care have resulted in a substantial decrease in acute allograft rejection, which previously led to significantly limited survival of transplant recipients. However, major impediments to long-term allograft survival exist, including rejection, infection, CAV, and malignancy. Nevertheless, through careful balance of immunosuppressive therapy and vigilant surveillance for complications, further advances in the long-term outcomes of heart transplant recipients are expected over the decades to come.

REFERENCES

1. Yancy CW, Jessup M, Bozkurt B, et al. 2013 ACCF/ AHA guideline for the management of heart failure: a report of the American College of Cardiology

Foundation/American Heart Association Task Force on Practice Guidelines. Circulation 2013. http://dx.doi.org/10.1161/CIR.0b013e31829e8776.

2. Stehlik J, Edwards LB, Kucheryavaya AY, et al. The registry of the International Society for Heart and Lung Transplantation: 29th official adult heart transplant report—2012. J Heart Lung Transplant 2012; 31(10):1052–64. http://dx.doi.org/10.1016/j.healun.2012.08.002.

3. Balady GJ, Arena R, Sietsema K, et al. Clinician's guide to cardiopulmonary exercise testing in adults: a scientific statement from the American Heart Association. Circulation 2010;122(2):191–225.

4. Mehra MR, Kobashigawa J, Starling R, et al. Listing criteria for heart transplantation: International Society for Heart and Lung Transplantation guidelines for the care of cardiac transplant candidates–2006. J Heart Lung Transplant 2006;25(9):1024–42.

5. Gustafsson F, Ross HJ. Renal-sparing strategies in cardiac transplantation. Curr Opin Organ Transplant 2009;14:566–70. http://dx.doi.org/10.1097/MOT.0b013e32832e6f7b.

6. Lindenfeld J, Miller GG, Shakar SF, et al. Drug therapy in the heart transplant recipient: part I: cardiac rejection and immunosuppressive drugs. Circulation 2004;110(24):3734–40.

7. Hershberger RE, Starling RC, Eisen HJ, et al. Daclizumab to prevent rejection after cardiac transplantation. N Engl J Med 2005;352:2705–13.

8. Lindenfeld J, Miller GG, Shakar SF, et al. Drug therapy in the heart transplant recipient: part II: immunosuppressive drugs. Circulation 2004; 110(25):3858–65.

9. Kobashigawa JA, Patel J, Furukawa H, et al. Five-year results of a randomized, single-center study of tacrolimus vs microemulsion cyclosporine in heart transplant patients. J Heart Lung Transplant 2006;25(4):434–9.

10. Kobashigawa JA, Miller LW, Russell SD, et al. Tacrolimus with mycophenolate mofetil (MMF) or sirolimus vs. cyclosporine with MMF in cardiac transplant patients: 1-year report. Am J Transplant 2006; 6(6):1377–86.

11. Baran DA, Zucker MJ, Arroyo LH, et al. A prospective, randomized trial of single-drug versus dual-drug immunosuppression in heart transplantation: the Tacrolimus in Combination, Tacrolimus Alone Compared (TICTAC) trial. Circ Heart Fail 2011;4(2):129–37. http://dx.doi.org/10.1161/circheartfailure.110.958520.

12. Eisen HJ, Kobashigawa J, Keogh A, et al. Three-year results of a randomized, double-blind, controlled trial of mycophenolate mofetil versus azathioprine in cardiac transplant recipients. J Heart Lung Transplant 2005;24(5):517–25.

13. Lehmkuhl H, Hummel M, Kobashigawa J, et al. Enteric-coated mycophenolate-sodium in heart transplantation: efficacy, safety, and pharmacokinetic compared with mycophenolate mofetil. Transplant Proc 2008;40(4):953–5. http://dx.doi.org/10.1016/j.transproceed.2008.03.046.

14. Keogh A, Richardson M, Ruygrok P, et al. Sirolimus in de novo heart transplant recipients reduces acute rejection and prevents coronary artery disease at 2 years: a randomized clinical trial. Circulation 2004;110(17):2694–700.

15. Eisen HJ, Tuzcu EM, Dorent R, et al. Everolimus for the prevention of allograft rejection and vasculopathy in cardiac-transplant recipients. N Engl J Med 2003;349(9):847–58.

16. Eisen HJ, Kobashigawa J, Starling RC, et al. Everolimus versus mycophenolate mofetil in heart transplantation: a randomized, multicenter trial. Am J Transplant 2013;13(5):1203–16. http://dx.doi.org/10.1111/ajt.12181.

17. Flechner SM, Kobashigawa J, Klintmalm G. Calcineurin inhibitor-sparing regimens in solid organ transplantation: focus on improving renal function and nephrotoxicity. Clin Transplant 2008; 22(1):1–15.

18. Stehlik J, Edwards LB, Kucheryavaya AY, et al. The Registry of the International Society for Heart and Lung Transplantation: twenty-seventh official adult heart transplant report—2010. J Heart Lung Transplant 2010;29(10):1089–103.

19. Saraiva F, Matos V, Goncalves L, et al. Complications of endomyocardial biopsy in heart transplant patients: a retrospective study of 2117 consecutive procedures. Transplant Proc 2011;43(5):1908–12.

20. Baraldi-Junkins C, Levin HR, Kasper EK, et al. Complications of endomyocardial biopsy in heart transplant patients. J Heart Lung Transplant 1993; 12(1 Pt 1):63–7.

21. Stewart S, Winters GL, Fishbein MC, et al. Revision of the 1990 working formulation for the standardization of nomenclature in the diagnosis of heart rejection. J Heart Lung Transplant 2005;24(11): 1710–20.

22. Billingham ME, Cary NR, Hammond ME, et al. A working formulation for the standardization of nomenclature in the diagnosis of heart and lung rejection: Heart Rejection Study Group. The International Society for Heart Transplantation. J Heart Transplant 1990;9(6):587–93.

23. Kobashigawa J, Crespo-Leiro MG, Ensminger SM, et al. Report from a consensus conference on antibody-mediated rejection in heart transplantation. J Heart Lung Transplant 2011;30(3):252–69.

24. Deng MC, Eisen HJ, Mehra MR, et al. Noninvasive discrimination of rejection in cardiac allograft recipients using gene expression profiling. Am J Transplant 2006;6(1):150–60.

25. Pham MX, Teuteberg JJ, Kfoury AG, et al. Gene-expression profiling for rejection surveillance after

cardiac transplantation. N Engl J Med 2010; 362(20):1890–900.

26. Jarcho JA. Fear of rejection—monitoring the heart-transplant recipient. N Engl J Med 2010;362(20): 1932–3.

27. Mehra MR, Parameshwar J. Gene expression profiling and cardiac allograft rejection monitoring: is IMAGE just a mirage? J Heart Lung Transplant 2010;29(6):599–602.

28. Kobashigawa J, Patel J, Kittleson M, et al. Results of a randomized trial of Allomap vs. heart biopsy in the first year after heart transplant: early invasive monitoring attenuation through gene expression trial. J Heart Lung Transplant 2013; 32(4):S203.

29. Mancini D, Pinney S, Burkhoff D, et al. Use of rapamycin slows progression of cardiac transplantation vasculopathy. Circulation 2003;108(1):48–53.

30. Kobashigawa JA, Stevenson LW, Moriguchi JD, et al. Is intravenous glucocorticoid therapy better than an oral regimen for asymptomatic cardiac rejection? A randomized trial. J Am Coll Cardiol 1993;21(5):1142–4.

31. Wu GW, Kobashigawa JA, Fishbein MC, et al. Asymptomatic antibody-mediated rejection after heart transplantation predicts poor outcomes. J Heart Lung Transplant 2009;28(5):417–22.

32. Kfoury AG, Stehlik J, Renlund DG, et al. Impact of repetitive episodes of antibody-mediated or cellular rejection on cardiovascular mortality in cardiac transplant recipients: defining rejection patterns. J Heart Lung Transplant 2006;25(11):1277–82.

33. Kfoury AG, Hammond ME, Snow GL, et al. Cardiovascular mortality among heart transplant recipients with asymptomatic antibody-mediated or stable mixed cellular and antibody-mediated rejection. J Heart Lung Transplant 2009;28(8): 781–4.

34. Arbustini E, Roberts WC. Morphological observations in the epicardial coronary arteries and their surroundings late after cardiac transplantation (allograft vascular disease). Am J Cardiol 1996; 78(7):814–20.

35. Fishbein MC, Kobashigawa J. Biopsy-negative cardiac transplant rejection: etiology, diagnosis, and therapy. Curr Opin Cardiol 2004;19(2):166–9.

36. Kittleson MM, Patel JK, Moriguchi JD, et al. Heart transplant recipients supported with extracorporeal membrane oxygenation: outcomes from a single-center experience. J Heart Lung Transplant 2011; 30(11):1250–6.

37. Patel JK, Kittleson M, Kobashigawa JA. Cardiac allograft rejection. Surgeon 2011;9(3):160–7.

38. Patel J, Everly M, Chang D, et al. Reduction of allo-antibodies via proteosome inhibition in cardiac transplantation. J Heart Lung Transplant 2011; 30(12):1320–6.

39. Kirklin JK, Brown RN, Huang ST, et al. Rejection with hemodynamic compromise: objective evidence for efficacy of photopheresis. J Heart Lung Transplant 2006;25(3):283–8.

40. Costanzo MR, Naftel DC, Pritzker MR, et al. Heart transplant coronary artery disease detected by coronary angiography: a multiinstitutional study of preoperative donor and recipient risk factors. Cardiac Transplant Research Database. J Heart Lung Transplant 1998;17(8):744–53.

41. Syeda B, Roedler S, Schukro C, et al. Transplant coronary artery disease: incidence, progression and interventional revascularization. Int J Cardiol 2005;104(3):269–74.

42. Kobashigawa JA, Tobis JM, Starling RC, et al. Multicenter intravascular ultrasound validation study among heart transplant recipients: outcomes after five years. J Am Coll Cardiol 2005;45(9): 1532–7.

43. Uretsky BF, Kormos RL, Zerbe TR, et al. Cardiac events after heart transplantation: incidence and predictive value of coronary arteriography. J Heart Lung Transplant 1992;11(3 Pt 2):S45–51.

44. Potluri SP, Mehra MR, Uber PA, et al. Relationship among epicardial coronary disease, tissue myocardial perfusion, and survival in heart transplantation. J Heart Lung Transplant 2005;24(8):1019–25.

45. Aranda JM Jr, Hill J. Cardiac transplant vasculopathy. Chest 2000;118(6):1792–800.

46. Stark RP, McGinn AL, Wilson RF. Chest pain in cardiac-transplant recipients. Evidence of sensory reinnervation after cardiac transplantation. N Engl J Med 1991;324(25):1791–4.

47. Ramsdale DB, Bellamy CM. Angina and threatened acute myocardial infarction after cardiac transplantation. Am Heart J 1990;119(5):1195–7.

48. Schroeder JS, Hunt SA. Chest pain in heart-transplant recipients. N Engl J Med 1991;324(25): 1805–7.

49. Gao SZ, Schroeder JS, Hunt SA, et al. Acute myocardial infarction in cardiac transplant recipients. Am J Cardiol 1989;64(18):1093–7.

50. Kapadia SR, Nissen SE, Tuzcu EM. Impact of intravascular ultrasound in understanding transplant coronary artery disease. Curr Opin Cardiol 1999; 14(2):140–50.

51. Kapadia SR, Nissen SE, Ziada KM, et al. Development of transplantation vasculopathy and progression of donor-transmitted atherosclerosis: comparison by serial intravascular ultrasound imaging. Circulation 1998;98(24):2672–8.

52. Rickenbacher P. Role of intravascular ultrasound versus angiography for diagnosis of graft vascular disease. Transplant Proc 1998;30(3):891–2.

53. Konig A, Theisen K, Klauss V. Intravascular ultrasound for assessment of coronary allograft vasculopathy. Z Kardiol 2000;89(Suppl 9):IX/45–9.

54. Kobashigawa JA, Katznelson S, Laks H, et al. Effect of pravastatin on outcomes after cardiac transplantation. N Engl J Med 1995;333(10): 621–7.

55. Sharifi M, Siraj Y, O'Donnell J, et al. Coronary angioplasty and stenting in orthotopic heart transplants: a fruitful act or a futile attempt? Angiology 2000;51(10):809–15.

56. Tanaka K, Li H, Curran PJ, et al. Usefulness and safety of percutaneous coronary interventions for cardiac transplant vasculopathy. Am J Cardiol 2006;97(8):1192–7.

57. Simpson L, Lee EK, Hott BJ, et al. Long-term results of angioplasty vs stenting in cardiac transplant recipients with allograft vasculopathy. J Heart Lung Transplant 2005;24(9):1211–7.

58. Smith JA, Ribakove GH, Hunt SA, et al. Heart retransplantation: the 25-year experience at a single institution. J Heart Lung Transplant 1995;14(5): 832–9.

59. Fishman JA. Infection in solid-organ transplant recipients. N Engl J Med 2007;357(25):2601–14.

60. Kowalski R, Post D, Schneider MC, et al. Immune cell function testing: an adjunct to therapeutic drug monitoring in transplant patient management. Clin Transplant 2003;17(2):77–88.

61. Kowalski RJ, Post DR, Mannon RB, et al. Assessing relative risks of infection and rejection: a meta-analysis using an immune function assay. Transplantation 2006;82(5):663–8.

62. Kobashigawa JA, Kiyosaki KK, Patel JK, et al. Benefit of immune monitoring in heart transplant patients using ATP production in activated lymphocytes. J Heart Lung Transplant 2011;29(5):504–8.

63. Mathew T, Kreis H, Friend P. Two-year incidence of malignancy in sirolimus-treated renal transplant recipients: results from five multicenter studies*. Clin Transplant 2004;18(4):446–9.

64. Campistol JM, Eris J, Oberbauer R, et al. Sirolimus therapy after early cyclosporine withdrawal reduces the risk for cancer in adult renal transplantation. J Am Soc Nephrol 2006;17:581–9.

65. Salgo R, Gossmann J, Schöfer H, et al. Switch to a sirolimus-based immunosuppression in long-term renal transplant recipients: reduced rate of (pre-) malignancies and nonmelanoma skin cancer in a prospective, randomized, assessor-blinded, controlled clinical trial. Am J Transplant 2010;10(6):1385–93.

Management of the ACC/AHA Stage D Patient
Mechanical Circulatory Support

David A. Baran, MD[a,b,*], Abhishek Jaiswal, MD[c]

KEYWORDS

- Mechanical circulatory support • Advanced heart failure • Device malfunction

KEY POINTS

- Mechanical circulatory support (MCS) patients must be prepared to accept responsibility for maintaining their device and taking lifelong anticoagulation.
- Physicians taking care of MCS patients must be cognizant of the various ways in which MCS devices may malfunction and how to recognize each.
- Understanding the risks and benefits of MCS therapy will allow clinicians to make better choices when deciding which patients should be referred for MCS.

INTRODUCTION

Heart failure is a progressive illness, in many ways like malignancies, and for this reason the American College of Cardiology and American Heart Association defined stages of heart failure in their pioneering guidelines on the management of chronic heart failure in 2001.[1,2] Heart failure spans a continuum from stage A patients at risk for heart failure but without pathologic abnormality to stage D, whereby patients have advanced symptomatic disease that is life threatening. In this article, the management of end-stage heart failure patients with mechanical circulatory support (MCS) is reviewed.

All mechanical circulatory support devices are designed to solve the fundamental problem of inadequate cardiac output (typically from failure of the left ventricle of the heart). These devices have an inflow and outflow limb, and a pumping chamber in between. Depending on the kind of pump, some devices have valves to prevent regurgitant flow, and the size of the pump dictates where it is placed in the patient (intracorporeal or extracorporeal). The inflow is most commonly from the left ventricular apex and the outflow is usually the ascending aorta, above the aortic valve. Technology has advanced significantly over time and most of the older devices are obsolete now, but their use saved countless lives and led to the current generation of smaller, more reliable, and commercially approved pumps.

Cardiopulmonary bypass was introduced in 1953 and ushered in the modern era of cardiac surgery.[3] Some patients failed to separate from bypass at the completion of the surgical procedure and were supported with cardiopulmonary bypass with varying success. This varying success spurred the development of mechanical devices to provide cardiac support for patients in this critical condition. Liotta first used a MCS device for a critically ill patient in 1963. This MCS device was a pulsatile tube device that connected the patient's left atrium and the descending aorta and provided a few days of support before the patient ultimately died. Funding by the National Institutes of Health

Disclosures: Dr D.A. Baran has been a research study investigator for Thoratec, Heartware, and Terumo.
[a] Heart Failure and Transplant Research, Newark Beth Israel Medical Center, 201 Lyons Avenue, L-4, Transplant Center, Newark, NJ 07112, USA; [b] Rutgers New Jersey Medical School, Newark, NJ 07103, USA; [c] Advanced Heart Failure and Transplant Medicine, Newark Beth Israel Medical Center, 201 Lyons Avenue, Newark, NJ 07112, USA
* Corresponding author.
E-mail address: dbaran@barnabashealth.org

Cardiol Clin 32 (2014) 113–124
http://dx.doi.org/10.1016/j.ccl.2013.09.013
0733-8651/14/$ – see front matter © 2014 Elsevier Inc. All rights reserved.

led to advances and several experimental devices to support critically ill patients. Devices continued to evolve but most were designed to support the left ventricle alone. Stewart and Givertz[4] recently published a comprehensive review of the history of MCS and they document the evolution of devices into the current age.

The first commercially successful ventricular assist device (VAD) was the HeartMate 1000 IP left ventricular assist system (Thoratec Corporation, Pleasanton, CA, USA), which was approved by the Food and Drug Administration (FDA) in 1994. The HeartMate 1000 IP was a relatively bulky metal device (570 g), which was surgically placed into the abdomen and pumped blood in a pulsatile manner from the left ventricular apex to the aorta, a couple of centimeters above the aortic valve. It had 2 tissue valves to prevent regurgitation of blood, and although it has been rendered obsolete by current technology, it was an amazing advance at the time. It was powered by a pneumatic driver console and connected to the patient by a very bulky tube that protruded from the abdomen. This connection or "driveline" is required in some form on every current VAD and represents one of the most critical quality-of-life issues for patients with MCS devices.

This pump was reliable as long as the pneumatic console was appropriately connected and patients routinely stayed in the hospital for months awaiting transplant while on support. The next iteration of this pump replaced the need for air pulses with a complicated system of cams and was known as the HeartMate Vented Electric (VE) (Thoratec Corporation, Pleasanton, CA, USA).[5] This device allowed patients to walk with batteries and a controller rather than being tethered to a bulky console and was used in many centers worldwide.

Mechanical modifications of the VE device were made and the device was renamed the HeartMate XVE. The system of cams produced a characteristic loud swish and bang sound that was clearly audible to patients and caregivers alike. Ultimately, the device was not durable beyond 1 to 2 years of support and often failed when the bearings wore down from 60 to 100 actuations per minute over many months. In addition, the pump was quite bulky and was implanted in the preperitoneal fat of the abdomen. The air hose driveline was replaced by a narrower driveline, which carried electricity for the motor/cam system, as well as an air vent hose to release air displaced by the pump with each beat. The device was constructed from titanium and the surface was sintered to promote the formation of a "neointimal" surface. Ultimately this proved to be fortuitous as this resulted in a very low risk of clots despite no anticoagulation.

The HeartMate pumps (VE and XVE) (Thoratec Corporation, Pleasanton, CA, USA) were able to generate a stroke volume of 83 mL, and typically ejected blood 50 to 100 times per minute, generating blood flow in the 4 to 10 L per minute range. The HeartMate XVE was approved by the FDA for patients awaiting a heart transplant in 1995 and was the dominant device used worldwide until the development of smaller, rotary blood pumps.

The major problems with the HeartMate XVE and similar pulsatile blood pumps were the large size, lack of long-term durability (pump malfunction requiring replacement was nearly universal by 2 years after implant), and skin infections at the site of the bulky driveline cable. A competing device, the Novacor VAD (WorldHeart Corporation, Salt Lake City, UT, USA), was significantly more reliable, although it was even bulkier and was still subject to driveline infections and an increased risk of cerebrovascular accidents.

The next generation of VADs was designed with a continuous-flow model instead of pulsatile flow. Devices of this generation included the MicroMed Debakey (MicroMed Technology Inc, Houston, TX, USA), Jarvik 2000 (Jarvik Heart, Inc., New York, NY, USA), and the HeartMate II (Thoratec Corporation, Pleasanton, CA, USA). In these type of pumps (axial flow or second-generation pumps) blood is moved by an impeller blade, which spins much like a propeller, at a high rate of speed (6000-12,000 rpm), resulting in a patient without a significant pulse, in contrast to first-generation pumps, which mimic the heart and keep pulsatile flow. Results with these pumps are reviewed later in **Table 2**, but have been sufficiently positive to lead to approval of some of these devices by the FDA for a variety of indications.

The third generation of VADs to be developed are the centrifugal flow devices. These devices are even smaller than the axial flow second-generation designs and examples include the Ventracor (defunct, company out of business) and the HeartWare (HeartWare, Framingham, MA, USA). The blood is delivered to the top of the device and a rapidly rotating impeller sends blood out of the pump at a 90° angle (tangential to the course of the impeller). As a result of this design, these devices are fairly sensitive to changes in the loading conditions (both delivery of blood to the machine and blood pressure, representing impedance to flow).

INDICATIONS FOR MCS

All of these pumps solve the basic problem of insufficient cardiac output, by shunting blood from the left ventricle to the aorta, distal to the aortic valve. All require energy to accomplish this and use some kind of a "driveline" of varying diameter depending on which device is placed. In the early days of MCS, the devices were very large, not very reliable, and usually not suitable for use outside of a health care facility. The initial indication for MCS was salvage when patients could not be weaned from cardiopulmonary bypass to await myocardial recovery, although survival was not high. Devices such as the Abiomed BVS 5000 (Abiomed, Danvers, MA, USA) and Centrimag are available for short-term circulatory support. These devices are temporary by design and the pump mechanism is external to the patient. These devices offer simple insertion in the operating room, no need to dissect a pump pocket, and lower initial costs than implanted VADs.

Over time, implanted devices such as the Thoratec HeartMate VE and Novacor were used as a "bridge to transplant," with patients increasingly sent home as waiting times increased and familiarity with the technology grew. In particular, with longer durations of support of a year or more, the idea that the technology should be limited to only those awaiting transplantation was questioned, with some centers extending the use to longer term support.[6,7]

To evaluate properly the question of whether MCS devices could improve outcomes for patients who were not listed for heart transplant, a prospective, randomized trial was required. The Randomized Evaluation of Mechanical Assistance for the Treatment of Congestive Heart Failure (REMATCH) trial (discussed in detail later) firmly established that MCS was associated with improved survival in comparison to optimal medical therapy in patients deemed ineligible for transplant.[8] Long-term support with MCS became known as "destination" therapy (as opposed to Bridge to Transplant therapy).

Some critically ill patients are difficult to classify and are not sufficiently evaluated to be approved for transplant, but are not clearly appropriate for long-term "destination therapy." For these cases, the indication for MCS may be deemed "Bridge to Decision." Such patients may improve sufficiently to allow approval for transplant listing, or a decision to implant a "destination therapy" durable device, or they may recover sufficient cardiac function (such as post-cardiotomy-shock patients) to allow successful removal of the device and survival.

Fig. 1 illustrates one possible "decision tree" for inpatients with severe heart failure. This decision

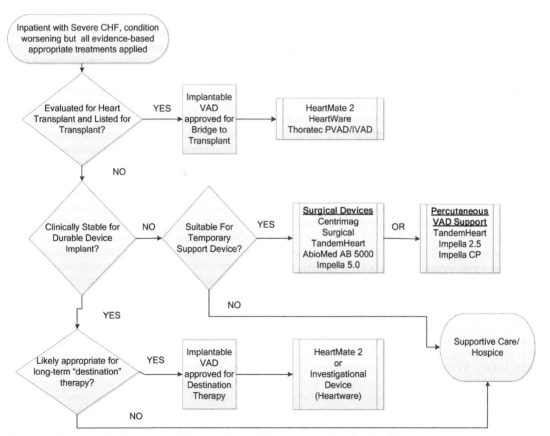

Fig. 1. Decision tree for inpatient with severe heart failure, worsening despite therapy.

tree is applicable for patients who have not responded to guideline/evidence-based therapies and who have a short life expectancy without intervention. The first decision is whether the patient is appropriate for cardiac transplantation. This decision is best made in collaboration with an affiliated heart transplant center. If the patient is listed for transplantation, there are multiple approved MCS options including HeartMate II, Heartware, as well as the older (rarely used) Thoratec paracorporeal ventricular assist device/implantable ventricular assist device systems.

In many cases, the patient may be too ill to undergo a full transplant workup and the team must decide whether the patient is stable enough to benefit from a durable MCS device. Durable devices such as the HeartMate II are quite costly, and the survival after implantation is carefully tracked via the INTERMACS database. Therefore, patients at high risk of death are usually not given durable devices due to the cost and the availability of less expensive temporary support options. For such critically ill patients, the Centrimag system (Thoratec Centrimag, Thoratec, Pleasanton, CA, USA) or Abiomed Impella 5.0 or AB5000 system (Abiomed, Danvers, MA, USA) is available for a surgical approach, or percutaneous support is available via the Abiomed Impella (2.5, or CP), or TandemHeart percutaneous VAD (Cardiac Assist, Pittsburgh, PA, USA). These percutaneous support devices may be placed in the catheterization laboratory by the interventional cardiologist and may facilitate recovery of the patient, potentially allowing further decisions to be made. This mode of MCS support is often called "bridge to decision."

If the patient is appropriately stable for a durable MCS device but has not yet been cleared for transplant, a "destination" durable device may be more appropriate. As of this writing, the only commercially available MCS system for destination therapy is the Thoratec HeartMate II, although the Heartware system is being considered for this indication as well.

BEYOND NEW YORK HEART ASSOCIATION CLASS: INTERMACS PROFILES

The Interagency Registry for Mechanically Assisted Circulatory Support (INTERMACS) is a North American registry established in 2005 to track patients who are receiving MCS devices to treat advanced heart failure. INTERMACS was established as a joint effort of the FDA, clinicians, scientists, and industry representatives in conjunction with Dr James K. Kirklin and the University of Alabama at Birmingham, the National Heart, Lung, and Blood Institute, and the Centers for Medicare and Medicaid. It is a prospective registry that collects clinical data, including follow-up, essentially as it happens. Post-implant follow-up data are collected at 1 week, 1 month, 3 months, 6 months, and every 6 months thereafter. Major outcomes after implant (eg, death, explant, rehospitalization, and adverse events) are entered as they occur and also a part of the defined follow-up at scheduled intervals (http://www.uab.edu/medicine/intermacs/).

As part of the design of the registry, the group realized that a new classification system was needed to classify patients undergoing support. New York Heart Association class is a common way of classifying patients with heart failure, but does not really apply when dealing with critically ill inpatients with decompensated heart failure. **Table 1** details this classification system, known as the INTERMACS Profiles.[9] Like any classification system, there is some subjectivity to this schema but studies have shown that the profiles correlate with differential outcomes between groups.[10,11]

KEY TRIALS IN MCS

Table 2 lists 4 key trials in the MCS field. A full review of the important trials in MCS is beyond the scope of this article however. The REMATCH[8] trial was the first trial to compare MCS with medical therapy in patients who were deemed not to be eligible for transplantation. The investigators randomized 129 patients with severe end-stage heart failure to the Heartmate VE VAD or continued medical therapy (68 in the VAD group and 61 with medical therapy). The trial showed a significant improvement in survival at 1 year after implant, but by 2 years most of the patients had died in both study groups (**Fig. 2**). There were a multitude of complications noted for the patients in the VAD cohort. Bleeding occurred in 42% of patients, and strokes occurred at a rate of 0.39 strokes per patient year. The Heartmate VE was not very reliable and 35% of the patients experienced device failure during the 2 years of the study.

This trial was a landmark because it ushered in a new era where MCS could be considered superior to medical therapy for severe heart failure. In addition, the high rate of device failure was vigorously pursued by device manufacturers as an opportunity to develop more reliable pumps.

Slaughter and colleagues[12] reported the trial experience with Thoratec's smaller, more reliable pump, the Heartmate II, applied to a destination therapy (not eligible for transplant) population. Two hundred patients were randomized in a 2:1 fashion to Heartmate II or Heartmate XVE (pulsatile flow). The Heartmate II group had a higher survival than those randomized to the XV pump (**Fig. 3**).

Table 1
INTERMACS levels

INTERMACS Level	"Shorthand Name"	Definition	Time Frame for Intervention
1	"Crash and burn"	Critical cardiogenic shock Patients with life-threatening hypotension despite rapidly escalating inotropic support, critical organ hypoperfusion, often confirmed by worsening acidosis and/or lactate levels	Definitive intervention needed within hours
2	"Sliding on inotropes"	Progressive decline Patient with declining function despite intravenous inotropic support, may be manifest by worsening renal function, nutritional depletion, inability to restore volume balance. Also describes declining status in patients unable to tolerate inotropic therapy.	Definitive intervention needed within few days
3	"Dependent stability"	Stable but inotrope dependent Patient with stable blood pressure, organ function, nutrition, and symptoms on continuous intravenous inotropic support (or a temporary circulatory support device or both), but demonstrating repeated failure to wean from support due to recurrent symptomatichypotension or renal dysfunction	Definitive intervention elective over a period of weeks to few months
4		Resting symptoms Patient can be stabilized close to normal volume status but experiences daily symptoms of congestion at rest or during activities of daily living. Doses of diuretics generally fluctuate at very high levels. More intensive management and surveillance strategies should be considered, which may in some cases reveal poor compliance that would compromise outcomes with any therapy. Some patients may shuttle between 4 and 5.	Definitive intervention elective over period of weeks to few months
5		Comfortable at rest and with activities of daily living but unable to engage in any other activity, living predominantly within the house. Patients are comfortable at rest without congestive symptoms, but may have underlying refractory elevated volume status, often with renal dysfunction. If underlying nutritional status and organ function are marginal, patient may be more at risk than INTERMACS 4, and require definitive intervention.	Variable urgency, depends on maintenance of nutrition, organ function, and activity

(continued on next page)

Table 1 *(continued)*			
INTERMACS Level	"Shorthand Name"	Definition	Time Frame for Intervention
6	Walking Wounded	Exertion limited Patient without evidence of fluid overload is comfortable at rest, and with activities of daily living and minor activities outside the home but fatigues after the first few minutes of any meaningful activity. Attribution to cardiac limitation requires careful measurement of peak oxygen consumption, in some cases with hemodynamic monitoring to confirm severity of cardiac impairment.	Variable, depends on maintenance of nutrition, organ function, and activity level
7		Advanced New York Heart Association III A placeholder for more precise specification in the future, this level includes patients who are without current or recent episodes of unstable fluid balance, living comfortably with meaningful activity limited to mild physical exertion.	Transplantation or circulatory support may not currently be indicated

From Stevenson LW, Pagani FD, Young JB, et al. INTERMACS profiles of advanced heart failure: the current picture. J Heart Lung Transplant 2009;28(6):535; with permission.

However, bleeding was similar between groups and was noted in approximately 80% of patients (most of this being perioperative bleeding). Stroke was much less common with Heartmate II (0.13 per patient-year compared to 0.22 per patient-year with Heartmate XVE). Despite anticoagulation with Heartmate II, 13 of 134 pumps needed replacement, largely because of pump thrombosis. This percentage compared favorably with the nearly 41% exchange rate with the older pulsatile pump (24/59 patients had pump exchange). Largely because this data, the FDA approved Heartmate II for destination therapy use.

Miller and colleagues[13] reported the results of the nonrandomized trial of Heartmate II for patients awaiting transplant (presumably a "healthier" cohort than patients who are not eligible for transplant). Three-quarters of patients in this study were alive at 6 months after implantation of the Heart-Mate 2, with 42% having undergone transplantation and the remainder on continued support (**Fig. 4**). Similar to other trials, bleeding was common (53% of patients required 2 or more units of blood transfusion). Strokes were noted in 8% of patients, along with 4% who suffered a transient ischemic attack.

Recently, Aaronson and colleagues[14] reported the results of the Heartware HVAD applied to a bridge to transplant cohort. One hundred forty patients who were listed for transplantation received the Heartware HVAD as support. The competing outcomes graph is shown in **Fig. 5**. An impressive 90% of patients were alive or transplanted at 6 months, with 86% alive at a year after implant. Bleeding requiring surgery was noted in 14.3% of patients. Stroke was noted in 12.8% of patients, along with 4.3% of patients suffering a transient ischemic attack. Although these statistics appear superior to the Heartmate II, it is difficult to compare trials as the definitions of key complications such as bleeding and stroke vary between investigators. Also, the exclusion criteria for each trial are different and this impacts the outcomes that are observed. In addition, this was not a randomized clinical trial but instead compared the outcomes of the study population who received the HVAD to patients in the INTERMACS registry who contemporaneously received VAD support (mainly Heartmate II). The use of the HVAD for destination therapy will be determined by the ENDURANCE trial, in which patients are randomized to receive the HVAD or the Heartmate II.

What can be learned from these 4 key trials in MCS? The clear message is that VAD therapy is here to stay, and that continued improvements in the safety and reliability of these devices will be a main thrust over the coming years. It is

Table 2
Key trials in MCS

First Author	Trial Name	No. of Patients/Devices	Length of Follow-up	Device	Indication	Comparison	Incidence of Bleeding	Incidence of Stroke	Incidence of Device Thrombosis/Replacement	Survival
Rose et al,[8] 2001	REMATCH	68 VAD, 61 Med Tx	2 y	Heartmate XVE	DT	DT VAD vs Medical therapy	42% within 6 mo of implant	0.39 per patient/y	35% device failure at 24 mo 10/68 (15%) device replacement	52% at 1 y and 23% at 2 y post-VAD
Slaughter et al,[12] 2009	Heartmate II DT Trial	134 HM 2, 66 HM XVE	2 y	Heartmate II vs Heartmate XVE	DT	Newer axial flow VAD vs older pulsatile system	Bleeding requiring transfusion HM2: 81% HM XVE 76%	0.13 per patient/y with HM2 0.22 per patient/y HM XVE	HM 2: 13 patients with replacement HM XVE: 24/59 patients had explant or replacement	68% 1 y, 58% 2 y HM2 55 B% 1 y, 24% 2 y HM XVE
Miller et al,[13] 2007	Heartmate II BTT Trial	133 Heartmate II	1 y	Heartmate II	BTT	Nonrandomized, no control group	2.09 bleeds per patient-year requiring only transfusion	0.19 per patient/y	2% device thrombosis, 4% replacement	75% alive or underwent transplant at 1 y
Aaronson et al,[14] 2012	ADVANCE Trial	140 Heartware	1 y	Heartware HVAD	BTT	Nonrandomized INTERMACS contemporaneous cohort	14.3% of patients with bleeding requiring surgery in Heartware group	0.2 per patient/y 12.8% of patients had stroke	10 patients with pump replacement	86% at 1 y

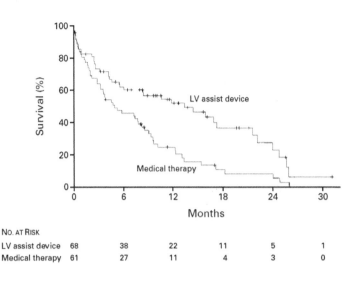

Fig. 2. Survival in the REMATCH trial. (*From* Rose EA, Gelijns AC, Moskowitz AJ, et al, for the Randomized Evaluation of Mechanical Assistance for the Treatment of Congestive Heart Failure (REMATCH) Study Group. Long-term use of a left ventricular assist device for end-stage heart failure. N Engl J Med 2001;345(20):1439; with permission.)

interesting that despite anticoagulation, and multiple different changes to pump design over the last 20 years, stroke remains a significant hazard. In addition, none of the MCS devices currently available have a long-term survival record that resembles heart transplant. There are no 10-year survivors on MCS devices, although it is a rapidly changing field and many devices from 10 years ago are retired and have been superseded by newer technology.

PATIENT PERSPECTIVE: LIFE WITH AN MCS DEVICE

From the patient's perspective, having an MCS device is a significant adjustment. The patient must always be cognizant of the time on the

batteries that power their life-saving pump, unless they are attached to the base unit via 2 wires (typically used when sleeping or stationary for long periods of time). The connections are relatively simple, but need to be practiced several times before they are completely mastered. The authors usually advise at least one main caregiver to be trained fully in the operation and troubleshooting of the MCS device. The MCS recipient also needs to carry 2 batteries and a controller and some wear special vests to carry and conceal the equipment.

One of the biggest issues is the need to change the sterile dressing on the driveline that traverses the skin and provides the power inlet for the MCS device. Each center has their particular protocol for cleansing the skin and providing a sterile dressing but all have the same goal, which is to

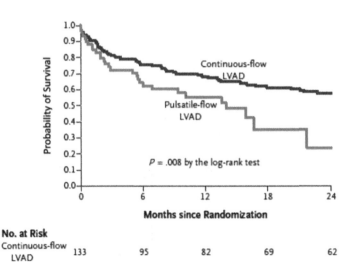

Fig. 3. Survival in the Heartmate II DT trial. (*From* Slaughter MS, Rogers JG, Milano CA, et al. Advanced heart failure treated with continuous-flow left ventricular assist device. N Engl J Med 2009;361(23):2247; with permission.)

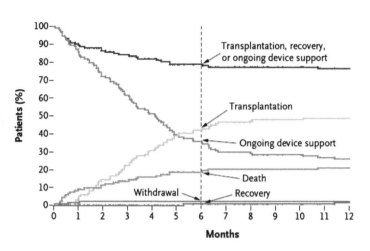

Fig. 4. Competing outcomes in the HeartMate II Bridge to Transplant trial. (*From* Miller LW, Pagani FD, Russell SD, et al. Use of a continuous-flow device in patients awaiting heart transplantation. N Engl J Med 2007; 357(9):893; with permission.)

prevent the driveline site from becoming infected. Driveline infections can be localized to the skin or may track infection into the area around the pump or even into the mediastinum. They are a significant cause of morbidity and mortality after MCS implant. There are several excellent reviews of this topic, which provide more information.[15–17]

Another issue is the need to avoid getting the electronic controller, driveline site, and batteries wet. Although there are workarounds for showers, MCS patients cannot use bathtubs, swim, nor sit in a pool. Balanced against the lifesaving benefits of the MCS device, it is a reasonable tradeoff but when the VAD is a permanent solution especially, these become important points to some patients. The patient with an MCS device may be discouraged from fishing in a boat because an accidental fall into the water could be fatal. Travel by airplane is possible, particularly with smaller controller base units that are available today, but it is still far from routine. Even the mundane act of driving a car is somewhat controversial. There are no published guidelines regarding driving a car while on MCS. Analogous to an implantable defibrillator, if there is a malfunction of the MCS device, the patient could lose consciousness while driving. Each team must individualize recommendations for patients but it is important for patients to understand the potential limitations before undergoing placement of an elective MCS device. In the authors' experience, these issues are less problematic when the patient is waiting for transplantation because the issues with the VAD are temporary.

The last major issue is anticoagulation. The Heartmate XVE did not require anticoagulation and simple oral aspirin was sufficient, but all currently available pumps require anticoagulation. Intensity of therapy is device-specific and also modified by patient factors. Warfarin is the most common agent used, with no information available about use of the novel anticoagulants. In addition, it is not likely that agents such as dabigatran will be used in an off-label fashion given the recent FDA warning involving use of dabigatran in mechanical

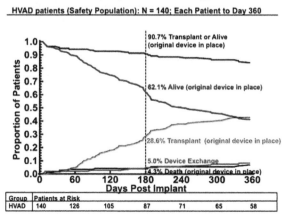

Fig. 5. Competing outcomes in the Heartware Bridge to Transplant trial. HVAD, HeartWare ventricular assist device. (*From* Aaronson KD, Slaughter MS, Miller LW, et al. Use of an intrapericardial, continuous-flow, centrifugal pump in patients awaiting heart transplantation. Circulation 2012;125: 3197; with permission.)

heart valve patients (http://www.fda.gov/drugs/drugsafety/ucm332912.htm). The Re-ALIGN trial[18] was recently stopped early because of a finding of excess clotting and stroke with dabigatran versus warfarin in a randomized trial. The findings have not been published but sound a cautionary note for use of nonwarfarin oral anticoagulants in patients with heart valves and, by logical extension, those with MCS devices.

WHAT COULD POSSIBLY GO WRONG? MODES OF FAILURE OF MCS DEVICES

As beneficial and lifesaving as MCS devices are, they can and do fail and it is important for the cardiologist to have familiarity with some specific ways that this may happen to allow proper recognition and management.[19–21] The comments focus on the currently available devices that are approved for a bridge to transplantation in the United States (Thoratec Heartmate II, Heartware Inc, Heartware HVAD).

The most basic mode of failure is lack of power for the device. If the batteries are running low, all approved devices have loud alarms that will sound to warn patients and caregivers of an impending emergency in sufficient time to replace the batteries or change to base unit power. The portable controller can malfunction and fail to energize the pump but often the result of a controller malfunction is an alarm but not actual cessation of the pump. The sole means of transmitting power to the implantable MCS device is the driveline, and there have been reports of patients accidentally cutting the driveline, although it is engineered to be very durable. Regardless of how it fails, complete cessation of pump support is often catastrophic and patients should be brought to a VAD center hospital as soon as possible and the center contacted by phone for emergency advice.

The next mode of failure can be more subtle and it is pump thrombosis. Neither the Heartmate II nor the HeartWare HVAD have a direct flow measurement probe and the parameters, which are reported on the main console, are indirect measures of VAD performance. Thrombosis can occur in partial degrees and coat the impeller of the device, reducing the effective flow through it. The flows that are reported are based on the power consumption of the machine, and complex formulae as opposed to direct measurement of the flow in the outflow limb of the pump. The diagnosis is suspected when the patient who was previously stable develops signs and symptoms of worsening congestive heart failure in the absence of obvious dysfunction of the MCS device. Echocardiography is extremely useful because it may allow visualization of decreased velocity going into the device or at the aortic outflow graft and is well reviewed elsewhere.[22–25]

An interesting side effect of continuous-flow MCS devices that was not seen in pulsatile pumps such as the Heartmate VE and XVE is the severe reduction or elimination of aortic valve opening. Pulsatile devices were usually out of sync with the native heart rhythm and so the aortic valve would periodically open when the left ventricle filled sufficiently. With continuous flow (both axial devices like the Heartmate II and centrifugal devices like the HeartWare), the heart is continuously drained and aortic valve motion is reduced or eliminated depending on the speed of the MCS device. It is possible that this contributes to the development of aortic insufficiency in previously normal valves, which is increasingly noted in MCS recipients.[26–28] This can begin as minor regurgitation and become severe in nature over time. Reoperation may be required in some cases but is associated with variable risk given the prior surgery. Transcatheter aortic valve replacement is not a good option for these patients given the lack of calcification in the regurgitant valve but there have been reports of sealing the aortic valve percutaneously with an Amplatz device.[29,30]

Another interesting problem that has only been reported in the era of continuous-flow MCS devices is that of gastrointestinal bleeding from arteriovenous malformations (AVMs). In many ways, the aortic pulse tracing resembles that of patients with severe aortic stenosis, and the association of aortic stenosis and AVMs is well known (Heyde syndrome).[31] It is interesting that some continuous-flow MCS patients develop AVMs as well, which is a particular problem because their device requires anticoagulation![32,33]

A related problem is that of acquired coagulopathy due to the destruction of von Willebrand multimers by the continuous-flow MCS device. A 2009 report highlighted the development of an acquired von Willebrand deficiency in a patient switched from a failing Heartmate XVE to a Heartmate II, where serial markers of hemostasis were being systematically studied.[34] Later work confirmed that the phenomenon is nearly universal after continuous-flow MCS implantation and contributes to the bleeding noted in these patients.[35–37] Strategies for dealing with these problems are in evolution and no clear answer exists at the moment except to reduce anticoagulation.

FUTURE TRENDS

Thoratec recently announced that more than 15,000 Heartmate II devices had been implanted worldwide, which is an incredible feat for a device first studied in 2005. Multiple companies are working in advance in MCS because the patient population that could potentially benefit from this technology is enormous.

One of the major focuses is on reducing the morbidities that are associated with MCS devices, in particular, the driveline. Both Thoratec (http://www.faqs.org/sec-filings/110803/THORATEC-CORP_8-K/v230675_ex99-1.htm) and Heartware (http://www.heartware.com/products-technology/technology-pipeline) are working on transcutaneous energy transfer to allow patients to have a fully implantable system without a driveline.[38] If these efforts are successful, the issue of driveline dressings and infections will no longer be relevant and will fade into memory like the venerable Heartmate XVE, which blazed the trail but is no longer in production.

The other major trend is on miniaturization of devices. The paradigm of the pulsatile MCS devices was to support the left ventricle completely and one of the compromises with continuous-flow devices is that the heart is not completely unloaded except at very high speeds in some cases. Nevertheless, the clinical outcomes have been excellent. Taking this one step further, companies are working on tiny MCS devices that cannot flow more than 2 to 3 litres per minute, but are very simple to implant and may represent an appropriate strategy for "partial ventricular support," particularly in patients who are not in florid cardiogenic shock. Examples include Heartware's MVAD (http://www.heartware.com/products-technology/technology-pipeline) and Circulite Inc's Synergy device (http://www.circulite.net/clinicians/synergy-information.php).

SUMMARY

Although stage D heart failure is a devastating diagnosis to give patients, given the poor prognosis it carries, it must be remembered that there are new treatments being developed and that robust, commercially available MCS devices exist for eligible patients available at an ever-expanding range of implant centers. This article has reviewed the field and provided a broad overview, along with references to allow the clinician to delve into the intricacies of individual aspects. The likelihood is that today's MCS devices will seem as antiquated as the primitive MCS devices of the 1980s in a few years. New challenges will undoubtedly be identified, and medical research will undoubtedly prevail. We stand in awe of the elegance, beauty, and efficiency of the human heart, which reliably lasts for 90 years or more, and hope that someday our mechanical devices might provide a reasonable fraction of that longevity.

REFERENCES

1. Hunt SA, Baker DW, Chin MH, et al. ACC/AHA guidelines for the evaluation and management of chronic heart failure in the adult: executive summary. A report of the American College of Cardiology/American Heart Association Task Force on practice guidelines (Committee to revise the 1995 guidelines for the evaluation and management of heart failure): developed in collaboration with the International Society for Heart and Lung Transplantation; endorsed by the Heart Failure Society of America. Circulation 2001; 104(24):2996–3007.

2. Hunt SA, Baker DW, Chin MH, et al. ACC/AHA guidelines for the evaluation and management of chronic heart failure in the adult: executive summary. A report of the American College of Cardiology/American Heart Association Task Force on practice guidelines (committee to revise the 1995 guidelines for the evaluation and management of heart failure). J Am Coll Cardiol 2001;38(7):2101–13.

3. Gibbon JH Jr. Application of a mechanical heart and lung apparatus to cardiac surgery. Minn Med 1954; 37(3):171–85 passim.

4. Stewart GC, Givertz MM. Mechanical circulatory support for advanced heart failure: patients and technology in evolution. Circulation 2012;125(10):1304–15.

5. Poirier VL. The heartmate left ventricular assist system: worldwide clinical results. Eur J Cardiothorac Surg 1997;11(Suppl):S39–44.

6. Shiono M, Takatani S, Sasaki T, et al. Baylor multipurpose circulatory support system for short- to long-term use. ASAIO J 1992;38(3):M301–5.

7. Weiss WJ, Rosenberg G, Snyder AJ, et al. Permanent circulatory support systems at the Pennsylvania State University. IEEE Trans Biomed Eng 1990; 37(2):138–45.

8. Rose EA, Gelijns AC, Moskowitz AJ, et al, for the Randomized Evaluation of Mechanical Assistance for the Treatment of Congestive Heart Failure (Rematch) Study Group. Long-term use of a left ventricular assist device for end-stage heart failure. N Engl J Med 2001;345(20):1435–43.

9. Stevenson LW, Pagani FD, Young JB, et al. INTERMACS profiles of advanced heart failure: the current picture. J Heart Lung Transplant 2009;28(6):535–41.

10. Kirklin JK, Naftel DC, Kormos RL, et al. Fifth INTERMACS annual report: risk factor analysis from more than 6,000 mechanical circulatory support patients. J Heart Lung Transplant 2013;32(2):141–56.

11. Boyle AJ, Ascheim DD, Russo MJ, et al. Clinical outcomes for continuous-flow left ventricular assist device patients stratified by pre-operative INTERMACS

classification. J Heart Lung Transplant 2011;30(4): 402–7.

12. Slaughter MS, Rogers JG, Milano CA, et al. Advanced heart failure treated with continuous-flow left ventricular assist device. N Engl J Med 2009; 361(23):2241–51.

13. Miller LW, Pagani FD, Russell SD, et al. Use of a continuous-flow device in patients awaiting heart transplantation. N Engl J Med 2007;357(9):885–96.

14. Aaronson KD, Slaughter MS, Miller LW, et al. Use of an intrapericardial, continuous-flow, centrifugal pump in patients awaiting heart transplantation. Circulation 2012;125(25):3191–200.

15. Pereda D, Conte JV. Left ventricular assist device driveline infections. Cardiol Clin 2011;29(4):515–27.

16. Califano S, Pagani FD, Malani PN. Left ventricular assist device-associated infections. Infect Dis Clin North Am 2012;26(1):77–87.

17. Schaffer JM, Allen JG, Weiss ES, et al. Infectious complications after pulsatile-flow and continuous-flow left ventricular assist device implantation. J Heart Lung Transplant 2011;30(2):164–74.

18. Van de Werf F, Brueckmann M, Connolly SJ, et al. A comparison of dabigatran etexilate with warfarin in patients with mechanical heart valves: THE Randomized, phase II study to evaluate the safety and pharmacokinetics of oral dabigatran etexilate in patients after heart valve replacement (RE-ALIGN). Am Heart J 2012;163(6):931–7.e1.

19. Potapov EV, Stepanenko A, Krabatsch T, et al. Managing long-term complications of left ventricular assist device therapy. Curr Opin Cardiol 2011; 26(3):237–44.

20. Feldman D, Pamboukian SV, Teuteberg JJ, et al. The 2013 International Society for Heart and Lung Transplantation Guidelines for mechanical circulatory support: executive summary. J Heart Lung Transplant 2013;32(2):157–87.

21. Klein T, Jacob MS. Management of implantable assisted circulation devices: emergency issues. Cardiol Clin 2012;30(4):673–82.

22. Estep JD, Stainback RF, Little SH, et al. The role of echocardiography and other imaging modalities in patients with left ventricular assist devices. JACC Cardiovasc Imaging 2010;3(10):1049–64.

23. Topilsky Y, Oh JK, Shah DK, et al. Echocardiographic predictors of adverse outcomes after continuous left ventricular assist device implantation. JACC Cardiovasc Imaging 2011;4(3):211–22.

24. Uriel N, Morrison KA, Garan AR, et al. Development of a novel echocardiography ramp test for speed optimization and diagnosis of device thrombosis in continuous-flow left ventricular assist devices: the Columbia ramp study. J Am Coll Cardiol 2012; 60(18):1764–75.

25. Horton SC, Khodaverdian R, Chatelain P, et al. Left ventricular assist device malfunction: an approach to diagnosis by echocardiography. J Am Coll Cardiol 2005;45(9):1435–40.

26. Rajagopal K, Daneshmand MA, Patel CB, et al. Natural history and clinical effect of aortic valve regurgitation after left ventricular assist device implantation. J Thorac Cardiovasc Surg 2013;145(5):1373–9.

27. Aggarwal A, Raghuvir R, Eryazici P, et al. The development of aortic insufficiency in continuous-flow left ventricular assist device-supported patients. Ann Thorac Surg 2013;95(2):493–8.

28. Morgan JA, Brewer RJ, Nemeh HW, et al. Management of aortic valve insufficiency in patients supported by long-term continuous flow left ventricular assist devices. Ann Thorac Surg 2012;94(5):1710–2.

29. Parikh KS, Mehrotra AK, Russo MJ, et al. Percutaneous transcatheter aortic valve closure successfully treats left ventricular assist device-associated aortic insufficiency and improves cardiac hemodynamics. JACC Cardiovasc Interv 2013;6(1):84–9.

30. Russo MJ, Freed BH, Jeevanandam V, et al. Percutaneous transcatheter closure of the aortic valve to treat cardiogenic shock in a left ventricular assist device patient with severe aortic insufficiency. Ann Thorac Surg 2012;94(3):985–8.

31. Batur P, Stewart WJ, Isaacson JH. Increased prevalence of aortic stenosis in patients with arteriovenous malformations of the gastrointestinal tract in Heyde syndrome. Arch Intern Med 2003;163(15): 1821–4.

32. Demirozu ZT, Radovancevic R, Hochman LF, et al. Arteriovenous malformation and gastrointestinal bleeding in patients with the HeartMate II left ventricular assist device. J Heart Lung Transplant 2011; 30(8):849–53.

33. Huang RJ, Wong RJ, Draper KV, et al. De novo arteriovenous malformations following implantation of the HeartMate II left ventricular assist device. Endoscopy 2012;44(Suppl 2 UCTN):E441.

34. Malehsa D, Meyer AL, Bara C, et al. Acquired von Willebrand syndrome after exchange of the HeartMate XVE to the HeartMate II ventricular assist device. Eur J Cardiothorac Surg 2009;35(6):1091–3.

35. Eckman PM, John R. Bleeding and thrombosis in patients with continuous-flow ventricular assist devices. Circulation 2012;125(24):3038–47.

36. Sponga S, Nalli C, Casonato A, et al. Severe upper gastrointestinal bleeding in Heartmate II induced by acquired von Willebrand deficiency: anticoagulation management. Ann Thorac Surg 2012;94(2):e41–3.

37. Suarez J, Patel CB, Felker GM, et al. Mechanisms of bleeding and approach to patients with axial-flow left ventricular assist devices. Circ Heart Fail 2011; 4(6):779–84.

38. Slaughter MS, Myers TJ. Transcutaneous energy transmission for mechanical circulatory support systems: history, current status, and future prospects. J Card Surg 2010;25(4):484–9.

Arrhythmias and Heart Failure

Heath E. Saltzman, MD, FACC

KEYWORDS

- Heart failure • Arrhythmia • Atrial fibrillation • Ventricular tachyarrhythmia

KEY POINTS

- Atrial fibrillation and ventricular tachyarrhythmias are frequently seen in patients with heart failure, and complicate the management of such patients.
- Both types of arrhythmia lead to increased patient morbidity and mortality.
- Many randomized studies have been performed in patients with these conditions and heart failure, and these have helped to guide clinicians in designing optimal treatment strategies.

Heart failure (HF) is a highly prevalent disorder, afflicting approximately 6 million individuals in the United States with an incidence of 10 per 1000 population after the age of 65 years.[1] Nearly 300,000 Americans are diagnosed with heart failure annually and, although overall survival has improved over time, the mortality remains high, as approximately 50% of patients die within 5 years from initial diagnosis.[2] The 2 most common arrhythmias dealt with in HF patients are atrial fibrillation (AF) and ventricular arrhythmias such as ventricular tachycardia (VT) and ventricular fibrillation (VF). These disorders cause considerable mortality and often prove to be challenging issues to manage.

ATRIAL FIBRILLATION
Prevalence

AF is by far the most common arrhythmia in North America, affecting an estimated 2.3 million people. In the last 20 years, hospital admissions attributable to AF have increased by 66%.[3] It is estimated that the prevalence of AF will increase by 2.5-fold by the end of the year 2050 and will affect 5.6 million Americans.[4]

Association Between Heart Failure and Atrial Fibrillation

AF and HF are thought to perpetuate each other. Both share common risk factors, such as:

- Advanced age
- Hypertension
- Diabetes mellitus
- Coronary artery disease
- Heart disease

Evidence also exists of a more complex relationship between the two that may be independent of mutually predisposing factors.

HF is the strongest predictor for the development of AF, with up to a 6-fold increase in risk seen in the Framingham study.[5] In the Framingham Heart Study, 1470 subjects developed either new AF or HF from 1948 to 1995, with 383 (26%) developing both.[6] In addition, lifetime risks for developing AF in men and in women who are 40 years or older is 1 in 6 in patients without congestive HF or myocardial infarction (MI), and 1 in 4 in the same population when patients with congestive HF or prior MI are included.[7]

The reported prevalence of AF in series of moderate HF patients ranges from 13% to 27%.[8–12] It has also been noted that prevalence of AF in patients with HF increases in parallel with the severity of HF, ranging from 5% in patients with mild HF, 10% to 26% among patients with moderate HF, and up to 50% patients with severe HF.[13] A study by Deedwania and Lardizabal[14] showed an almost identical parallel association. The prevalence of AF in the setting of preexisting HF increases in patients with worsening HF class: 4% at functional

The author has no disclosures.

Division of Cardiology, Cardiac Electrophysiology, and Pacing, Drexel University College of Medicine, 245 North 15th Street, Mail Stop 470, Philadelphia, PA 19102, USA

E-mail address: heath.saltzman@drexelmed.edu

Cardiol Clin 32 (2014) 125–133

http://dx.doi.org/10.1016/j.ccl.2013.09.005

class I, 27% at functional class II and III, and 50% at functional class IV.

Middlekauff and colleagues[8] found that patients with advanced HF and AF had a significantly reduced 1-year survival when compared with patients in sinus rhythm. However, AF seems to be a stronger predictor of negative outcome in patients with mild to moderate HF in comparison with patients with severe HF. A study by Corell and colleagues[15] found that the presence of AF in patients with HF was associated with increased morbidity and mortality in patients with better cardiac function.

Atrial Fibrillation Precipitating Heart Failure

AF may directly facilitate the development and/or progression of HF in several ways. First, the increase in resting heart rate and an exaggerated heart-rate response to exercise results in shorter diastolic filling times, which lead to a reduction in cardiac output. The irregular ventricular response leads to a reduction in left ventricular filling during short cycles. In addition, the loss of an effective atrial contraction is a contributing factor, as the contribution of left atrial systole in left ventricular filling can be up to 50%.[16,17]

The onset of AF is often accompanied by cardiac decompensation and deterioration in functional class in patients with HF. In a study by Pozzoli and colleagues,[18] 344 patients with previously diagnosed HF, initially in sinus rhythm, were found to have worsening of New York Heart Association (NYHA) functional class, peak oxygen consumption, and cardiac index, as well as increased mitral and tricuspid regurgitation and cardiac chamber dimensions, corresponding to the onset of AF.

Restoration of sinus rhythm improves cardiac output, exercise capacity, and maximal oxygen consumption.[19] In the Valsartan in Acute Myocardial Trial (VALIANT) of 14,703 patients with acute MI complicated by HF, AF was associated with greater long-term mortality and morbidity.[19]

In the Trandolapril Cardiac Evaluation (TRACE) study, long-term mortality was found to be increased in all groups of patients in AF except those with the most advanced disease.[20]

The presence of AF, while serving as a marker for outcomes, may not necessarily directly affect the prognosis of patients with HF. For example, post hoc analysis of data from the Veterans Affairs Vasodilator Heart Failure Trials (V-HeFT),[9] which enrolled more than 1300 patients with mild to moderate HF, found that the rates of mortality, hospitalization, and other adverse events in patients with AF were no different from those in sinus rhythm. Similarly, in severe HF, AF has not been shown to be independently associated with adverse outcomes in the Prospective Randomized Study of Ibopamine on Mortality and Efficacy (PRIME) study.[21] Ahmed and Perry[22] found that among 944 elderly patients hospitalized with HF, onset of new AF carried a significantly higher risk of death when compared with patients with no AF or those in chronic AF. In fact, more than 80% of patients hospitalized with HF and found to have new-onset AF died within 4 years of discharge, compared with only 61% to 66% of those without AF or with persistent AF, respectively.

A post hoc analysis of data from the Carvedilol Or Metoprolol European Trial (COMET), which enrolled more than 3000 patients with symptomatic systolic HF, showed that patients who were in AF on baseline electrocardiogram had significantly higher risks of all-cause and cardiovascular mortality and hospitalization rates over a 5-year period. However, after adjustment for patient-related variables (eg, age and gender), the presence of AF at baseline was no longer independently associated with mortality. Serial electrocardiography was performed throughout the COMET follow-up period to screen for subsequent development of AF. Of the nearly 2500 patients who were in sinus rhythm at baseline, 580 developed new-onset AF during the study. In this subset of patients, new-onset AF was an independent predictor of subsequent all-cause mortality, and remained so regardless of treatment and changes in functional class over time.[23] In summary, although preexisting chronic AF has not been definitively shown to independently affect the rates of mortality or morbidity in patients with HF, the onset of new AF is certainly associated with adverse outcomes in chronic HF.

Pathophysiology

Under normal circumstances, atrial systole may contribute up to 25% of cardiac output. In the setting of ventricular dysfunction, atrial contribution to the total cardiac output may be 50%. The onset of AF abolishes the "atrial kick," leading to a reduction in cardiac output, and peak oxygen uptake in exercise tolerance.[16,17] Rapid ventricular rates during periods of uncontrolled AF lead to inadequate ventricular filling forward blood flow. An irregular ventricular response, even if independent of heart rate, causes a decrease in cardiac output, increased pulmonary wedge pressures, and elevation of right atrial pressures.[24–27]

AF also plays a direct role in the development of a cardiomyopathy, namely a tachycardia-induced cardiomyopathy. Studies have shown that chronic persistent tachycardias can cause HF, and that elimination of these arrhythmias frequently reverses the hemodynamic and clinical manifestations associated with these syndromes of both canines and humans.[28-32] The mechanism for the development of a tachycardia-induced cardiomyopathy is not fully understood; however, animal models suggest that myocardial ischemia, depletion in myocardial energy, and abnormalities in calcium regulation may all contribute. High heart rates and longer tachycardia durations lead to more severe ultrastructural cardiac remodeling, which is characterized by cytoskeleton alteration, matrix metalloproteinase distribution, completion of high-energy stores, and induction of abnormal tissue-remodeling process.[33-35]

Heart Failure Precipitating Atrial Fibrillation

Alternatively, HF can increase the risk for developing AF in many ways, including elevation of intracardiac filling pressures, dysregulation of intracellular calcium, and autonomic and neuroendocrine dysfunction. Atrial stretch results in activation of stretch-activated ionic currents, leading to increased dispersion of refractoriness as well as alterations in anisotropic and conduction properties, thus facilitating AF.[36] HF has also been associated with increased interstitial fibrosis, which creates substrate for AF in animal models.[37-39]

Therapeutic Considerations

Rate or rhythm control

Despite multiple studies, controversy still exists as to whether patients with HF respond better to rhythm restoration or control of ventricular rate. The Atrial Fibrillation Follow-up Investigation of Rhythm Management (AFFIRM) and the Rate Control Versus Electrical Cardioversion for Atrial Fibrillation (RACE)[40,41] studies looked at a rhythm-control strategy in comparison with a focused rate-controlling strategy in the general population of patients. The results showed no benefit, and a trend toward harm, with a rhythm-control strategy. Three other prospective, randomized trials[42-44] compared rate and rhythm control in patients. Each showed similar findings of equivalent outcomes in the study arms. Of note, only 23% to 64% patients assigned to the rhythm-control group remained in sinus rhythm. When interpreting these studies, it is important to remember that they included older patients or young patients with increased risk for stroke who were sufficiently tolerant of AF to be randomized. Moreover, left ventricular function was normal in

three-quarters of the AFFIRM patients, and only 9% had an NYHA functional class of II or greater.

Subsequent studies have also examined rhythm control in patients with both AF and HF. Ina study by Talajic and colleagues,[45] 1376 patients with AF, an ejection fraction less than 35%, and HF symptoms were randomized to rhythm-control or rate-control strategy. The investigators showed that neither a rhythm-control strategy nor the presence of sinus rhythm is associated with better outcomes in patients with both AF and congestive HF.

Ventricular-rate control

Treatment targets for heart rate in AF previously had been defined as between 60 and 80 beats/min at rest and 80 to 110 beats/min with moderate exercise. These targets have been recently challenged by the results of the Rate Control Efficacy in Permanent Atrial Fibrillation (RACE-II) trial.[46] The study enrolled more than 600 patients with AF, who were randomized to either lenient (target resting heart rate <110 beats/min) or strict rate control (target heart rate <80 beats/min at rest, <110 beats/min on moderate exercise). After 3 years, there was no significant difference seen in the composite rates of death, HF hospitalization, or major cardiovascular events between the two groups.

Rhythm restoration or control

There are numerous antiarrhythmic agents available for the treatment of AF in patients with a structurally normal heart, but HF patients have a more limited list of acceptable medications, in large part because of an increased susceptibility to side effects of antiarrhythmic medications.

The Cardiac Arrhythmia Suppression Trial (CAST) was a randomized, placebo-controlled study that examined the effect of class IC antiarrhythmic medications on ventricular ectopy after MI. This study showed that therapy with either flecainide or encainide was associated with increased mortality in these patients.[47] The applicability of the CAST results to other populations, such as those with HF and no active ischemia or with other class IC antiarrhythmic medications such as propafenone, is uncertain. However, currently it is prudent to consider any class IC rhythmic medications to confer a significant risk in patients with structural heart disease. Class IA agents should also be avoided in patients with HF because of the increased risk of ventricular arrhythmias.

In patients with advanced HF, the Antiarrhythmic Trial with Dronedarone in Moderate to Severe CHF Evaluating Morbidity Decrease (ANDROMEDA) found a 2-fold excess in mortality with dronedarone compared with placebo, primarily because of worsening HF, prompting the early termination of this study after just 2 months of clinical follow-up.[48]

The cornerstone of antiarrhythmic therapy in patients with HF is the use of amiodarone, sotalol, and dofetilide. Amiodarone, a class III agent with some overlap activity of class I, is among the most effective antiarrhythmic agents for suppression of AF,[49] and seems to be safe and effective in patients with HF. Despite its effectiveness, the use of amiodarone in patients with HF is associated with an increased risk for symptomatic bradycardia requiring implantation of a permanent pacemaker.[50]

Dofetilide is a relatively new class III antiarrhythmic agent, used to suppress AF. In the Danish Investigations of Arrhythmia and Mortality on Dofetilide (DIAMOND), a congestive HF substudy, dofetilide was significantly more effective than placebo in restoring and maintaining sinus rhythm in patients with AF and HF.[51] In addition, dofetilide therapy was associated with reduced hospitalizations for HF. Therapy with dofetilide is usually initiated in the hospital, with close monitoring of the QT interval. Even with careful monitoring, dofetilide has been associated with an increased risk for torsades de pointes, particularly in elderly patients.

In addition to specific antiarrhythmic medications, other medications commonly used in HF may also be of benefit. Studies have shown a reduction in the incidence of AF with inhibition of the renin-angiotensin-aldosterone system.[52–55] Therapy with β-blockers also was associated with reduced risk for AF. In the midanalysis of 7 randomized placebo-controlled trials including 11,952 patients with HF already taking angiotensin-converting enzyme inhibitors, β-blockers significantly reduced the incidence of new AF from 39 to 28 per 1000 patient-years, a relative risk (RR) reduction of 27%.[56]

Recent studies also suggest that 3-hydroxy-3-methylglutaryl coenzyme A reductase inhibitors (statin) therapy may reduce the incidence of recurrence of AF in patients with HF.[57] A recent meta-analysis of randomized trials of statins showed a significant decrease in the risk of AF in comparison with control patients.[58] In addition, the benefit of statin therapy seemed more marked in secondary prevention and for new-onset or postoperative AF.

Atrial Fibrillation and Pacemaker Therapy

In patients with symptomatic AF and rapid ventricular responses that are refractory to pharmacologic therapy, radiofrequency ablation of the atrioventricular node and subsequent pacemaker placement can improve cardiac performance.

A meta-analysis by Wood and colleagues[59] reviewed 21 studies with 1181 patients, and found that for patients with AF, atrial pacing improved a broad range of clinical outcomes. The 1-year mortality rate was low and comparable with medical therapy.

Ganesan and colleagues[60] performed a meta-analysis of 6 studies and 768 patients, and found that atrioventricular node ablation in patients with cardiac resynchronization therapy (CRT) and both AF and HF was associated with a reduction in all-cause mortality and cardiovascular mortality, and improvement in NYHA functional class when compared with medical therapy in patients with CRT.

Other options for the management of AF in patients with HF include radiofrequency ablation of the AF. A meta-analysis by Dagres and colleagues[61] looked at 9 studies and 354 patients with left ventricular dysfunction. Following ablation, patients experienced a pooled absolute improvement in left ventricular ejection fraction (LVEF) of 11.1%. A large multicenter trial to evaluate AF ablation in HF patients, the Catheter Ablation versus Standard Conventional Treatment in Patients with Left Ventricular Dysfunction and Atrial Fibrillation (CASTLE-AF) trial, is currently under way.

VENTRICULAR ARRHYTHMIAS

Ventricular arrhythmias are frequently encountered in patients with left ventricular dysfunction and HF. Nonsustained VT occurs in anywhere from 20% to 80% of patients with HF. Patients with HF carry a 5-fold increased risk of sudden cardiac death (SCD). Studies have found that approximately 30% to 50% of all cardiac deaths in patients with HF are attributable to SCD.[62–67]

Multiple randomized trials over the past 15 years have shown that mortality is reduced by implantable cardioverter-defibrillator (ICD) implantation, either for primary prevention of SCD in patients with HF and left ventricular systolic dysfunction, or for secondary prevention in patients with a history of prior ventricular arrhythmias or aborted SCD.[68–74]

The first major trial was the Multicenter Automatic Defibrillator Implantation Trial (MADIT),[68] which randomized 196 patients with a prior MI, nonsustained VT on ambulatory monitoring, LVEF less than 35%, and inducible sustained VT during electrophysiology study to prophylactic ICD or medical therapy alone. After 27 months, those treated with an ICD had significantly lower total mortality (15 vs 39 deaths in the medical therapy group, hazard ratio [HR] 0.46, 95% confidence interval [CI] 0.26–0.82; $P = .009$), as well as lower rates of cardiac death and SCD.

The Multicenter Unsustained Tachycardia Trial (MUSTT)[72] randomized 704 patients with a prior MI (>1 month prior), asymptomatic nonsustained VT, and LVEF of 40% or less to placebo versus electrophysiologic study (EPS)-guided medical therapy with ICD after failure of at least 1 medical agent. A lower risk of cardiac arrest or death from arrhythmia was found among those receiving EPS-guided therapy (25% vs 32% without therapy, RR 0.73, 95% CI 0.53–0.99), which was largely attributed to ICD therapy in many of these patients (RR 0.24 for ICD vs without ICD, 95% CI 0.13–0.45; $P<.001$).

MADIT II[70] evaluated patients with no evidence of arrhythmia inducibility. This study randomized 1232 patients with an MI more than 30 days before enrollment and an LVEF of 30% or less to a prophylactic ICD or medical therapy.[11] Unlike MADIT-I, nonsustained VT was not a precondition of enrollment. During a mean follow-up of 20 months, the mortality rates were significantly lower in the ICD group (14.2% vs 19.8% in the medical therapy group, HR 0.69, 95% CI 0.51–0.93; $P<.016$).

The largest of the primary prevention ICD trials published was the Sudden Cardiac Death in Heart Failure Trial (SCD-HeFT),[73] which also evaluated patients with nonischemic cardiomyopathy. SCD-HeFT evaluated 2521 patients with an LVEF of 35% or less (48% ischemic) and NYHA class II or III HF, and at a median follow-up of 45.5 months. There was significantly lower mortality in the ICD group (29% vs 22% in the placebo group, HR 0.77, 97.5% CI 0.62–0.96; $P = .007$). In a subgroup, there was no evidence that the etiology of the cardiomyopathy modified the effect of ICDs on mortality. This study also identified no adverse consequences of ICD therapy on quality of life.

Theuns and colleagues[75] performed a meta-analysis of ICD therapy for primary prevention of SCD in patients with ischemic cardiomyopathy focusing on the MADIT, MADIT II, and SCD-HeFT trials. This pooled analysis showed significant reductions in all-cause mortality with RR reductions ranging from 22% to 59%. The pooled results using a random-effects model showed a 33% RR reduction in all-cause mortality with ICD therapy (95% CI 12%–49%; $P = .004$).

Medical Therapy for Ventricular Arrhythmias in Heart Failure

Despite optimal ICD usage and programming, a significant proportion of HF patients will have sustained ventricular arrhythmias and ICD shocks. In such cases, an antiarrhythmic medication is often considered. These medications are often discussed using the modified Vaughn-Williams classification.

The different classes of antiarrhythmic drugs (AADs) are: class I, sodium-channel blockers; class II, β-blockers; class III, potassium-channel blockers; and class IV, calcium-channel blockers.

β-Blockers are one of the central medications used in the management of HF. Several studies have demonstrated reduction in SCD and mortality with β-blockers in patients with both ischemic and nonischemic cardiomyopathy. This clear mortality benefit is unique to this class of antiarrhythmic therapy, and most patients with left ventricular dysfunction should already be on optimal dosing of β-blocker therapy from a heart rate and hemodynamic standpoint. Carvedilol has unique properties, being a nonselective β-blocker and α1-blocker. It can also block potassium (HERG), calcium, and sodium currents, and modestly prolong the duration of action potential. The Carvedilol Prospective Randomized Cumulative Survival (COPERNICUS) and Carvedilol Postinfarct Survival Control in Left Ventricular Dysfunction (CAPRICORN) trials demonstrated the benefit of carvedilol in reducing VT and VF in patients with HF.[76,77]

The Metoprolol CR/XL Randomized Intervention Trial in Congestive Heart Failure (MERIT-HF)[66] and the Cardiac Insufficiency Bisoprolol Study II (CIBIS-II)[78] showed the benefits of metoprolol succinate and bisoprolol, respectively, in preventing arrhythmic deaths in CHF. For patients with continued VT/VF episodes and ICD therapy despite β-blockade, an additional medical treatment option may be necessary to suppress ventricular arrhythmias. The class III agents most commonly added to β blocker therapy to suppress ventricular arrhythmias are amiodarone and sotalol. These drugs block potassium channels and prolong the duration of action potential, and therefore the refractory period. Amiodarone also shares mechanisms similar to those of multiple classes of antiarrhythmic drugs. A meta-analysis of trials comparing the efficacy of amiodarone in patients with MI and HF demonstrated reduction in incidence of SCD but not in the absolute risk for all-cause mortality.[79] Amiodarone also had no mortality benefit in patients with an LVEF of less than 35% when compared with placebo in primary prevention of SCD.[73]

Amiodarone administered with β-blocker was more effective in preventing ICD shocks in secondary-prevention patients with a mean LVEF of 34%.[80]

Sotalol has been shown to reduce time to delivery of the first ICD shock, and the frequency of shocks in patients with an ICD.[81] The prophylactic use of sotalol had no improvement on mortality and may, in fact, increase overall mortality.[82] Sotalol initiation in patients with structural heart disease must be closely monitored, given the increased risk of torsades de pointes.

Among the class I drugs, lidocaine and mexiletine are used to treat ventricular arrhythmias. These agents act by blocking sodium channels, inhibiting phase-0 depolarization, and reducing conduction velocity. Lidocaine is usually a secondary option to amiodarone for the control of unstable ventricular arrhythmias in HF. Mexiletine is an oral medication with electrophysiologic effects similar to but weaker than those of lidocaine. Mexiletine is typically used for suppression of chronic VT/VF as an adjunctive medication when a patient is already taking a β-blocker and/or amiodarone.

Class IV drugs comprise the calcium-channel blockers, which add little benefit to the treatment of ventricular arrhythmias in HF; in fact, they can be harmful because of their negative inotropic effects.

REFERENCES

1. National Heart, Lung, and Blood Institute. NHLBI fiscal year 2009 factbook. Bethesda (MD): National Institutes of Health; 2009.
2. American Heart Association Heart Disease, Stroke Statistics Writing Group. Executive summary: heart disease and stroke statistics—2011 update: a report from the American Heart Association. Circulation 2011;123(4):459–63.
3. Friberg J, Buch P, Scharling H, et al. Rising rates of hospital admissions for atrial fibrillation. Epidemiology 2003;14:666–72.
4. Go AS, Hylek EM, Phillips KA, et al. Prevalence of diagnosed atrial fibrillation in adults: national implications for rhythm management and stroke prevention: the AnTicoagulation and Risk Factors in Atrial Fibrillation (ATRIA) Study. JAMA 2001;285:2370–5.
5. Benjamin EJ, Levy D, Vaziri SM, et al. Independent risk factors for atrial fibrillation in a population-based cohort: the Framingham Heart Study. JAMA 1994;271(11):840–4.
6. Wang TJ, Larson MG, Levy D, et al. Temporal relations of atrial fibrillation and congestive heart failure and their joint influence on mortality: the Framingham Heart Study. Circulation 2003;107:2920–5.
7. Lloyd-Jones D, Larson M, Leip E, et al. Lifetime risk for developing congestive heart failure: the Framingham Heart Study. Circulation 2002;106:3068.
8. Middlekauff HR, Stevenson WG, Stevenson LW. Prognostic significance of atrial fibrillation in advanced heart failure: a study of 390 patients. Circulation 1991;84:40–8.
9. Carson PE, Johnson GR, Dunkman WB, et al. The influence of atrial fibrillation on prognosis in mild to moderate heart failure. The V-HeFT Studies. The V-HeFT VA Cooperative Studies Group. Circulation 1993;87(Suppl 6):VI102–10.
10. Mahoney P, Kimmel S, DeNofrio D, et al. Prognostic significance of atrial fibrillation in patients at a tertiary medical center referred for heart transplantation because of severe heart failure. Am J Cardiol 1999;83:1544–7.
11. Senni M, Tribouilloy CM, Rodeheffer RJ, et al. Congestive heart failure in the community: a study of all incident cases in Olmsted County, Minnesota, in 1991. Circulation 1998;98:2282–9.
12. Deedwania PC, Singh BN, Ellenbogen K, et al. Spontaneous conversion and maintenance of sinus rhythm by amiodarone in patients with heart failure and atrial fibrillation: observations from the Veterans Affairs Congestive Heart Failure Survival Trial of Antiarrhythmic Therapy (CHF-STAT): the Department of Veterans Affairs CHF-STAT investigators. Circulation 1998;98:2574–9.
13. Maisel WH, Stevenson LW. Atrial fibrillation in heart failure: epidemiology, pathophysiology, and rationale for therapy. Am J Cardiol 2003;91:2D–8D.
14. Deedwania PC, Lardizabal JA. Atrial fibrillation in heart failure: a comprehensive review. Am J Med 2010;123(3):198–204.
15. Corell P, Gustafsson F, Schou M, et al. Prevalence and prognostic significance of atrial fibrillation in outpatients with heart failure due to left ventricular systolic dysfunction. Eur J Heart Fail 2007;9:258–65.
16. Leonard JJ, Shaver J, Thompson M. Left atrial transport function. Trans Am Clin Climatol Assoc 1981;92:133–41.
17. Rahimtoola SH, Ehsani A, Sinno MZ, et al. Left atrial transport function in myocardial infarction. Importance of its booster pump function. Am J Med 1975;59(5):686–94 Atrial Fibrillation in Heart Failure 1997.
18. Pozzoli M, Cioffi G, Traversi E, et al. Predictors of primary atrial fibrillation and concomitant clinical and hemodynamic changes in patients with chronic heart failure: a prospective study in 344 patients with baseline sinus rhythm. J Am Coll Cardiol 1998;32(1):197–204.
19. Gosselink AT, Crijns HJ, van den Berg MP, et al. Functional capacity before and after cardioversion of atrial fibrillation: a controlled study. Br Heart J 1994;72:161–6.
20. Pedersen OD, Bagger H, Køber L, et al, TRACE Study Group. Impact of congestive heart failure and left ventricular systolic function on the prognostic significance of atrial fibrillation and atrial

flutter following acute myocardial infarction. Int J Cardiol 2005;100:65–71.

21. Crijns HJ, Tjeerdsma G, de Kam PJ, et al. Prognostic value of the presence and development of atrial fibrillation in patients with advanced chronic heart failure. Eur Heart J 2000;21(15):1238–45.

22. Ahmed A, Perry GJ. Incident atrial fibrillation and mortality in older adults with heart failure. Eur J Heart Fail 2005;7:1118–21.

23. Swedberg K, Olsson LG, Charlesworth A, et al. Prognostic relevance of atrial fibrillation in patients with chronic heart failure on long-term treatment with beta-blockers: results from COMET. Eur Heart J 2005;26(13):1303–8.

24. Raymond RJ, Lee AJ, Messineo FC, et al. Cardiac performance early after cardioversion from atrial fibrillation. Am Heart J 1998;136(3):435–42.

25. Shite J, Yokota Y, Yokoyama M. Heterogeneity and time course of improvement in cardiac function after cardioversion of chronic atrial fibrillation: assessment of serial echocardiographic indices. Br Heart J 1993;70(2):154–9.

26. Pardaens K, Van Cleemput J, Vanhaecke J, et al. Atrial fibrillation is associated with a lower exercise capacity in male chronic heart failure patients. Heart 1997;78:564–8.

27. Clark DM, Plumb VJ, Epstein AE, et al. Hemodynamic effects of an irregular sequence of ventricular cycle lengths during atrial fibrillation. J Am Coll Cardiol 1997;30(4):1039–45.

28. Zupan I, Rakovec P, Budihna N, et al. Tachycardia induced cardiomyopathy in dogs: relation between chronic supraventricular and chronic ventricular tachycardia. Int J Cardiol 1996;56:75–81.

29. Armstrong PW, Stopps TP, Ford SE, et al. Rapid ventricular pacing in the dog: pathophysiologic studies of heart failure. Circulation 1986;74:1075–84.

30. Wilson JR, Douglas P, Hickey WF, et al. Experimental congestive heart failure produced by rapid ventricular pacing in the dog: cardiac effects. Circulation 1987;75:857–67.

31. Zipes DP. Atrial fibrillation: a tachycardia-induced atrial cardiomyopathy. Circulation 1997;95:562–4.

32. Van Gelder IC, Crijns HJ, Blanksma PK, et al. Time course of hemodynamic changes and improvement of exercise tolerance after cardioversion of chronic atrial fibrillation unassociated with cardiac valve disease. Am J Cardiol 1993;72:560–6.

33. Shinbane JS, Wood MA, Jensen DN, et al. Tachycardia-induced cardiomyopathy: a review of animal models and clinical studies. J Am Coll Cardiol 1997;29(4):709–15.

34. Byrne MJ, Raman JS, Alferness CA, et al. An ovine model of tachycardia-induced degenerative dilated cardiomyopathy and heart failure with prolonged onset. J Card Fail 2002;8(2):108–15.

35. Nerheim P, Birger-Botkin S, Piracha L, et al. Heart failure and sudden death in patients with tachycardia-induced cardiomyopathy and recurrent tachycardia. Circulation 2004;110:247–52.

36. Solti F, Vecsey T, Kékesi V, et al. The effect of atrial dilatation on the genesis of atrial arrhythmias. Cardiovasc Res 1989;23:882–6.

37. Li D, Fareh S, Leung TK, et al. Promotion of atrial fibrillation by heart failure in dogs: atrial remodeling of a different sort. Circulation 1999;100:87–95.

38. Guerra JM, Everett TH 4th, Lee KW, et al. Effects of the gap junction modifier rotigaptide (ZP123) on atrial conduction and vulnerability to atrial fibrillation. Circulation 2006;114:110–8.

39. Lee KW, Everett TH 4th, Rahmutula D, et al. Pirfenidone prevents the development of a vulnerable substrate for atrial fibrillation in a canine model of heart failure. Circulation 2006;114:1703–12.

40. Wyse DG, Waldo AL, DiMarco JP, et al, Atrial Fibrillation Follow-up Investigation of Rhythm Management (AFFIRM) Investigators. A comparison of rate control and rhythm control in patients with atrial fibrillation. N Engl J Med 2002;347:1825–33, 59.

41. Van Gelder IC, Hagens VE, Bosker HA, et al, Rate Control Versus Electrical Cardioversion for Persistent Atrial Fibrillation Study Group. A comparison of rate control and rhythm control in patients with recurrent persistent atrial fibrillation. N Engl J Med 2002;347:1834–40.

42. Opolski G, Torbicki A, Kosior DA, et al, Investigators of the Polish How to Treat Chronic Atrial Fibrillation Study. Rate control vs rhythm control in patients with nonvalvular persistent atrial fibrillation: the results of the polish how to treat chronic atrial fibrillation (HOT CAFE) study. Chest 2004;126:476–86.

43. Al-Khatib SM, Shaw LK, Lee KL, et al. Is rhythm control superior to rate control in patients with atrial fibrillation and congestive heart failure? Am J Cardiol 2004;94:797–800.

44. Hohnloser SH, Kuck KH, Lilienthal J. Rhythm or rate control in atrial fibrillation: pharmacological intervention in atrial fibrillation (PIAF): a randomised trial. Lancet 2000;356:1789–94.

45. Talajic M, Khairy P, Levesque S, et al. Maintenance of sinus rhythm and survival in patients with heart failure and atrial fibrillation. J Am Coll Cardiol 2010;55(17):1796–802.

46. Van Gelder IC, Groenveld HF, Crijns HJ, et al. Lenient versus strict rate control in patients with atrial fibrillation. N Engl J Med 2010;362(15):1363–73.

47. Echt DS, Liebson PR, Mitchell LB, et al, the CAST Investigators. Mortality and morbidity in patients receiving encainide, flecainide, or placebo: the cardiac arrhythmia suppression trial. N Engl J Med 1991;324:781–8.

48. Køber L, Torp-Pedersen C, McMurray JJ, et al. Increased mortality after dronedarone therapy for severe heart failure. N Engl J Med 2008;358(25): 2678–87.

49. Roy D, Talajic M, Dorian P, et al. Amiodarone to prevent recurrence of atrial fibrillation: Canadian trial of atrial fibrillation. N Engl J Med 2000;342:913–20.

50. Weinfeld MS, Drazner MH, Stevenson WG, et al. Early outcome of initiating amiodarone for atrial fibrillation in advanced heart failure. J Heart Lung Transplant 2000;19:638–43.

51. Pedersen OD, Bagger H, Keller N, et al. Efficacy of dofetilide in the treatment of atrial fibrillation-flutter in patients with reduced left ventricular function: a Danish Investigation of Arrhythmia and Mortality on Dofetilide (DIAMOND) substudy. Circulation 2001;104:292–6.

52. Burstein B, Nattel S. Atrial fibrosis: mechanisms and clinical relevance in atrial fibrillation. J Am Coll Cardiol 2008;51:802–9.

53. Pedersen OD, Bagger H, Kober L, et al. Trandolapril reduces the incidence of atrial fibrillation after acute myocardial infarction in patients with left ventricular dysfunction. Circulation 1999;100:376–80.

54. Madrid AH, Bueno MG, Rebollo JM, et al. Use of irbesartan to maintain sinus rhythm in patients with long-lasting persistent atrial fibrillation: a prospective and randomized study. Circulation 2002; 106:331–6.

55. Vermes E, Tardif JC, Bourassa MG, et al. Enalapril decreases the incidence of atrial fibrillation in patients with left ventricular dysfunction: insight from the Studies Of Left Ventricular Dysfunction (SOLVD) trials. Circulation 2003;107:2926–31.

56. Nasr IA, Bouzamondo A, Hulot JS, et al. Prevention of atrial fibrillation onset by beta-blocker treatment in heart failure: a meta-analysis. Eur Heart J 2007; 28:457–62.

57. Young-Xu Y, Jabbour S, Goldberg R, et al. Usefulness of statin drugs in protecting against atrial fibrillation in patients with coronary artery disease. Am J Cardiol 2003;92:1379–83.

58. Fauchier L, Pierre B, de Labriolle A, et al. Antiarrhythmic effect of statin therapy and atrial fibrillation: a metaanalysis of randomized controlled trials. J Am Coll Cardiol 2008;51:828–35.

59. Wood MA, Brown-Mahoney C, Kay GN, et al. Clinical outcomes after ablation and pacing therapy for atrial fibrillation. Circulation 2000;101:1138–44.

60. Ganesan AN, Brooks AG, Roberts-Thomson KC, et al. Role of AV nodal ablation in cardiac resynchronization in patients with coexistent atrial fibrillation and heart failure: a systematic review. J Am Coll Cardiol 2012;59(8):719–26.

61. Dagres N, Varounis C, Gaspar T, et al. Catheter ablation for atrial fibrillation in patients with left ventricular systolic dysfunction. A systematic review and meta-analysis. J Card Fail 2011; 17(11):964–70.

62. Kannel WB, Wilson PW, D'Agostino RB, et al. Sudden coronary death in women. Am Heart J 1998; 136(2):205–12.

63. Mosterd A, Cost B, Hoes AW, et al. The prognosis of heart failure in the general population: the Rotterdam Study. Eur Heart J 2001;22(15):1318–27.

64. Effect of enalapril on survival in patients with reduced left ventricular ejection fractions and congestive heart failure. The SOLVD investigators. N Engl J Med 1991;325(5):293–302.

65. Effect of enalapril on mortality and the development of heart failure in asymptomatic patients with reduced left ventricular ejection fractions. The SOLVD investigators. N Engl J Med 1992;327(10):685–91.

66. MERIT-HF Study Group. Effect of metoprolol CR/XL in chronic heart failure: Metoprolol CR/XL Randomised Intervention Trial in congestive Heart Failure (MERIT-HF). Lancet 1999;353(9169):2001–7.

67. Pfeffer MA, Braunwald E, Moye LA, et al. Effect of captopril on mortality and morbidity in patients with left ventricular dysfunction after myocardial infarction. Results of the survival and ventricular enlargement trial. The SAVE investigators. N Engl J Med 1992;327(10):669–77.

68. Moss AJ, Hall WJ, Cannom DS, et al. Improved survival with an implanted defibrillator in patients with coronary disease at high risk for ventricular arrhythmia. Multicenter Automatic Defibrillator Implantation Trial investigators. N Engl J Med 1996; 335(26):1933–40.

69. Moss AJ, Fadl Y, Zareba W, et al. Survival benefit with an implanted defibrillator in relation to mortality risk in chronic coronary heart disease. Am J Cardiol 2001;88(5):516–20.

70. Moss AJ, Zareba W, Hall WJ, et al. Prophylactic implantation of a defibrillator in patients with myocardial infarction and reduced ejection fraction. N Engl J Med 2002;346(12):877–83.

71. Greenberg H, Case RB, Moss AJ, et al. Analysis of mortality events in the Multicenter Automatic Defibrillator Implantation Trial (MADIT-II). J Am Coll Cardiol 2004;43(8):1459–65.

72. Buxton AE, Lee KL, Fisher JD, et al. A randomized study of the prevention of sudden death in patients with coronary artery disease. Multicenter Unsustained Tachycardia Trial investigators. N Engl J Med 1999;341(25):1882–90.

73. Bardy GH, Lee KL, Mark DB, et al. Amiodarone or an implantable cardioverter-defibrillator for congestive heart failure. N Engl J Med 2005; 352(3):225–37.

74. Bristow MR, Saxon LA, Boehmer J, et al. Cardiac-resynchronization therapy with or without an implantable defibrillator in advanced chronic heart failure. N Engl J Med 2004;350(21):2140–50.

75. Theuns DA, Smith T, Hunink MG, et al. Effectiveness of prophylactic implantation of cardioverter defibrillators without cardiac resynchronization therapy in patients with ischaemic or nonischaemic heart disease: a systematic review and meta-analysis. Europace 2010;12(11):1564–70.

76. Packer M, Coats AJ, Fowler MB, et al. Effect of carvedilol on survival in severe chronic heart failure. N Engl J Med 2001;344:1651–8.

77. Dargie HJ. Effect of carvedilol on outcome after myocardial infarction in patients with left-ventricular dysfunction: the CAPRICORN randomized trial. Lancet 2001;357:1385–90.

78. CIBIS-II Investigators and Committees. The Cardiac Insufficiency Bisoprolol Study II (CIBIS-II): a randomised trial. Lancet 1999;353:9–13.

79. Piccini JP, Berger JS, O'Conner CM, et al. Amiodarone for the prevention of sudden cardiac death: a meta-analysis of randomised controlled trials. Eur Heart J 2009;30:1245–53.

80. Connolly SJ, Dorian P, Roberts RS, et al. Comparison of beta-blockers, amiodarone plus beta-blockers, or sotalol for prevention of shocks from implantable cardioverter defibrillators. JAMA 2006;295:165–71.

81. Pacifico A, Hohnloser SH, Williams JH, et al. Prevention of implantable defibrillator shocks by treatment with sotalol. D,L-Sotalol Implantable Cardioverter-Defibrillator Study group. N Engl J Med 1999;340:1855–62.

82. Waldo AL, Camm AJ, Deruyter H, et al. Effect of d-sotalol on mortality in patients with left ventricular dysfunction after recent and remote myocardial infarction. The SWORD investigators. Survival with oral D-sotalol. Lancet 1996;348: 7–12.

Sudden Cardiac Death in Heart Failure

Liviu Klein, MD, MS[a], Henry Hsia, MD[b],*

KEYWORDS

- Heart failure • Implantable cardiac defibrillators • Ischemic heart disease
- Nonischemic cardiomyopathy • Sudden death • Ventricular tachycardia

KEY POINTS

- Sudden cardiac death is common in patients with heart failure and depends on ejection fraction.
- Although several techniques exist for risk stratification, they are imperfect.
- Several pharmacologic strategies exist to prevent sudden death in patients with heart failure.
- Implantable cardioverter-defibrillators, cardiac resynchronization therapy defibrillators, and wearable cardioverter-defibrillators are the most effective tools to prevent sudden death in patients with heart failure and systolic dysfunction.

INTRODUCTION

Heart failure (HF) is a clinical syndrome resulting from structural and functional myocardial abnormalities leading to impaired ability to circulate blood at a rate sufficient to maintain the metabolic needs of internal organs and peripheral tissues. These abnormalities are consequences of long-standing ischemia caused by coronary artery disease or loss of myocardial mass because of prior infarction, myocardial remodeling, and structural damage from long-standing hypertension, valvular disease, or direct toxin exposure (eg, alcohol abuse, illicit substances, chemotherapeutic agents).[1] The prevalence of HF in the United States is around 5.7 million patients, of whom approximately 45% have reduced ejection fraction/systolic dysfunction.[2] There are more than half a million cases of HF newly diagnosed every year and there are more than 1 million hospitalizations yearly with HF as the primary diagnosis.[3] More than 80% of deaths in patients with HF have cardiovascular causes, with most being either sudden cardiac deaths (SCDs) or deaths caused by progressive pump failure.[4]

In general, SCD events are defined as unexpected deaths from cardiovascular causes that are preceded by a witnessed collapse, occur within 1 hour of an acute change in clinical condition, or occur not more than 24 hours after the deceased individuals were known to be in their usual state of health.[5] It is estimated that 350,000 to 380,000 SCD cases occur every year in the adult population in the United States, and that most of these individuals have preexisting heart disease.[6] If the American College of Cardiology/American Heart Association stage-based system for the classification of HF were applied, most patients presenting with SCD could be classified as stage A to D (**Fig. 1**). This classification adds a useful dimension to the understanding of the magnitude of SCD in HF by recognizing that there

Disclosures: Liviu Klein is a consultant for Boston Scientific, and Zoll Medical; and has received research grants from St. Jude Medical. Henri Hsia is a consultant for VytronUS, Inc; is on the Advisory Board for Biosense Webster, Medtronic, Inc; and has received research support from Medtronic, Inc.

[a] Division of Cardiology, University of California San Francisco, San Francisco, CA 94143, USA; [b] Division of Cardiology, San Francisco Veterans Affairs Medical Center, University of California San Francisco, Building 203, 111C-6, Room 2A-52A, 4150 Clement Street, San Francisco, CA 94121, USA
* Corresponding author.
E-mail address: henry.hsia@ucsf.edu

Cardiol Clin 32 (2014) 135–144
http://dx.doi.org/10.1016/j.ccl.2013.09.008
0733-8651/14/$ – see front matter Published by Elsevier Inc.

cardiology.theclinics.com

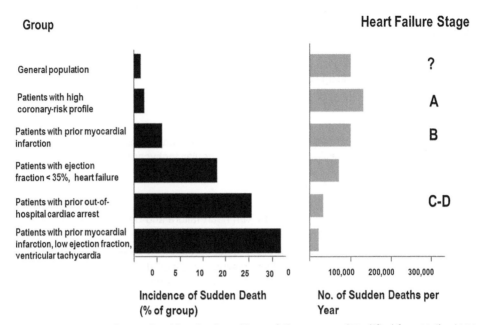

Fig. 1. Relation between incidence of sudden death and heart failure stages. (*Modified from* Huikuri HV, Castellanos A, Myerburg RJ. Sudden death due to cardiac arrhythmias. N Engl J Med 2001;345:1474; with permission.)

are established risk factors and structural prerequisites for the development of SCD and that therapeutic interventions used early after the development of left ventricular dysfunction can prevent the occurrence of SCD.

PATHOPHYSIOLOGY

The mechanisms of SCD in patients with HF are complex and require the chance interaction between a transient event and underlying pathologic substrate. In arrhythmic SCD, the process induces electrical instability and ventricular arrhythmias followed by hemodynamic collapse and death. This event happens more frequently in patients with ischemic cardiomyopathy, and can occur in 2 settings: (1) acute myocardial ischemia (with or without infarction), and (2) structural alterations (scar formation) secondary to prior myocardial infarction or chronic myocardial ischemia. In the setting of acute myocardial ischemia, the electrical instability generates ventricular fibrillation that degenerates to asystole over the course of several minutes. Thus, most SCD cases show asystole or pulseless electric activity when first examined by the emergency medical response teams. In cases in which there has been a short time between collapse and the initial rhythm determination, the proportion with documented ventricular tachycardia/fibrillation increases to 75% to 80%.[7] After experiencing an acute coronary event, women and men have a 4-fold and 10-fold higher

risk of SCD, respectively.[8] Although the absolute rate of SCD is highest in the first 30 days after the event and decreases gradually with time,[9] rates are still high in certain subsets of postinfarction patients, and the degree of left ventricular systolic dysfunction and symptoms (New York Heart Association [NYHA] class) are powerful predictors for SCD in these patients.[10] In the chronic stage of ischemic cardiomyopathy (months and years after the initial infarction), the presumed mechanism of SCD is an electrical event caused by ventricular arrhythmias often originating from areas of prior infarcted myocardium that are adjacent to dense scar that has formed over time. Residual endomyocardial fibers survive, probably because of perfusion from the ventricular cavity or retrograde perfusion through sinusoidal channels. These surviving myocytes become embedded within regions of fibrosis that constitute substrate for abnormal nonuniform anisotropy with conduction block and propagation barrier that promote reentry and the ensuing ventricular arrhythmias.

In patients with systolic dysfunction after a myocardial infarction, nonarrhythmic SCD occurs frequently during the first 4 to 6 weeks. Within hours of infarction, extracellular matrix is digested and results in wall thinning and infarct expansion that may result in ventricular rupture that can manifest as SCD.[11] In addition, autopsy data from Optimal Trial in Myocardial Infarction with Angiotensin II Antagonist Losartan (OPTIMAAL), Assessment of Treatment with Lisinopril and Survival

(ATLAS), and Valsartan In Acute myocardial Infarction Trial (VALIANT) showed that recurrent myocardial infarctions may account for as much as 40% to 50% of the SCD in this population.[12–14] It seems that the proportions of arrhythmic and nonarrhythmic SCD cases become equivalent approximately 1 to 3 months after the initial infarct.[14] These observations are important, because they influence the choice of therapy to prevent SCD after myocardial infarction and explain the time differential effect of therapies (ie, β-blockers and mineralocorticoid receptor blockers vs implantable cardioverter-defibrillators [ICDs]) in this setting.

In contrast with ischemic cardiomyopathy, ventricular myocardium in nonischemic cardiomyopathy often has multiple patchy areas of fibrosis and myofibril disarray with various degrees of myocyte hypertrophy and atrophy. Autopsy studies in patients with idiopathic dilated cardiomyopathy showed that there was a high incidence of myocardial fibrosis without significant visible scar.[15] Myocardial scar-based reentry accounts for only half of the mechanisms of ventricular arrhythmias in patients with nonischemic cardiomyopathy, with the rest having focal initiation of ventricular tachycardia from triggered activity with early afterdepolarizations and delayed afterdepolarizations.[16] Irrespective of the HF cause, patients with advanced HF (stage D) have a different distribution of arrhythmias that may be triggered primarily by pump failure. One series showed that 62% of such patients had severe bradycardia or electromechanical dissociation as the underlying cause for their SCD and only 38% had ventricular tachycardia/ventricular fibrillation.[17]

In other uncommon causes of nonischemic cardiomyopathies, such as infiltrative (sarcoidosis), genetic (arrhythmogenic right ventricular cardiomyopathy), and inflammatory/immunologic (acute myocarditis or Chagas disease), SCD is almost always caused by ventricular arrhythmias. In patients with sarcoidosis, myocardial involvement may be multifocal and the sarcoid granulomas become foci of abnormal automaticity and increase the likelihood of reentrant arrhythmias.[18] In arrhythmogenic right ventricular cardiomyopathy, the infiltration of fibrous tissue and fat into regions of normal myocardium, analogous to infarct-related aneurysms in ischemic heart disease, forms the arrhythmogenic basis for development of reentrant ventricular tachycardia.[19] The anatomic substrate for ventricular tachycardia in Chagas disease is primarily located epicardially and/or at the inferolateral base of the left ventricle. Histologic examinations show patches of focal and diffuse fibrosis of the myocardium, suggesting that VT resulting from this disease may also be caused by a reentrant mechanism.[20]

EPIDEMIOLOGY

Compared with the general population, SCD occurs 6 to 9 times more frequently in patients with HF and is present in patients with both depressed and preserved ejection fraction.[21] Before effective therapies became available, the incidence of SCD in patients with HF and ejection fraction less than 30% was greater than 20% per year.[22] However, with current medical and nonpharmacologic interventions, the incidence of SCD has decreased to about 3% per year.[1] In patients with systolic HF, SCD accounts for about 40% to 45% of all deaths[23] and the proportion of SCD is higher in patients with milder symptoms; two-thirds of patients with NYHA functional class II experience SCD, compared with only a third of those with NYHA functional class IV symptoms, who die preponderantly from progressive pump failure.[24]

Although for a long time patients with diastolic HF were thought to be at low risk for SCD, recent studies have shown an increased risk in this population as well. In the Irbesartan in Heart Failure With Preserved Ejection Fraction Study (I-PRESERVE) trial[25] and the Candesartan in Heart Failure Assessment of Reduction in Mortality (CHARM) Preserved study,[26] a little more than a quarter of the deaths were deemed to be arrhythmic SCD, highlighting the need for strategies to prevent the high burden of SCD in these patients with diastolic HF.

RISK STRATIFICATION

The highest risk for SCD seems to be in patients who have a depressed ejection fraction and HF symptoms. Several risk factors for SCD have been identified and proposed in patients who have structural heart disease, but developing a comprehensive risk stratification strategy remains a challenging task (**Table 1**).

Left Ventricular Ejection Fraction

Left ventricular ejection fraction remains the most consistent predictor of SCD in patients with structural heart disease, irrespective of the cause. For instance, patients after myocardial infarction enrolled in the Multicenter Automatic Defibrillator Implantation Trial (MADIT-II) with ejection fractions less than 30% had an annual rate of SCD of approximately 5.5%,[27] whereas patients after myocardial infarction with ejection fractions greater than 35% had a risk of SCD of only 1.8%.[28] Although left ventricular ejection fraction has a powerful role in predicting future ventricular arrhythmia and sudden death, it remains an imperfect tool for risk stratification because most

Table 1
Summary of risk stratification tools for sudden death in patients with heart failure

Technique	Findings
Left ventricular ejection fraction	Most studied and proven predictor of sudden death
	Imperfect in identifying the patients who will benefit most from defibrillators
MTWA	Several trials suggest limited use to direct decisions on defibrillator implantation
	Combination of MTWA and electrophysiologic studies seem to have some predictive value but limited clinical applicability
Ambulatory electrocardiography	Conflicting data on the predictive value of nonsustained ventricular tachycardia in patient with heart failure
	Heart rate variability, baroreflex sensitivity, and signal-averaged ECG do not reliably predict sudden death and have limited applicability in the absence of clinical trials
Cardiac imaging	Presence and extent of scar on cardiac magnetic resonance imaging have predictive value
	Abnormal washout rate of I-123 metaiodobenzylguanidine is associated with arrhythmic events

Abbreviations: ECG, electrocardiogram; MTWA, microvolt T-wave alternans.

patients enrolled in MADIT-II or Sudden Cardiac Death in Heart Failure trial (SCD-HeFT) did not receive ICD therapy for primary prevention.[27,29]

Ventricular Ectopy

The presence of ventricular ectopy in patients with HF also has prognostic significance. In patients with prior myocardial infarction, frequent premature ventricular complexes (>10/h) or nonsustained ventricular tachycardia were associated with an increased risk of SCD.[30] Nonsustained ventricular tachycardia was associated with SCD in patients with nonischemic cardiomyopathy in the Grupo de Estudio de la Sobrevida en la Insuficiencia Cardiaca en Argentina (GESICA) trial.[31]

Microvolt T-wave Alternans

Microvolt T-wave alternans (MTWA) is a noninvasive test that detects beat-to-beat oscillations in the T-wave amplitude recorded on electrocardiogram (ECG) for the purpose of detecting arrhythmia vulnerability. Although MTWA has been promoted as a predictor of ventricular events, its value is controversial because prospective trial results have been inconsistent[32–34] and the optimal population in which it can be used for risk stratification is yet to be determined.

Heart Rate Variability and Baroreflex Sensitivity

Depressed heart rate variability (HRV) and baroreflex sensitivity (BRS) reflect the autonomic nervous system health, and have been shown in some

studies to be predictors of arrhythmic events in patients who have myocardial infarctions.[35,36] However, such altered autonomic parameters have been associated with increased total non–sudden death mortality in most studies. Because of the inconsistent results, they are not routinely used in clinical practice.

Signal-averaged ECG

The signal-averaged ECG (SAECG) is a high-resolution recording technique designed to measure the low-amplitude, high-frequency surface ECG signals in the terminal QRS complex that cannot be detected by a standard ECG machine. These late potentials have been correlated with localized areas of delayed endocardial activation and reflect the substrate for ventricular reentry. In patients with ischemic cardiomyopathy, SAECG has a high negative predictive value (more than 96%), but its usefulness as prognostic tool remains controversial in patients who have idiopathic nonischemic cardiomyopathy.[37,38]

Electrophysiology Studies

The prognostic value of electrophysiology studies and programmed ventricular stimulation depends on the underlying substrate and the arrhythmia presentations. The inducibility of monomorphic ventricular tachycardia is a powerful marker of risk for SCD only in patients who have a history of prior myocardial infarction and reduced ejection fraction or syncope. In patients with nonischemic cardiomyopathies, the usefulness of electrophysiology studies to determine prognosis and to guide therapy remains limited. The clinical outcomes do not correlate with arrhythmia inducibility, and suppression of induced arrhythmia does not predict a good prognosis.[39,40]

Cardiac Magnetic Resonance Imaging

Cardiac magnetic resonance imaging has provided unique capabilities to identify morphologic changes in the cardiac structure in both ischemic and nonischemic cardiomyopathies. Applications of gadolinium-enhanced imaging provide detailed characterization of cardiac tissues and identification of areas of scar, with several studies showing inducibility of ventricular arrhythmias and appropriate defibrillator discharge in patients with higher scar burden.[41]

I-123 Metaiodobenzylguanidine

Abnormal washout rate of I-123 metaiodobenzylguanidine (MIBG) (an analog of norepinephrine used for estimating cardiac adrenergic nerve activity) has been correlated with increased risk of SCD and appropriate defibrillator shocks.[42,43]

PREVENTION AND TREATMENT OF SUDDEN DEATH
Pharmacologic Therapies

The most striking benefit of therapies with angiotensin-converting enzyme (ACE) inhibitors is the dramatic increase in survival seen in patients with NYHA functional class II to IV and in all patients with systolic dysfunction after an acute myocardial infarction, even in those without symptoms or signs of HF. Although all the ACE inhibitors studied decreased mortality caused by progressive HF, in patients after myocardial infarction, these agents decreased the SCD rate in only 2 studies, by 24% and 30%.[44,45] The angiotensin receptor blockers (ARBs) have been shown to increase SCD mortality by 30% compared with ACE inhibitors, especially in the post–myocardial infarction setting.[46,47]

In addition to the neurohormonal modulation benefits in the management of patients with HF, β-blockers have been shown to be antiarrhythmic. The total mortality reduction with these agents is approximately 35%, with approximately a 40% to 45% reduction in the incidence of SCD in patients with chronic HF and around 25% in the immediate post–myocardial infarction period.[48–50]

The mineralocorticoid receptor blockers spironolactone and eplerenone have been shown not only to decrease total mortality across the HF spectrum (patients with NYHA functional class II-IV) but also to significantly decrease the risk for SCD by 21% to 29%.[51–53] Even more importantly, starting eplerenone within a week after a myocardial infarction led to a significant 30% decrease in SCD within 2 weeks after the initiation of therapy. These data are of paramount importance, because this represents the vulnerable period in which the ICDs have been shown not to reduce mortality.[54,55]

All antiarrhythmic drugs possess potential proarrhythmic toxicity and class IA and IC drugs, as well as dronedarone, are contraindicated in patients with HF. Amiodarone is the only antiarrhythmic drug that may reduce the risk of SCD in patients after myocardial infarction and represents a viable alternative in patients who are not eligible for, refuse, or who do not have access to ICD therapy for the prevention of SCD.[56]

Although a post hoc analysis from the Multicenter Automatic Defibrillator Implantation Trial (MADIT-II) showed that, among patients treated with ICD, those with background statin therapy had a lower rate of ventricular arrhythmias,[57] 2 prospective studies of statins in systolic HF showed no benefit in terms of preventing or reducing SCD compared with placebo.[58,59] In addition, although it was thought that fish oil containing omega-3 polyunsaturated fatty acids could reduce SCD in patients with ischemic HF by reducing the risk of recurrent acute coronary syndrome, this hypothesis was not confirmed in a large randomized trial.[60]

Coronary Revascularization

It is clear that immediate revascularization decreases the risk of SCD in the setting of ST elevation myocardial infarction. Recently, analyses from the Surgical Treatment for Ischemic Heart Failure (STICH) trial showed that in patients with ischemic systolic HF, surgical revascularization decreases the risk of SCD by 27%.[61] Interestingly, there was time dependency on the protective effect of surgical revascularization, with the SCD risk being significantly affected only 24 months after coronary artery bypass grafting.

ICDs

The initial studies using ICDs were targeted at survivors of SCD (secondary prevention) and showed a significant survival benefit in total mortality and SCD mortality. When combined, the results of the Antiarrhythmics Versus Implantable Defibrillators (AVID) trial,[62] Canadian Implantable Defibrillator Study (CIDS),[63] and the Cardiac Arrest Study Hamburg (CASH)[64] showed a 57% decrease in the risk of arrhythmic death along with a 30% decrease in all-cause mortality in survivors of SCD. Over the last 15 years, several major trials have evaluated the role of ICDs in the primary prevention of SCD in patients with ischemic and non-ischemic cardiomyopathies with reduced ejection fraction (**Table 2**). All these trials showed a clear reduction in SCD and in all-cause mortality in patients with HF and reduced ejection fraction. Based on these trial results, the current guidelines recommend ICD as primary prevention in all patients with systolic dysfunction, NYHA functional class II and III symptoms and ejection fraction less than 35%, or NYHA functional class I and ejection fraction less than 30%.[65]

Although ICDs improve survival in these high-risk patients, there is the potential morbidity associated with inappropriate shocks and the significant increase in the rate of hospitalization for worsening HF. As such, judicious programming is needed to minimize the untoward side effects and improve survival.[66] Simple clinical variables, such as NYHA functional class greater than II, age greater than 70 years, BUN greater than 26 mg/dL, QRS duration greater than 0.12 seconds, and atrial fibrillation, can be used to identify the subset of patients with ischemic ventricular dysfunction who may not benefit from primary ICD implantation.[67] In addition, careful timing is needed for ICD implantation to avoid the early lack of benefit in the immediate post–myocardial infarction period.

Cardiac Resynchronization Therapy

In patients with systolic HF and electrical dyssynchrony (QRS >120 milliseconds), cardiac resynchronization therapy (CRT) has been used successfully to improve ventricular remodeling, patients' symptoms, functional capacity, and survival. The Comparison of Medical Therapy, Pacing, and Defibrillation in Heart Failure (COMPANION) and the Cardiac Resynchronization Heart Failure (CARE-HF) trials have shown a 36% and 46% decrease in SCD, respectively.[68,69]

Table 2
Implantable cardioverter defibrillator trials for prevention of sudden death

Trial	Inclusion Criteria	Intervention	Results
Primary Prevention			
DEFINITE	Nonischemic cardiomyopathy, EF <36%, NSVT	Placebo vs ICD	80% decrease in SCD Insignificant decrease in all-cause mortality
MADIT-I	MI, EF <35%, NSVT, inducible/ nonsuppressible arrhythmias	Placebo vs ICD	54% decrease in overall mortality
MADIT-II	MI, EF <30%	Placebo vs ICD	31% decrease in overall mortality
MUSTT	CAD, EF <40%, NSVT	EP vs non–EP-guided treatment, antiarrhythmic drugs vs ICD	55%–60% decrease in all-cause mortality in ICD vs drugs at 39 mo 73%–76% decrease in SCD in ICD vs drugs
SCD-HeFT	EF <35% and NYHA functional class II and III	Placebo vs amiodarone vs ICD	23% decrease in all-cause mortality in ICD vs drugs at 5 y Amiodarone does not improve survival
Secondary Prevention			
AVID	VF, VT/syncope, VT with EF ≤40%	Amiodarone vs sotalol vs ICD	31% decrease in all-cause mortality in ICD vs drugs at 3 y
CASH	Survivors of VF (no EF requirement)	Metoprolol vs amiodarone vs propafenone vs ICD	37% decrease all-cause mortality in ICD vs drugs at 2 y 85% decrease in SCD in ICD vs drugs
CIDS	VF, VT/syncope, VT/EF ≤35%, CL <400 ms	Amiodarone vs ICD	20% decrease all-cause mortality in ICD group vs amiodarone at 3 y

Abbreviations: CAD, coronary artery disease; CL, cycle length; DEFINITE, Defibrillators in Nonischemic Cardiomyopathy Treatment Evaluation; EF, ejection fraction; ICD, implantable cardioverter defibrillator; MADIT, Multicenter Automatic Defibrillator Implantation Trial; MI, myocardial infarction; MUSTT, Multicenter Unsustained Tachycardia Trial; NSVT, nonsustained ventricular tachycardia; SCD, sudden cardiac death; SCD-HeFT, Sudden Cardiac Death in Heart Failure Trial; VF, ventricular fibrillation; VT, ventricular tachycardia.

Table 3
Summary of pharmacologic, electrical and surgical treatment strategies for sudden death in patients with heart failure

Strategy	Decreases Sudden Death (Clinical Trials)	No Effect on Sudden Death (Clinical Trials)
ACE inhibitors	AIRE, TRACE	CONSENSUS, SAVE, SOLVD, SMILE
Mineralocorticoid receptor blocker	EMPHASIS, EPHESUS, RALES	—
β-Blockers	CAPRICORN, CIBIS II; MERIT-HF	—
Statins	—	CORONA, GISSI-HF
Fish oil	—	GISSI-HF
ICDs	AVID, CIDS, CASH DEFINITE, MADIT I and II, MUSTT, SCD-HeFT	—
CRT	CARE-HF, COMPANION	—
Surgical coronary revascularization	STICH	—

Abbreviations: ACE, angiotensin converting enzyme; AIRE, Acute Infarction Ramipril Efficacy; CAPRICORN, Carvedilol Post-Infarct Survival Control in Left Ventricular Dysfunction; CARE-HF, Cardiac Resynchronization Heart Failure; CIBIS II, Cardiac Insufficiency Bisoprolol Study II; COMPANION, Comparison of Medical Therapy, Pacing, and Defibrillation in Heart Failure; CONSENSUS, Cooperative North Scandinavian Enalapril Survival Study; CORONA, Controlled Rosuvastatin Multinational Trial in Heart Failure; CRT, cardiac resynchronization therapy; EMPHASIS-HF, Eplerenone in Mild Patients Hospitalization and Survival Study in Heart Failure; EPHESUS, Eplerenone Post-Acute Myocardial Infarction Heart Failure Efficacy and Survival Study; GISSI-HF, Gruppo Italiano per lo Studio della Sopravvivenza nell'Insuffi cienza cardiaca; ICD, implantable cardioverter defibrillator; MERIT-HF, Metoprolol CR/XL Randomised Intervention Trial in Congestive Heart Failure; RALES, Randomized Aldactone Evaluation Study; SAVE, Survival and Ventricular Enlargement; SMILE, Survival of Myocardial Infarction Long-Term Evaluation; SOLVD, Studies of Left Ventricular Dysfunction; STICH, Surgical Treatment for Ischemic Heart Failure; TRACE, Trandolapril Cardiac Evaluation.

Based on these benefits, CRT is recommended in the guidelines for patients with systolic HF, ejection fraction less than 35%, NYHA functional class II to IV, left bundle branch block, and QRS (preferably) more than 150 milliseconds.[65]

Wearable Cardioverter-Defibrillators

The wearable cardioverter defibrillator represents an alternative approach to prevent SCD until either ICD implantation is clearly indicated or the arrhythmic risk is considered significantly lower or absent. Recent studies show a benefit in the early post–myocardial infarction period or after revascularization, with about 1.5% of patients having an appropriate defibrillation.[70] Because it has been shown that as many as 28% of patients can improve their function significantly using appropriate neurohormonal antagonists,[71] it is reasonable to use this strategy as SCD protection while giving the chance for myocardial recovery. A summary of pharmacologic and electrical treatment strategies for SCD prevention in patients with heart failure is listed in **Table 3**.

SUMMARY

Sudden death is responsible for most deaths in patients with HF, irrespective of the ejection fraction. In most cases, SCD is arrhythmic, but it can be caused by recurrent myocardial infarction or myocardial rupture. Although several strategies have been developed for risk assessment and to improve patient selection for ICDs, left ventricular ejection fraction is still the best qualifier. Besides ICDs and CRTs, pharmacologic therapy plays an important role in reducing the risk of SCD.

REFERENCES

1. Yancy CW, Jessup M, Bozkurt B, et al. 2013 American College of Cardiology Foundation/American heart Association guidelines for the management of heart failure: a report of the American College of Cardiology Foundation/American Heart Association Task Force on Practice Guidelines. J Am Coll Cardiol 2013;62:1495–539.
2. Go AS, Mozaffarian D, Roger VL, et al, American Heart Association Statistics Committee and Stroke Statistics Subcommittee. Heart disease and stroke statistics - 2013 update: a report from the American Heart Association. Circulation 2013;127:e6–245.
3. Chen J, Dharmarajan K, Wang Y, et al. National trends in heart failure hospital stay rates, 2001 to 2009. J Am Coll Cardiol 2013;61:1078–88.
4. Ye S, Grunnert M, Thune JJ, et al. Circumstances and outcomes of sudden unexpected death in

patients with high-risk myocardial infarction: implications for prevention. Circulation 2011;123: 2674–80.

5. Deo R, Albert CM. Epidemiology and genetics of sudden cardiac death. Circulation 2012;125:620–37.

6. Stecker EC, Vickers C, Waltz J, et al. Population-based analysis of sudden cardiac death with and without left ventricular systolic dysfunction: two-year findings from the Oregon Sudden Unexpected Death Study. J Am Coll Cardiol 2006;47: 1161–6.

7. Gang UJ, Jons C, Jorgensen RM, et al. Heart rhythm at the time of death documented by an implantable loop recorder. Europace 2010;12: 254–60.

8. Albert CM, McGovern BA, Newell JB, et al. Sex differences in cardiac arrest survivors. Circulation 1996;93:1170–6.

9. Solomon SD, Zelenkofske S, McMurray JJ, et al. Sudden death in patients with myocardial infarction and left ventricular dysfunction, heart failure, or both. N Engl J Med 2005;352:2581–8.

10. Adabag AS, Therneau TM, Gersh BJ, et al. Sudden death after myocardial infarction. JAMA 2008;300: 2022–9.

11. Yousef ZR, Redwood SR, Marber MS. Postinfarction left ventricular remodeling: a pathophysiological and therapeutic review. Cardiovasc Drugs Ther 2000;14:243–52.

12. Orn S, Cleland JG, Romo M, et al. Recurrent infarction causes the most deaths following myocardial infarction with left ventricular dysfunction. Am J Med 2005;118:752–8.

13. Uretsky BF, Thygesen K, Armstrong PW, et al. Acute coronary findings at autopsy in heart failure patients with sudden death: results from the Assessment of Treatment with Lisinopril and Survival (ATLAS) trial. Circulation 2000;102:611–6.

14. Pouleur AC, Barkoudah E, Uno H, et al, VALIANT Investigators. Pathogenesis of sudden unexpected death in a clinical trial of patients with myocardial infarction and left ventricular dysfunction, heart failure, or both. Circulation 2010;122:597–602.

15. Roberts WC, Siegel RJ, McManus BM. Idiopathic dilated cardiomyopathy: analysis of 152 necropsy patients. Am J Cardiol 1987;60:1340–55.

16. Pogwizd SM, Hoyt RH, Saffitz JE, et al. Reentrant and focal mechanisms underlying ventricular tachycardia in the human heart. Circulation 1992; 86:1872–87.

17. Luu M, Stevenson WG, Stevenson LW, et al. Diverse mechanisms of unexpected cardiac arrest in advanced heart failure. Circulation 1989;80: 1675–80.

18. Roberts WC, McAllister HA, Ferrans VJ. Sarcoidosis of the heart. A clinic-pathologic study of 35 necropsy patients and review of 78 previously described necropsy patients. Am J Med 1977;63: 86–108.

19. Marcus FI, Fontaine GH, Guiraudon G, et al. Right ventricular dysplasia: a report of 24 adult cases. Circulation 1982;65:384–98.

20. Maguire JH, Hoff R, Sherlock I, et al. Cardiac morbidity and mortality due to Chagas' disease: prospective electrocardiographic study of a Brazilian community. Circulation 1987;75:1140–5.

21. Huikuri HV, Castellanos A, Myerburg RJ. Sudden death due to cardiac arrhythmias. N Engl J Med 2001;345:1473–82.

22. Stevenson WG, Stevenson LW, Middlekauff HR, et al. Sudden death prevention in patients with advanced ventricular dysfunction. Circulation 1993;88:2953–61.

23. Carson P, Anand I, O'Connor C, et al. Mode of death in advanced heart failure: the Comparison of Medical, Pacing, and Defibrillation Therapies in Heart Failure (COMPANION) trial. J Am Coll Cardiol 2005;46:2329–34.

24. Effect of metoprolol CR/XL in chronic heart failure: Metoprolol CR/XL Randomised Intervention Trial in Congestive Heart Failure (MERIT-HF). Lancet 1999;353:2001–7.

25. Zile MR, Gaasch WH, Anand IS, et al. Mode of death in patients with heart failure and a preserved ejection fraction. Results from the Irbesartan in Heart Failure with Preserved Ejection Fraction study (I-PRESERVE) trial. Circulation 2010;121: 1393–405.

26. Solomon SD, Wang D, Finn P, et al. Effect of candesartan on cause-specific mortality in heart failure patients: the Candesartan in Heart Failure Assessment of Reduction in Mortality and Morbidity (CHARM) program. Circulation 2004;110:2180–3.

27. Moss AJ, Zareba W, Hall WJ, et al. Prophylactic implantation of a defibrillator in patients with myocardial infarction and reduced ejection fraction. N Engl J Med 2002;346:877–83.

28. Makikallio TH, Barthel P, Schneider R, et al. Prediction of sudden cardiac death after acute myocardial infarction: role of Holter monitoring in the modern treatment era. Eur Heart J 2005;26:762–9.

29. Bardy GH, Lee KL, Mark DB, et al. Amiodarone or an implantable cardioverter-defibrillator for congestive heart failure. N Engl J Med 2005;352: 225–37.

30. Bigger JT, Fleiss JL, Kleiger R, et al. The relationships among ventricular arrhythmias, left ventricular dysfunction, and mortality in the 2 years after myocardial infarction. Circulation 1984;69:250–8.

31. Doval HC, Nul DR, Grancelli HO, et al. Non-sustained ventricular tachycardia in severe heart failure: independent marker of increased mortality due to sudden death. GESICA-GEMA investigators. Circulation 1996;94:3198–203.

32. Costantini O, Hohnloser SH, Kirk MM, et al. The ABCD (Alternans before Cardioverter Defibrillator) Trial: strategies using T-wave alternans to improve efficiency of sudden cardiac death prevention. J Am Coll Cardiol 2009;53:471–9.

33. Chow T, Kereiakes DJ, Onufer J, et al. Does microvolt T-wave alternans testing predict ventricular tachyarrhythmias in patients with ischemic cardiomyopathy and prophylactic defibrillators? The MASTER (Microvolt T Wave Alternans Testing for Risk Stratification of Post-Myocardial Infarction Patients) trial. J Am Coll Cardiol 2008;52:1607–15.

34. Salerno-Uriarte JA, De Ferrari GM, Klersy C, et al. Prognostic value of T-wave alternans in patients with heart failure due to non-ischemic cardiomyopathy: results of the ALPHA Study. J Am Coll Cardiol 2007;50:1896–904.

35. La Rovere MT, Bigger JT, Marcus FI, et al. Baroreflex sensitivity and heart-rate variability in prediction of total cardiac mortality after myocardial infarction. ATRAMI (Autonomic Tone and Reflexes after Myocardial Infarction) Investigators. Lancet 1998;351:478–84.

36. La Rovere MT, Pinna GD, Maestri R, et al. Short-term heart rate variability strongly predicts sudden cardiac death in chronic heart failure patients. Circulation 2003;107:565–70.

37. Borggrefe M, Fetsch T, Martinez-Rubio A, et al. Prediction of arrhythmia risk based on signal averaged ECG in post infarction patients. Pacing Clin Electrophysiol 1997;20:2566–76.

38. Mancini DM, Wong KL, Simson MB. Prognostic value of an abnormal signal-averaged electrocardiogram in patients with non-ischemic congestive cardiomyopathy. Circulation 1993;87:1083–92.

39. Naccarella F, Lepera G, Rolli A. Arrhythmic risk stratification of post-myocardial infarction patients. Curr Opin Cardiol 2000;15:1–6.

40. Hsia HH, Marchlinski FE. Electrophysiology studies in patients with dilated cardiomyopathies. Card Electrophysiol Rev 2002;6:472–81.

41. Scott PA, Rosengarten JA, Curzen NP, et al. Late gadolinium enhancement cardiac magnetic resonance imaging for the prediction of ventricular tachyarrhythmic events: a meta-analysis. Eur J Heart Fail 2013;15:1019–27.

42. Tamaki S, Yamada T, Okuyama Y, et al. Cardiac iodine-123 metaiodobenzylguanidine imaging predicts sudden cardiac death independently of left ventricular ejection fraction in patients with chronic heart failure and left ventricular systolic dysfunction. J Am Coll Cardiol 2009;53:426–35.

43. Koutelou M, Katsikis A, Flevari P, et al. Predictive value of cardiac autonomic indexes and MIBG washout in ICD recipients with mild to moderate heart failure. Ann Nucl Med 2009;23:677–84.

44. Effect of ramipril on mortality and morbidity of survivors of acute myocardial infarction with clinical evidence of heart failure. The Acute Infarction Ramipril Efficacy (AIRE) Study Investigators. Lancet 1993;342:821–8.

45. Kober L, Torp-Pedersen C, Carlsen JE, et al, for the Trandolapril Cardiac Evaluation (TRACE) Study Group. A clinical trial of the angiotensin-converting enzyme inhibitor trandolapril in patients with left ventricular dysfunction after myocardial infarction. N Engl J Med 1995;333:1670–6.

46. Pitt S, Poole-Wilson PA, Segal R, et al. Randomised trial of losartan versus captopril on mortality in patients with symptomatic heart failure: the Losartan Heart Failure Survival Study, ELITE II. Lancet 2000;355:1582–7.

47. Dickstein K, Kjekshus J, the OPTIMAAL Steering Committee for the OPTIMAAL Study Group. Effects of losartan and captopril on mortality and morbidity in high-risk patients after acute myocardial infarction: the OPTIMAAL randomised trial. Lancet 2002;360:752–60.

48. CIBIS II Investigators and Committees. The Cardiac Insufficiency Bisoprolol study II (CIBIS II): a randomised trial. Lancet 1999;353:9–13.

49. Hjalmarson A, Goldstein S, Fagerberg B, et al, for the MERIT-HF Study Group. Effects of controlled-release metoprolol on total mortality, hospitalizations, and well-being in patients with heart failure: the Metoprolol CR/XL Randomized Intervention Trial in Congestive Heart Failure (MERIT-HF). JAMA 2000;283:1295–302.

50. The CAPRICORN Investigators. Effect of carvedilol on outcome after myocardial infarction in patients with left ventricular dysfunction: the CAPRICORN randomised trial. Lancet 2001;357:1385–90.

51. Pitt B, Zannad F, Remme WJ, et al, for the Randomized Aldactone Evaluation Study Investigators. The effect of spironolactone on morbidity and mortality in patients with severe heart failure. N Engl J Med 1999;341:709–17.

52. Pitt B, Remme W, Zannad F, et al, for the Eplerenone Post-Acute Myocardial Infarction Heart Failure Efficacy and Survival Study Investigators. Eplerenone, a selective aldosterone blocker, in patients with left ventricular dysfunction after myocardial infarction. N Engl J Med 2003;348:1309–21.

53. Zannad F, McMurray JJ, Krum H, et al. Eplerenone in patients with systolic heart failure and mild symptoms. N Engl J Med 2011;364:11–21.

54. Hohnloser SH, Kuck KH, Dorian P, et al. Prophylactic use of an implantable cardioverter-defibrillator after acute myocardial infarction. N Engl J Med 2004;351:2481–8.

55. Steinbeck G, Andresen D, Seidl K, et al. Defibrillator implantation early after myocardial infarction. N Engl J Med 2009;361:1427–36.

56. Piccini JP, Berger JS, O'Connor CM. Amiodarone for the prevention of sudden cardiac death: a meta-analysis of randomized controlled trials. Eur Heart J 2009;30:1245–53.

57. Vyas AK, Guo H, Moss AJ, et al, MADIT-II Research Group. Reduction in ventricular tachyarrhythmias with statins in the multicenter automatic defibrillator implantation trial (MADIT)-II. J Am Coll Cardiol 2006;47:769–73.

58. Kjekshus J, Apetrei E, Barrios V, et al, CORONA Group. Rosuvastatin in older patients with systolic heart failure. N Engl J Med 2007;357:2248–61.

59. GISSI-HF Investigators, Tavazzi L, Maggioni AP, et al. Effect of rosuvastatin in patients with chronic heart failure (the GISSI-HF trial): a randomised, double-blind, placebo-controlled trial. Lancet 2008;372:1231–9.

60. GISSI-HF Investigators, Tavazzi L, Maggioni AP, et al. Effect of n-3 polyunsaturated fatty acids in patients with chronic heart failure (the GISSI-HF trial): a randomised, double-blind, placebo-controlled trial. Lancet 2008;372:1223–30.

61. Carson P, Wertheimer J, Miller A, et al. STICH Investigators. Surgical treatment for ischemic heart failure: mode of death results. J Am Coll Cardiol HF 2013;1:400–8.

62. The Antiarrhythmics Versus Implantable Defibrillators (AVID) investigators. A comparison of antiarrhythmic-drug therapy with implantable defibrillators in patients resuscitated from near-fatal ventricular arrhythmias. The Antiarrhythmics versus Implantable Defibrillators (AVID) investigators. N Engl J Med 1997;337:1576–83.

63. Connolly SJ, Gent M, Roberts RS, et al. Canadian Implantable Defibrillator Study (CIDS): a randomized trial of the implantable cardioverter defibrillator against amiodarone. Circulation 2000;101:1297–302.

64. Kuck KH, Cappato R, Siebels J, et al. Randomized comparison of antiarrhythmic drug therapy with implantable defibrillators in patients resuscitated from cardiac arrest: the Cardiac Arrest Study Hamburg (CASH). Circulation 2000;102:748–54.

65. Epstein AE, DiMarco JP, Ellenbogen KA, et al, American College of Cardiology Foundation, American Heart Association Task Force on Practice Guidelines, Heart Rhythm Society. 2012 ACCF/AHA/HRS focused update incorporated into the ACCF/AHA/HRS 2008 guidelines for device-based therapy of cardiac rhythm abnormalities: a report of the American College of Cardiology Foundation/American Heart Association Task Force on Practice Guidelines and the Heart Rhythm Society. J Am Coll Cardiol 2013;61:e6–75.

66. Moss AJ, Schuger C, Beck CA, et al, for the MADIT-RIT Trial Investigators. Reduction in inappropriate therapy and mortality through ICD programming. N Engl J Med 2012;367:2275–83.

67. Goldenberg I, Moss AJ, Hall WJ, et al. Causes and consequences of heart failure after prophylactic implantation of a defibrillator in the multicenter automatic defibrillator implantation trial II. Circulation 2006;113:2810–7.

68. Bristow MR, Saxon LA, Boehmer J, et al. Cardiac resynchronization therapy with or without an implantable defibrillator in advanced chronic heart failure. N Engl J Med 2004;350:2140–50.

69. Cleland JG, Daubert JC, Erdmann E, et al, on behalf of the CARE-HF Study Investigators. Longer-term effects of cardiac resynchronization therapy on mortality in heart failure [the Cardiac REsynchronization-Heart Failure (CARE-HF) trial extension phase. Eur Heart J 2006;27:1928–32.

70. Zishiri ET, Williams S, Cronin EM, et al. Early risk of mortality after coronary artery revascularization in patients with left ventricular dysfunction and potential role of the wearable cardioverter defibrillator. Circ Arrhythm Electrophysiol 2013;6:117–28.

71. Wilcox JE, Fonarow GC, Yancy CW, et al. Factors associated with improvement in ejection fraction in clinical practice among patients with heart failure: findings from IMPROVE HF. Am Heart J 2012;163:49–56.

Managing Acute Decompensated Heart Failure

Daniel F. Pauly, MD, PhD

KEYWORDS

- Heart failure • Myocardial infarction • Cardiomyopathy • Hospitalizations

KEY POINTS

- In patients with acute decompensated heart failure, an important first step is to determine the factors that precipitated the deterioration in cardiac function or increased the body's demand.
- Such factors can include myocardial ischemia, poorly controlled hypertension, atrial fibrillation, anemia, thyroid disease, noncompliance with medications, excessive salt or fluid intake, as well as deterioration in kidney function.
- Patients often require management in an intensive care unit setting, which allows for gradual volume removal, telemetric monitoring, and ongoing electrolyte replacement.
- Patients with end-stage heart failure may progressively deteriorate despite maximal medical therapy.
- Some patients with end-stage heart failure are candidates for a ventricular assist device or cardiac transplantation; for those who are not, end-of-life care should be openly discussed.
- Precipitants of heart failure can include systolic dysfunction, diastolic dysfunction, acute dysrhythmia, or valvular heart disease.
- Vigilance for the triggers of heart failure exacerbations gives the physician the best chance of recognizing the occasional patient with a reversible cause.

INTRODUCTION: NATURE OF THE PROBLEM

Acute decompensated heart failure (ADHF) refers to the sudden onset of fatigue, breathlessness, and edema that occurs when cardiac function cannot keep pace with the body's demand. This may occur due to impaired contractility during systole, impaired relaxation during diastole, acute abnormalities of rhythm, or valve dysfunction. ADHF may occur de novo, as for example with acute myocardial infarction. Most cases, however, occur due to exacerbation of an underlying chronic cardiomyopathy.

ADHF is a growing medical problem. It is the leading reason for hospital admission among patients over age 65.[1] It is the most costly cardiovascular disorder in Western countries, and the short-term mortality following hospital admission in most studies exceeds 10%.[2]

In evaluating the patient with ADHF caused by cardiomyopathy, consideration of the cause may help the physician identify treatable, reversible causes. Depending on the patient population studied, cases of cardiomyopathy generally segregate with one-third due to hypertensive heart disease, one-third due to ischemic heart disease, and one-third due to myocyte heart disease (**Fig. 1**). Myocyte heart disease is predominantly made up of patients with idiopathic cardiomyopathy. However, it also includes such diverse causes as genetic familial cardiomyopathies, peripartum cardiomyopathy, coxsackie viral cardiomyopathy, and exposure-related cardiomyopathies including

The author has nothing to disclose.

Section of Cardiology, Department of Medicine, Truman Medical Centers, School of Medicine, University of Missouri Kansas City, 2301 Holmes Street, Kansas City, MO 64108, USA

E-mail address: paulydf@tmcmed.org

Cardiol Clin 32 (2014) 145–149

http://dx.doi.org/10.1016/j.ccl.2013.09.011

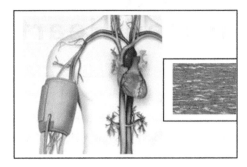

1/3 hypertensive heart disease

1/3 myocyte heart disease

1/3 ischemic heart disease

Fig. 1. Cardiomyopathy-related heart failure. The 3 principal etiologies are shown. Hypertensive heart disease is illustrated by the blood pressure cuff. Ischemic heart disease is shown by the heart's coronary arteries. Myocyte heart disease is indicated with the close-up histologic section of cardiac muscle. (Source: American Heart Association.)

those due to alcohol, cocaine, or chemotherapeutic agents.

ADHF is generally precipitated by a new disturbance that places hemodynamic load on an already failing ventricle. Such precipitants can include tachyarrhythmias, acute anemia, or systemic infection. The most common cause, however, of reversible cardiac decompensation is noncompliance: either with diet, salt restriction, medications, or a combination. Even a small increase in dietary sodium, a change in fluid intake, or intermittent failure to take a medication can trigger a heart failure exacerbation in this population. Use of drugs such as nonsteroidal anti-inflammatory agents may blunt diuresis and the vasodilatory effects of the renin-angiotension-aldosterone antagonists, thus resulting in ADHF.[3] For treatment, coronary revascularization can be an effective approach if active angina accompanies the heart failure. The benefit of revascularization is most pronounced when large amounts of viable myocardium are suitable for revascularization. Indeed, the most common contributing comorbidities are active myocardial ischemia, poorly controlled hypertension, or initiation of atrial fibrillation. Any of these can contribute to ADHF. In addition, patients are now being treated more commonly for diuretic resistance and the cardiorenal syndrome. Kidney dysfunction is now recognized as a late-stage exacerbating factor that plays a larger role as patients become more refractory to medication therapy. This has led to an increasing use of ultrafiltration for diuretic-resistant patients[4] and hemodialysis for patients with progressive kidney disease. Each of these strategies can play a role in re-establishing a new set point for the heart failure patient's fluid balance and hemodynamic stability.

MANAGEMENT GOALS

Patients with ADHF generally present with some combination of dyspnea, fatigue, volume overload, hypotension, and end-organ dysfunction. The first goal is to relieve symptoms, especially in patients who have signs of congestion. The goals of medical treatment are to bring the ventricular filling pressures down to the normal range and optimize end-organ perfusion. While hospitalized, there is the ability to assess the patient's often complex medication regimen and the patient's ability to comply. Similarly, hospitalization allows for a period of patient education focused on salt and fluid restriction and on daily monitoring of body weight as a surrogate for fluid retention.

Finally, the time in hospital allows the physician to readdress advanced treatment options. These may include antiarrhythmic therapy or cardioversion for atrial tachyarrhythmias, coronary revascularization for patients with treatable ischemic heart disease, or cardiac resynchronization therapy for patients with significant dyssynchrony as evidenced by QRS duration on electrocardiogram (ECG) greater than 120 to 130 milliseconds. Still more aggressive treatments, including support with ventricular assist device or pursuing cardiac transplantation, can be entertained.

PHARMACOLOGIC STRATEGIES

Intravenous diuretics, especially furosemide and bumetanide, have remained the primary first-line treatment for ADHF for many decades. The optimal dosing of diuretic therapy remains controversial. A randomized study published in 2011 studied high-dose and low-dose strategies and studied continuous infusions versus intermittent dosing.[5] This study showed no significant difference in the patient global assessment of symptoms. There was also no difference in the change in renal function. For this reason, the dosing of loop diuretics continues to remain a matter of personal preference.

Vasodilators are a longstanding bellwether of treatment for ADHF. These include intravenous and oral nitrates, hydralazine, angiotensin-converting enzyme inhibitors, angiotensin II receptor blockers, and intravenous sodium nitroprusside. The combination of nitrates and hydralazine is particularly beneficial for patients with impaired kidney function (serum creatinine >2.5) and for African-American patients with heart failure.[6] Nitroprusside has the distinct advantage of decreasing neurohormonal activation, although the need for invasive hemodynamic monitoring during its use has been a substantial impediment to its more widespread use.

Intravenous nesiritide (human B-type natriuretic peptide) acts to cause natriuresis and vasodilation. It is approved for relief of dyspnea in patients with acute heart failure. The ASCEND-HF (Acute Study of Clinical Effectiveness of Nesiritide in Decompensated Heart Failure) study randomly assigned patients with acute heart failure to nesiritide or placebo.[7] The patients received 24 to 168 hours of treatment on top of standard medical care. The primary endpoints were a dyspnea scale, rehospitalization for heart failure, or death within 30 days. This study showed that nesiritide was not associated with a change in the rate of death and rehospitalization. It also was not associated with a change in kidney function. Following the publication of the study, the use of nesiritide has lessened. However, it is not clear whether a 24-hour treatment course as was used in the study is really long enough to obtain the benefit.

Vasopressin receptor antagonists are a class of medications that produce selective water aquaresis, and thus ameliorate hyponatremia. The EVEREST (Efficacy of Vasopressin Antagonism in Heart Failure Outcome Study with Tolvaptan) study enrolled 4133 heart failure patients in a randomized, double-blind, placebo-controlled fashion.[8] At the median follow-up of 9.9 months, there was no mortality benefit or rehospitalization benefit for patients treated with the vasopressin receptor antagonist tolvaptan. Most patients in the study, however, had heart failure without hyponatremia. Chronic hyponatremia in association with heart failure can be a significant source of morbidity. Features can include gait instability, unsteadiness, propensity for falls, chronic mental confusion, and increased burden on caregivers.[9] Because hyponatremia in heart failure generally portends a pathologic, low output cardiac state, the aquaretic medications may still have a role in patients with heart failure and symptomatic hyponatremia.

Intravenous positive inotropic agents have enjoyed a long history of use for ADHF. Dobutamine is a mixed beta1 and beta2 receptor agonist. It is the most widely used of these agents. There are, however, few randomized controlled trial data evaluating this drug. In contrast, intravenous milrinone is a phosphodiesterase-3 inhibitor. The randomized controlled OPTIME-CHF (Outcomes of a Prospective Trial of Intravenous Milrinone for Exacerbations of Chronic Heart Failure) trial assessed patients in whom inotropic therapy was indicated but not required.[10] The patients who randomized to milrinone developed more hypotension, atrial arrhythmias, and early treatment failure. The endpoints of death and rehospitalization showed a disadvantage to milrinone as compared with placebo, especially in patients with cardiomyopathy caused by an ischemic rather than nonischemic etiology. This has led to a general recommendation against use of this medication except in patients who present with signs of cardiogenic shock, end-organ hypoperfusion, acidosis, or cognition impaired by low cardiac output.

HEMODYNAMIC STRATEGIES

Direct measurement of cardiac hemodynamics is one way to choose and regulate medication treatment in ADHF. The ESCAPE (Evaluation Study of Congestive Heart Failure and Pulmonary Artery Catheterization Effectiveness) trial randomized patients such that 1 group received clinical medical therapy based on symptoms and physical examination signs. They were compared against patients in another group who received a pulmonary artery catheter-guided approach.[11] Therapies to vasodilate, to diurese, and to provide inotropic support were guided clinically in 1 arm and guided by the invasive hemodynamic assessments in the other arm. Surprisingly, the study demonstrated no significant difference in the primary endpoint of days alive and out of the hospital over a 6-month follow-up period. For this reason, routine management of ADHF using invasive hemodynamic assessment is now reserved for patients with worsening end-organ dysfunction due to hypoperfusion, hypotension, or kidney failure.

For most patients, a clinical assessment of filling pressure (dry vs wet) and systemic perfusion (warm vs cold) will provide the same information as an invasive pulmonary artery catheter for selecting treatment medications (**Fig. 2**). Identification of high filling pressures (wet) is judged by symptoms

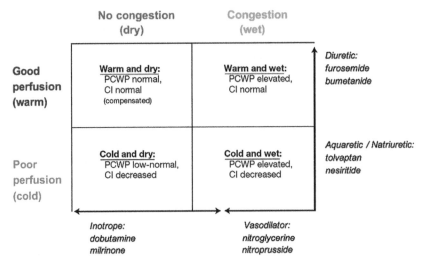

Fig. 2. Hemodynamic schema for heart failure assessment. The patient's volume status is shown across the top. The perfusion status is shown down the left side. Arrows indicate the three hemodynamic quadrants that make up decompensated heart failure. Medications are shown next to the hemodynamic profiles that they most benefit. CI, cardiac index; PCWP, pulmonary capillary wedge pressure.

of orthopnea and edema and by signs of jugulovenous distension and S3 gallop. Rales on pulmonary examination have a poor negative predictive value. Patients with longstanding elevation in filling pressures often have no rales at all. Identification of reduced cardiac output and poor perfusion (cold) is evidenced by cool extremities, hypotension, and impaired cognition. This assessment is important for determining an initial strategy of treatment. Optimal treatment generally includes diuretics for wet patients, vasodilators for cool wet patients, and positive inotropes for cool dry patients.

SELF-MANAGEMENT STRATEGIES

Hospitalizations for ADHF are currently estimated to exceed $1 million annually in the United States. In addition, the 30-day readmission rate for patients with ADHF is estimated at 27%.[12] This is the highest readmission rate among all medical conditions. Most the health care costs for ADHF are generated by inpatient hospital care. This is a large economic burden likely to grow larger as the US population's mean age continues to rise.

Strategies to improve outcomes now include self-care and self-management. Self-care refers to a patient's commitment to adhere to medications. It also focuses on following dietary restrictions and exercise recommendations. Self-management then extends this concept to a patient who can determine his or her own volume status and adjust diuretic medications accordingly.

Strategies of self-management can then be advanced to multidisciplinary teams for home visitation, structured telephone support, and telemonitoring from a remote location. Telemonitoring aims to transfer physiologic patient information, such as body weight, blood pressure, and oxygen saturation through telephone or wireless networks. Recent studies, including TIM-HF (Telemedical Interventional Monitoring in Heart Failure), have been unable to show an impact of remote monitoring on rehospitalization rates or on mortality.[13]

EVALUATION AND ADJUSTMENT

The unreliability of patients collecting their own data has led to more automated methods. Implantable devices have been developed that allow transmission of recorded data through a transmitter to a central database. The information is then made available to the physician, who can interpret the data and make needed medication adjustments. An implantable pulmonary artery sensor has been developed for this purpose. The CHAMPION (Cardiomems Heart Sensor Allows Monitoring of Pressure to Improve Outcomes in NYHA Class III Patients) trial evaluated its effectiveness. This trial showed a reduction in hospitalizations for heart failure by nearly 30% in the class III heart failure subgroup.[14] With the large number of heart failure patients in the United States, the potential benefit for home monitoring to reduce the episodes of ADHF seems enormous.

The current monitoring methods for patients with ADHF all require ongoing input from the physician. The physician is expected to diagnose any clinical deterioration and make the appropriate medical decisions to avoid rehospitalization. These devices and their implantation are expected to be costly. However, it is hoped that strategies of this type will ultimately be cost-effective by reducing the financial burden of repeated episodes of heart failure.

SUMMARY

ADHF occurs when cardiac function falls below the demands of the body. In patients with ADHF, an important first step is to determine the factors that precipitated the deterioration in cardiac function or increased the body's demand. Such factors can include myocardial ischemia, poorly controlled hypertension, atrial fibrillation, anemia, thyroid disease, noncompliance with medications, excessive salt or fluid intake, and deterioration in kidney function. Patients often require management in an intensive care unit setting. This allows for gradual volume removal, telemetric monitoring, and ongoing electrolyte replacement. Patients with end-stage heart failure may progressively deteriorate despite maximal medical therapy. Some patients are then candidates for implantation of a ventricular assist device or for cardiac transplantation. For those who are not, end-of-life care should be openly discussed.

The precipitants of heart failure can include systolic dysfunction, diastolic dysfunction, acute dysrhythmia, or valvular heart disease. The cardiomyopathies generally occur due to a fairly even split among hypertensive disease, coronary disease, and myocyte disease. Vigilance for the triggers of heart failure exacerbations gives the physician the best chance of recognizing the occasional patient with a reversible cause.

The current health care system is placing an ever-increasing premium on avoiding recurrent hospitalizations for heart failure. Thus, specialists in this field are likely to be increasingly in demand. Physicians are being asked to improve systems of care to the point where heart failure can be managed with frequent outpatient adjustments, rather than repeated exacerbations requiring hospitalization. As such, today's paradigm is to repeatedly reoptimize the patient's hemodynamic neurohormonal set point, and thus minimize the decompensations.

REFERENCES

1. Dec GW. Management of acute decompensated heart failure. Curr Probl Cardiol 2007;32:321–66.

2. Allen LA, O'Connor CM. Management of acute decompensated heart failure. CMAJ 2007;176(6): 797–805.

3. Page J, Henry D. Consumption of NSAIDs and the development of congestive heart failure in elderly patients: an underrecognized public health problem. Arch Intern Med 2000;160:777–84.

4. Costanzo MR, Saltzberg M, O'Sullivan J, et al. Early ultrafiltration in patients with decompensated heart failure and diuretic resistance. J Am Coll Cardiol 2005;46:2047–51.

5. Felker GM, Lee KL, Bull DA, et al. Diuretic strategies in patients with acute decompensated heart failure. N Engl J Med 2011;364(9):797–805.

6. Taylor AL, Ziesche S, Yancy C, et al, for the African-American Heart Failure Trial Investigators. Combination of isosorbide dinitrate and hydralazine in blacks with heart failure. N Engl J Med 2004;351:2049–57.

7. O'Connor CM, Starling RC, Hernandez AF, et al. Effect of nesiritide in patients with acute decompensated heart failure. N Engl J Med 2011;365:32–43.

8. Konstam MA, Gheorghiade M, Burnett JC Jr, et al. Effects of oral tolvaptan in patients hospitalized for worsening heart failure: The EVEREST Outcome Trial. JAMA 2007;297:1319–31.

9. Renneboog B, Musch W, Vandemergel X, et al. Mild chronic hyponatremia is associated with falls, unsteadiness, and attention deficits. Am J Med 2006; 119(1):71.e1–8.

10. Felker GM, Benza RL, Chandler AB, et al, for the OPTIME-CHF Investigators. Heart failure etiology and response to milrinone in decompensated heart failure: results from the OPTIME-CHF study. J Am Coll Cardiol 2003;41:997–1003.

11. Binanay C, Califf RM, Hasselblad V, et al, ESCAPE Investigators and Study Coordinators. Evaluation study of congestive heart failure and pulmonary artery catheterization effectiveness. The ESCAPE Trial. JAMA 2005;294:1625–33.

12. Bui AL, Fonarow GC. Home monitoring for heart failure management. J Am Coll Cardiol 2012;59(2): 97–104.

13. Koehler F, Winkler S, Schieber M, et al. Impact of remote telemedical management on mortality and hospitalizations in ambulatory patients with chronic heart failure: the telemedical interventional monitoring in heart failure study. Circulation 2011;123: 1873–80.

14. Abraham WT, Adamson PB, Bourge RC, et al. Wireless pulmonary artery haemodynamic monitoring in chronic heart failure: a randomized controlled trial. Lancet 2011;377:658–66.

Heart Failure with Preserved Ejection Fraction
An Ongoing Enigma

Lisa J. Rose-Jones, MD, John J. Rommel, MD,
Patricia P. Chang, MD, MHS*

KEYWORDS

- Heart failure • Preserved ejection fraction • Diastolic dysfunction • HFpEF • Review

KEY POINTS

- Heart failure with preserved ejection fraction (HFpEF) is an increasing epidemic with mortality and morbidity similar to heart failure with reduced ejection fraction, but is more multifactorial in cause and has limited evidence-based therapies.
- Its pathophysiology may be induced by a systemic proinflammatory state, resulting in combined ventricular and arterial stiffness and impaired chronotropic and cardiac output reserve.
- At present, recommended therapy for patients with HFpEF includes symptom relief and management of related comorbidities such as hypertension, atrial fibrillation, and coronary artery disease.
- Medications endorsed by the most recent American College of Cardiology Foundation/American Heart Association guidelines for HFpEF include only diuretics, β-blockers, angiotensin-converting enzyme inhibitors, angiotensin receptor blockers, and omega-3 fatty acids.
- Ongoing investigations of potential HFpEF therapies include aldosterone antagonists, phosphodiesterase-5 inhibitors, advanced glycation end product crosslink breakers, physical exercise, and rate-adaptive pacing from implantable cardiac devices.

INTRODUCTION

With an estimated 50% (range 40%–71%) of all patients with clinical symptoms of heart failure (HF) having normal or near normal left ventricular (LV) ejection fractions (LVEF),[1–5] there has been an increasing need to understand and treat the complex syndrome of HF with preserved ejection fraction (HFpEF). The diagnosis of HFpEF requires a patient to have the typical symptoms of HF, such as dyspnea and fatigue, with normal LV volumes and contractility but increased LV filling pressure. HFpEF used to be called diastolic HF[6]; however, the terminology was controversial and has been updated over the past 8 years, initially to HF with normal ejection fraction (HFnEF),[7–11] then to

HFpEF because the pathogenesis of HFpEF is not exclusively based on diastolic dysfunction. It is imperative to isolate the terminology diastolic dysfunction to describe an abnormality in LV relaxation or chamber compliance.[12] Diastolic dysfunction can be present regardless of the LVEF or symptoms. The threshold for defining preserved LVEF varies greatly, from LVEF greater than 40% to greater than or equal to 55%, with greater than or equal to 50% becoming more widely accepted.[1,11] Patients with LVEF of 40% to 49% represent an intermediate or borderline HFpEF group and may also be considered as HF with improved or recovered LVEF. In practice, the diagnosis of HFpEF is often established after echocardiography reveals preserved LV systolic function

Disclosure Statement: The authors have no relevant conflict of interests to disclose.

Division of Cardiology, Department of Medicine, University of North Carolina at Chapel Hill, 160 Dental Circle, 6th Floor Burnett-Womack Building, Chapel Hill, NC 27599-7075, USA

* Corresponding author.

E-mail address: patricia_chang@med.unc.edu

http://dx.doi.org/10.1016/j.ccl.2013.09.006
0733-8651/14/$ – see front matter © 2014 Elsevier Inc. All rights reserved.

with signs of HF on examination and without valvular disease, pericardial disease, or other noncardiac causes accounting for dyspnea, edema, and fatigue.

EPIDEMIOLOGY

Over time, the proportion of patients with HFpEF has increased.[3,13] Although HF symptoms unify patients with HFpEF, there is marked heterogeneity in the clinical characteristics that potentially confer risk for this syndrome. Patients with HFpEF are typically older, more likely to be female, with higher body mass index and prevalence rates of hypertension and atrial fibrillation, and lower rates of coronary artery disease (CAD) and valve disease.[13,14] Hypertension (chronic pressure overload) remains the single most important predictor of HFpEF across multiple HF registries, epidemiologic trials, and large controlled trials.[15] Because patients with HFpEF have important comorbidities that strongly influence outcomes, the focus of HFpEF therapy is often on comorbid conditions (eg, hypertension, atrial fibrillation, diabetes, chronic kidney disease).

PATHOPHYSIOLOGY

Substantial attention has been devoted to better define the pathogenesis that leads to HFpEF in order to potentially target more effective treatment. Patients with HFpEF, even when well compensated, are characterized as having chronically increased left-sided filling pressures, reduced LV chamber distensibility (compliance), and increased diastolic wall stress. The classic paradigm is based on chronic LV afterload or pressure overload resulting in decreased LV compliance. Although impaired LV relaxation is usually present in patients with HFpEF, it is also considered part of the normal aging process, present in otherwise healthy seniors. What the HF community has not understood is why abnormal myocardial relaxation does not always indicate HFpEF.

Over the past decade, the pathogenesis of HFpEF has been shown to be related to ventricular stiffness combined with arterial or vascular stiffness.[16,17] Ventricular and arterial stiffness increases with advancing age[18] and is further amplified by comorbidities such as hypertension, diabetes, and chronic kidney disease.[19] However, increased end-diastolic static ventricular stiffness may not be a universal finding in patients with HFpEF compared with healthy, sedentary, age-matched controls.[20] In addition, left atrial stiffness has been reported as a predictor of discriminating patients with HFpEF from those with LV

hypertrophy without HF symptoms.[19,21] It has been hypothesized that titan, the third myofilament of cardiac muscle, also plays an important role in diastolic function by defining cardiomyocyte passive stiffness.[22] Although there is ongoing debate regarding the degree and prevalence of primary myocardial stiffness in this syndrome, it seems that additional contributive mechanisms must be present in order for HF to manifest.

The cardiac interstitium has been of increasing interest in this conundrum. In particular, fibroblasts and changes in the extracellular matrix (ECM) can cause myocardial fibrosis and thus myocardial remodeling. In a cohort of symptomatic patients with HFpEF, compared with patients with asymptomatic LV hypertrophy, plasma biomarkers that indicate ongoing ECM collagen changes were present, suggesting that a disruption of collagen homeostasis may be related to the pressure overload–LV remodeling phenomenon.[23] The panel of biomarkers (matrix metalloproteinases [MMPs]) was a more powerful predictor of HFpEF than N-terminal-pro-B-type natriuretic peptide, and a few of these biomarkers (MMP-2, MMP-7, MMP-8) showed patterns that were specific to patients with HFpEF compared with patients with only LV hypertrophy. Endomyocardial biopsy samples of patients with HFpEF have shown increased cardiac inflammatory cells that expressed profibrotic transforming growth factor beta, resulting in substantially more cardiac collagen production (type I and III).[24] These findings suggest that inflammation may be a key trigger in the accumulation of ECM that leads to fibrosis and HFpEF.

Other cardiovascular abnormalities, namely impaired chronotropic and cardiac output reserve, have been observed and likely contribute to the pathogenesis and presentation of HFpEF.[16] Chronotropic incompetence, defined as an inadequate heart rate response to exercise, is exaggerated in patients with HFpEF compared with healthy or hypertensive controls.[25,26] Patients with HFpEF also had significantly delayed heart rate recovery, more impaired exercise tolerance and systemic vasodilation, and lower increase in cardiac output with exercise.[25,26] Although diastolic dysfunction promotes congestion and pulmonary hypertension with stress in HFpEF, reduction in exercise capacity is predominantly related to inadequate cardiac output relative to metabolic needs.[27]

As in HF with reduced ejection fraction (HFrEF), neurohormonal imbalances have also been implicated in HFpEF. The renin-angiotensin-aldosterone system (RAAS) is considered an important contributor to the development of HFpEF.[28] The neurohormones angiotensin II and aldosterone have effects on vascular tone, water retention, and renal tubular sodium retention. These instigators lead to hypertensive remodeling with extensive ECM turnover and eventual ventricular fibrosis.[29] Recent data suggest that patients with HFpEF may also have a deficit of cyclic guanosine monophosphate (cGMP)–dependent protein kinase (PKG) activity.[30]

With evolving understanding of the potential mechanisms for HFpEF, based on myocardial structure, endothelial function, and cell signaling, a novel paradigm for the development of HFpEF has been suggested that is based on a systemic proinflammatory state induced by comorbidities. In this new paradigm, HFpEF occurs after the following sequence of events: (1) a high prevalence of comorbidities (such as hypertension, obesity, diabetes mellitus, and chronic obstructive pulmonary disease) induce a systemic proinflammatory state; (2) a systemic proinflammatory state causes coronary microvascular endothelial inflammation; (3) coronary microvascular endothelial inflammation reduces nitric oxide bioavailability, cGMP content, and PKG activity in adjacent cardiomyocytes; (4) low PKG activity favors hypertrophy development and raises resting tension because of hypophosphorylation of titin; and (5) both stiff cardiomyocytes and interstitial fibrosis contribute to high diastolic LV stiffness and development of HF.[31]

DIFFERENTIAL DIAGNOSIS

Dyspnea, reduced exertional tolerance, edema, and orthopnea are classic symptoms of HF. When present in the setting of a preserved LVEF and absence of valvular abnormalities on noninvasive imaging, HFpEF is presumed. However, other common conditions share some of these complaints. Pulmonary disease (including obstructive sleep apnea), obesity, and myocardial ischemia need to be excluded as the cause of symptoms. Documentation of increased B-type natriuretic peptide can be helpful in determining whether increased LV diastolic pressures are contributing to the symptoms.[32] Perhaps newer biomarkers such as MMP[23] will become more commonly used in the future.

Multiple diagnostic algorithms exist for the workup of HFpEF. In the simplest strategy, after noncardiac causes are ruled out, causes of HF can be divided into high output, nonmyocardial, and myocardial (**Fig. 1**).[11] Chronic anemia, chronic liver disease, thyrotoxicosis, or arteriovenous shunts (such as fistulas for hemodialysis) may all lead to LV volume overload and high-output HF. Pericardial diseases from constriction or tamponade and valvular diseases comprise the nonmyocardial causes that are important to distinguish. The myocardial category contains the broadest differential.

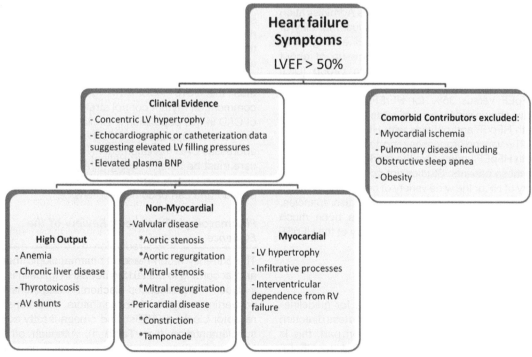

Fig. 1. Diagnostic algorithm for working up HF symptoms (dyspnea, fatigue, edema) in patients with documented LVEF greater than 50%. AV, arteriovenous; BNP, B-type natriuretic peptide; RV, right ventricular.

Although hypertensive LV hypertrophy is the most common cause of HFpEF, CAD is also common. Infiltrative disorders such as cardiac amyloidosis, sarcoidosis, and associated storage disorders like hemachromatosis all need to be considered. In addition, interventricular dependence, from right ventricular enlargement and dysfunction, must be excluded. Careful history and physical examination coupled with a thorough diagnostic evaluation are important to eliminate other conditions that may present in a similar manner. In some cases, invasive hemodynamic evaluation can be useful for diagnosis and to guide therapy.[33]

OUTCOMES

Although it is often reassuring to have an LVEF reported as normal, substantial morbidity and mortality still exist in HFpEF. Patients with preserved ejection fraction presenting with an acute HF decompensation may have a 50% chance of rehospitalization within 6 months.[34] Functional decline, as measured by an activities of daily living scale, occurred in more than a quarter of survivors. Both readmission and functional decline were statistically similar compared with those patients with reduced LVEF.

Survival with HFpEF may or may not be different than that of HFrEF. There are varying survival rates reported for patients with HFpEF depending on the population studied, how HFpEF was defined, and severity of disease.[35] The Veterans Administration Heart Failure Trial showed an annual mortality of 8% for HFpEF compared with 19% among those with HFrEF.[36] Over a mean follow-up of about 3 years, the Digitalis Intervention Group (DIG) study revealed a mortality approaching 23% for HFpEF versus 35% for HFrEF.[37] Other studies have shown similar survival rates between patients with HFpEF and patients with HFrEF.[3,13,38]

The varying prognoses reported among patients with HFpEF underscore the marked heterogeneity of these patients. Studies not controlling for a history of HF or the wide variety of comorbidities likely account for some of the observed discrepancies. Despite the differences, there has been much insight gained into the natural history of the HFpEF syndrome.

TREATMENT

Unlike the overwhelming evidence for guideline-based HFrEF therapy, there has been less direction on the best treatment of HFpEF. In part, this is because of the recent recognition of the HFpEF epidemic and consequently the limited number of studies over the past decade. Most of the

recommendations for treating HFpEF are extracted from smaller studies and expert opinion.[1,7,10,11] The newly released 2013 American College of Cardiology Foundation (ACCF)/American Heart Association (AHA) recommendations continue to focus on therapies directed at symptoms and comorbidities that can worsen HFpEF.[1] No current therapy recommendation was given a level of evidence A (data derived from multiple randomized controlled trials or meta-analyses). The few large-scale trials on HFpEF treatment have been neutral. The current treatment options that have been evaluated for HFpEF are summarized later.

Controlling Comorbid Conditions

In the latest versions of the 2013 ACCF/AHA guidelines and the 2010 HFSA guidelines on treatment of HFpEF, managing comorbid conditions remains a top priority.[1,11] These conditions include managing hypertension, atrial fibrillation, and CAD. **Table 1** summarizes the recommended approach and rationale for the management of the related comorbidities. Although no set blood pressure goal has been established in the most recent HF guidelines,[1] the 2009 ACC/AHA guidelines suggest a goal systolic pressure less than 130 mm Hg and diastolic pressure less than 80 mm Hg with potentially multiple agents with different mechanisms of action.[10] Because atrial fibrillation decreases LV filling and diastolic relaxation, rate control is highly recommended. Although some experts have suggested that restoring sinus rhythm might also improve patients, because of the reliance of LV filling on atrial contraction[7] there are no randomized controlled trials evaluating the benefits of sinus rhythm in patients with HFpEF; thus the 2013 ACCF/AHA guidelines do not comment on rhythm control strategies. Treatment of CAD in this population is similar to treatment in the general population, although no specific study addresses CAD management in HFpEF. However, care must be taken in using nitrates because patients with HFpEF tend to be more dependent on preload and can become hypotensive.

Pharmacologic Treatment: Review of the Evidence

The currently recommended pharmacologic therapy, according to the 2013 ACCF/AHA guidelines,[1] includes diuretics, β-blockers, angiotensin-converting enzyme (ACE) inhibitors, angiotensin receptor blockers (ARBs), and omega-3 fatty acid supplementation (see **Table 1**). Although other HF medications, such as calcium channel blockers, digoxin, aldosterone antagonists, and phosphodiesterase-5 (PDE5) inhibitors, are not

Table 1
Management of HFpEF by comorbidity and pharmacologic therapy

Strategy	Recommendation[a]	Class[a]	Level of Evidence[a]	Rationale/Evidence
Hypertension	Blood pressure should be controlled according to published clinical practice guidelines	I	B	↓ LV hypertrophy[44,70] ↓ Hospitalizations[71] ↑ Exercise tolerance[72]
Atrial fibrillation	Managing atrial fibrillation according to published clinical practice guidelines is reasonable to improve HF symptoms	IIa	C	Patients with HFpEF rely more heavily on the atria's contribution to stroke volume
CAD	Coronary revascularization for patients with CAD is reasonable if documented myocardial ischemia or anginal symptoms is present despite guideline-directed medical therapy	IIa	C	Ischemia impedes LV relaxation
Diuretics	Should be used to treat symptoms caused by volume overload	I	C	Hong Kong Diastolic HF study (n = 150, LVEF >45%): ↑ QoL[39]
β-Blockers	Reasonable for controlling hypertension and atrial fibrillation	IIa	C	SENIORS trial: HFpEF subgroup (n = 1359, LVEF >35%); nebivolol vs placebo, ↓ mortality/CV hospitalizations[45]
ACE inhibitors	Reasonable for controlling hypertension	IIa	C	PEP-CHF (n = 850, LVEF >40%), perindopril vs placebo: no difference on combined outcome mortality/HF hospitalization; ↑ functional status and 6MWT[40]
ARBs	Reasonable for controlling hypertension	IIa	C	I-PRESERVE (n = 4128, LVEF >45%), irbesartan vs placebo: no difference on mortality, hospitalization, or QoL[41]
	Might be considered for decreased hospitalizations	IIb	B	CHARM-PRESERVED (n = 3023, LVEF >40%), candesartan vs placebo: no difference on CV mortality/hospitalization; ↓ hospitalization[42]
Omega-3 fatty acid	Reasonable to use as adjunctive therapy	IIa	B	GISSI-HF (n = 6975), omega-3 fatty acid vs placebo: ↓ mortality and CV hospitalization regardless of whether LVEF > or ≤40%[56]
Other nutritional supplements	Routine use of other nutritional supplements is not recommended	III	C	—

(continued on next page)

Table 1
(continued)

Strategy	Recommendation[a]	Class[a]	Level of Evidence[a]	Rationale/Evidence
Calcium channel blockers	—	—	—	Verapamil (n = 15–20, LVEF >45%): ↓ HF symptoms, ↑ exercise capacity[47,48]
Digoxin	—	—	—	DIG Ancillary study (n = 988, LVEF >45%); digoxin vs placebo, no difference in mortality/hospitalization[53]
Aldosterone antagonist	—	—	—	RAAM-PEF (n = 44, LVEF ≥50%) eplerenone vs placebo: improved diastolic function by echo, ↓ biomarkers; no difference in 6MWT[49] ALDO-DHF (n = 422, LVEF >50%), spironolactone vs placebo: improved diastolic function by echo; no difference in exercise tolerance, symptoms, or QoL[50] TOPCAT (n = 3445, LVEF >45%), spironolactone vs placebo: ongoing[52]
PDE5 inhibitors	—	—	—	RELAX (n = 216, LVEF ≥50%), sildenafil vs placebo: ↓ mPA, ↑ QoL, no difference in peak Vo_2 or 6MWT[55]

Abbreviations: 6MWT, 6-minute walk test; ACE, angiotensin-converting enzyme; ALDO-DHF, Aldosterone Receptor Blockade in Diastolic Heart Failure; ARB, angiotensin receptor blocker; CHARM-Preserved, Candesartan in Heart Failure - Assessment of Reduction in Mortality and Morbidity; CV, cardiovascular; DIG, Digitalis Intervention Group; echo, echocardiography; GISSI-HF, Gruppo Italiano per lo Studio della Sopravvivenza nell'Infarto miocardico – heart failure; HF, heart failure; HFpEF, heart failure with preserved ejection fraction; I-PRESERVE, Irbesartan in Heart Failure with Preserved Ejection Fraction; LV, left ventricular; LVEF, left ventricular ejection fraction; mPA, mean pulmonary artery pressure; PDE5, phosphodiesterase-5; PEP-CHF, Perindopril in Elderly People with Chronic Heart Failure; QoL, Quality of life; RAAM-PEF, Randomized Aldosterone Antagonism in Heart Failure With Preserved Ejection Fraction; RELAX, Phosphodiesterase-5 Inhibition to Improve Clinical Status and Exercise Capacity in Heart Failure with Preserved Ejection Fraction; SENIORS, Study of Effects of Nebivolol Intervention on Outcomes and Rehospitalization in Seniors With Heart Failure; TOPCAT, Treatment of Preserved Cardiac Function with an Aldosterone Antagonist; Vo_2, oxygen consumption.

[a] Based on the 2013 ACCF/AHA Heart Failure Guidelines (Yancy CW, Jessup M, Bozkurt B, et al. 2013 ACCF/AHA guideline for the management of heart failure: a report of the American College of Cardiology Foundation/American Heart Association Task Force on Practice Guidelines. J Am Coll Cardiol 2013. pii:S0735-1097(13)02114-1. http://dx.doi.org/10.1016/j.jacc.2013.05.019).

recommended in the most recent ACCF/AHA guidelines, there have been mixed data and ongoing investigations regarding their effectiveness. Nevertheless, the evidence supporting these different medications is based mostly on a limited number of clinical trials, which are summarized in **Table 1**, many of which are of modest size.

Although loop and thiazide diuretics remain widely accepted therapy for decongesting patients with HFpEF, there are no randomized controlled trials comparing diuretics with placebo. Only 1 study, the Hong Kong Diastolic HF study, revealed significant improvement in quality of life at 52 weeks in patients treated with diuretic therapy that did not improve further with addition of an ACE inhibitor or ARB.[39]

Although ACE inhibitors have not been shown to improve mortality in HFpEF compared with placebo, the PEP-CHF (Perindopril in Elderly People with Chronic Heart Failure) trial did show that perindopril improved functional class and 6-minute walk distances in patients with HFpEF more than the age of 70 years.[40] ARBs have been the most studied in the HFpEF population. Although the large trials (I-PRESERVE [Irbesartan in Heart Failure with Preserved Ejection][41] and CHARM-Preserved [Candesartan in Heart Failure - Assessment of Reduction in Mortality and Morbidity][42]) failed to show significant survival benefits for patients with HFpEF taking ARBs, candesartan was associated with a significant decrease in hospitalizations.[42]

β-Blockers have been shown to improve diastolic function in patients with HFpEF,[43] induce left ventricular hypertrophy regression[44] and are standard therapy for hypertension, atrial fibrillation, and CAD. However, the evidence for β-blockers in patients with HFpEF has been mixed and is based on comparative data from combined populations of patients with HFpEF and HFrEF: the SENIORS trial (Study of Effects of Nebivolol Intervention on Outcomes and Rehospitalization in Seniors With Heart Failure) showed some benefit,[45] but the OPTIMIZE-HF (Organized Program to Initiate Lifesaving Treatment in Hospitalized Patients with Heart Failure) registry showed no benefit.[46]

Calcium channel blockers have been mentioned in previous treatment guidelines as treatment of hypertension, symptom-limit angina, and rate control of atrial fibrillation,[7,10,11] but are not specifically addressed in the 2013 ACCF/AHA guidelines.[1] Data supporting calcium channel blockers in this population remain limited to small patient samples (n = 20 or less) but they were associated with symptomatic improvement.[47,48]

Aldosterone antagonists are also not currently recommended in the 2013 ACCF/AHA guidelines but are actively being investigated as therapy for HFpEF. Although spironolactone may improve diastolic function and LV mass index by echocardiographic measures,[49,50] improved clinical outcomes have not been observed.[49–51] TOPCAT (Treatment of Preserved Cardiac Function with an Aldosterone Antagonist) is currently underway, comparing spironolactone versus placebo in 3445 patients with HFpEF with LVEF greater than 45% and controlled blood pressure.[52]

Digoxin has not been specifically recommended for HFpEF. An ancillary study of the DIG trial enrolled HF patients with LVEF greater than 45% but showed no statistical difference in mortality or hospitalization.[53] Although there was a trend toward decreased HF hospitalizations for patients with HFpEF on digoxin, this was offset by an increase in hospitalizations for unstable angina.

PDE5 inhibitors have emerged as a new class of medications for pulmonary hypertension and may be useful in patients with HFpEF with pulmonary hypertension. Although sildenafil effectively decreases pulmonary artery pressures and has been associated with improved quality of life in patients with HFpEF,[54] the RELAX (Phosphodiesterase-5 Inhibition to Improve Clinical Status and Exercise Capacity in Heart Failure with Preserved Ejection Fraction) study did not show any change in peak oxygen consumption during cardiopulmonary testing or in 6-minute walk distances at 24 weeks.[55] However, the short follow-up period may not have allowed enough time for differences to become apparent.

The only other medication endorsed by the ACCF/AHA guidelines for patients with HFpEF is omega-3 polyunsaturated fatty acids, based primarily on the GISSI-HF (Gruppo Italiano per lo Studio della Sopravvivenza nell'Infarto miocardico – heart failure) trial.[56] However, other nutritional supplements are not recommended.

OTHER ONGOING INVESTIGATIONS

Reduced exercise tolerance in patients with HFpEF is generally attributed to inadequate chronotropic response. It is currently unknown whether rate-adaptive pacing from implantable cardiac devices may have a role in patients with HFpEF. Adjustment of pacemaker sensor parameters has been shown to improve chronotropic response in patients who do not have HF.[57] The RESET (Restoration of Chronotropic Competence in Heart Failure Patients with Normal Ejection Fraction) trial is currently investigating whether pacemaker implantation with rate-adaptive pacing may be beneficial in patients with symptomatic HFpEF with an impaired chronotropic response.[58]

Although physical exercise is encouraged, the largest exercise training trial in patients with chronic HF (HF-ACTION [Heart Failure: A Controlled Trial Investigating Outcomes of Exercise Training]) did not show significant reductions in clinical outcomes.[59] However, smaller studies of patients with HFpEF have at least confirmed improved exercise capacity after medically supervised exercise training,[60,61] and a randomized study of 64 patients with HFpEF additionally showed that exercise was associated with atrial reverse remodeling and improved LV diastolic function.[62]

Another area of active drug investigation involves advanced glycation end products (AGEs), which are formed by a reaction between reducing sugars and biologic amines, which accumulate slowly over time and can contribute to age-associated cardiovascular changes such as increased vascular and myocardial stiffness, endothelial dysfunction, altered vascular injury responses, and atherosclerotic plaque formation.[63] Early investigational studies in patients with HFpEF suggested that alagebrium, an AGE-crosslink breaker, can decrease LV mass and improve LV diastolic filling and quality of life in patients with HFpEF.[64]

Other potential novel pharmacologic agents in ongoing research include a dual angiotensin receptor and neprilysin inhibitor (LCZ696).[65,66] Future research, based on animal models, may evaluate the efficacy of and ʟ-carnitine supplementation,[67] the I(f)-inhibitor ivabradine,[68] and MMP-9 inhibitors and nitroxyl donors.[69]

SUMMARY

HFpEF was initially thought to be a syndrome resulting from abnormalities of diastolic function from chronic pressure overload. However, further research suggests that there is much more at play. Its pathophysiology may be related to abnormalities of the endothelium, cardiomyocyte, and interstitium, and may be induced by a systemic proinflammatory state, resulting in combined ventricular and arterial stiffness, impaired chronotropic and cardiac output reserve, and increased filling pressures. This multifaceted syndrome is frequently encountered with an increasing prevalence and is associated with considerable mortality and morbidity, similarly to HFrEF. Although much effort has focused on establishing effective therapy, none of the evidence-based therapies for HFrEF have shown clear benefit in clinical outcomes for HFpEF. At present, management of volume overload with diuretics, control of hypertension, and therapy for comorbid conditions are the mainstay of therapy. With a projected 50% increase in the number of patients with HF by 2030, HFpEF will remain a focus of research for years to come.

REFERENCES

1. Yancy CW, Jessup M, Bozkurt B, et al. 2013 ACCF/AHA guideline for the management of heart failure: a report of the American College of Cardiology Foundation/American Heart Association Task Force on Practice Guidelines. J Am Coll Cardiol 2013. http://dx.doi.org/10.1016/j.jacc.2013.05.019. pii:S0735-1097(13)02114-1.

2. Bursi F, Weston SA, Redfield MM, et al. Systolic and diastolic heart failure in the community. JAMA 2006;296(18):2209-16.

3. Bhatia RS, Tu JV, Lee DS, et al. Outcome of heart failure with preserved ejection fraction in a population-based study. N Engl J Med 2006; 355(3):260-9.

4. Cleland JG, Swedberg K, Follath F, et al. The Euro-Heart Failure survey programme – a survey on the quality of care among patients with heart failure in Europe. Part 1: patient characteristics and diagnosis. Eur Heart J 2003;24(5):442-63.

5. Hogg K, Swedberg K, McMurray J. Heart failure with preserved left ventricular systolic function; epidemiology, clinical characteristics, and prognosis. J Am Coll Cardiol 2004;43(3):317-27.

6. Zile MR, Baicu CF, Bonnema DD. Diastolic heart failure: definitions and terminology. Prog Cardiovasc Dis 2005;47(5):307-13.

7. Hunt SA, Abraham WT, Chin MH, et al. ACC/AHA 2005 guideline update for the diagnosis and management of chronic heart failure in the adult: a report of the American College of Cardiology/American Heart Association Task Force on Practice Guidelines (Writing Committee to Update the 2001 Guidelines for the Evaluation and Management of Heart Failure): developed in collaboration with the American College of Chest Physicians and the International Society for Heart and Lung Transplantation: endorsed by the Heart Rhythm Society. Circulation 2005;112(12):e154-235.

8. Kass DA. Is heart failure with decent systole due to bad diastole? J Card Fail 2005;11(3):188-90.

9. Maurer MS, King DL, El-Khoury Rumbarger L, et al. Left heart failure with a normal ejection fraction: identification of different pathophysiologic mechanisms. J Card Fail 2005;11(3):177-87.

10. Hunt SA, Abraham WT, Chin MH, et al. 2009 Focused update incorporated into the ACC/AHA 2005 guidelines for the diagnosis and management of heart failure in adults a report of the American College of Cardiology Foundation/American Heart Association Task Force on Practice Guidelines Developed in Collaboration with the International Society for Heart and Lung Transplantation. J Am Coll Cardiol 2009;53(15):e1-90.

11. Heart Failure Society of America, Lindenfeld J, Albert NM, et al. HFSA 2010 comprehensive heart failure practice guideline. J Card Fail 2010;16(6):e1-194.

12. Miller AB, Pina IL. Understanding heart failure with preserved ejection fraction: clinical importance and future outlook. Congest Heart Fail 2009;15(4):186-92.

13. Owan TE, Hodge DO, Herges RM, et al. Trends in prevalence and outcome of heart failure with preserved ejection fraction. N Engl J Med 2006; 355(3):251-9.

14. Lee DS, Gona P, Vasan RS, et al. Relation of disease pathogenesis and risk factors to heart failure with preserved or reduced ejection fraction: insights from the Framingham Heart Study of the National Heart, Lung, and Blood Institute. Circulation 2009;119(24):3070-7.

15. Nohria A, Tsang SW, Fang JC, et al. Clinical assessment identifies hemodynamic profiles that predict outcomes in patients admitted with heart failure. J Am Coll Cardiol 2003;41(10):1797-804.

16. Kawaguchi M, Hay I, Fetics B, et al. Combined ventricular systolic and arterial stiffening in patients with heart failure and preserved ejection fraction: implications for systolic and diastolic reserve limitations. Circulation 2003;107(5):714-20.

17. Kass DA, Bronzwaer JG, Paulus WJ. What mechanisms underlie diastolic dysfunction in heart failure? Circ Res 2004;94(12):1533-42.

18. Redfield MM, Jacobsen SJ, Borlaug BA, et al. Age- and gender-related ventricular-vascular stiffening:

a community-based study. Circulation 2005; 112(15):2254–62.

19. Borlaug BA, Kass DA. Ventricular-vascular interaction in heart failure. Cardiol Clin 2011;29(3): 447–59.

20. Prasad A, Hastings JL, Shibata S, et al. Characterization of static and dynamic left ventricular diastolic function in patients with heart failure with a preserved ejection fraction. Circ Heart Fail 2010; 3(5):617–26.

21. Kurt M, Wang J, Torre-Amione G, et al. Left atrial function in diastolic heart failure. Circ Cardiovasc Imaging 2009;2(1):10–5.

22. LeWinter MM, Granzier H. Cardiac titin: a multifunctional giant. Circulation 2010;121(19):2137–45.

23. Zile MR, Desantis SM, Baicu CF, et al. Plasma biomarkers that reflect determinants of matrix composition identify the presence of left ventricular hypertrophy and diastolic heart failure. Circ Heart Fail 2011;4(3):246–56.

24. Westermann D, Lindner D, Kasner M, et al. Cardiac inflammation contributes to changes in the extracellular matrix in patients with heart failure and normal ejection fraction. Circ Heart Fail 2011;4(1): 44–52.

25. Borlaug BA, Melenovsky V, Russell SD, et al. Impaired chronotropic and vasodilator reserves limit exercise capacity in patients with heart failure and a preserved ejection fraction. Circulation 2006; 114(20):2138–47.

26. Phan TT, Shivu GN, Abozguia K, et al. Impaired heart rate recovery and chronotropic incompetence in patients with heart failure with preserved ejection fraction. Circ Heart Fail 2010; 3(1):29–34.

27. Abudiab MM, Redfield MM, Melenovsky V, et al. Cardiac output response to exercise in relation to metabolic demand in heart failure with preserved ejection fraction. Eur J Heart Fail 2013; 15(7):776–85.

28. Yamamoto K, Masuyama T, Sakata Y, et al. Roles of renin-angiotensin and endothelin systems in development of diastolic heart failure in hypertensive hearts. Cardiovasc Res 2000;47(2):274–83.

29. Gonzalez A, Lopez B, Querejeta R, et al. Regulation of myocardial fibrillar collagen by angiotensin II. A role in hypertensive heart disease? J Mol Cell Cardiol 2002;34(12):1585–93.

30. van Heerebeek L, Hamdani N, Falcao-Pires I, et al. Low myocardial protein kinase G activity in heart failure with preserved ejection fraction. Circulation 2012;126(7):830–9.

31. Paulus WJ, Tschope C. A novel paradigm for heart failure with preserved ejection fraction: comorbidities drive myocardial dysfunction and remodeling through coronary microvascular endothelial inflammation. J Am Coll Cardiol 2013;62(4):263–71.

32. Yamamoto K, Burnett JC Jr, Jougasaki M, et al. Superiority of brain natriuretic peptide as a hormonal marker of ventricular systolic and diastolic dysfunction and ventricular hypertrophy. Hypertension 1996;28(6):988–94.

33. Borlaug BA, Kass DA. Invasive hemodynamic assessment in heart failure. Cardiol Clin 2011;29(2): 269–80.

34. Smith GL, Masoudi FA, Vaccarino V, et al. Outcomes in heart failure patients with preserved ejection fraction: mortality, readmission, and functional decline. J Am Coll Cardiol 2003;41(9):1510–8.

35. Vasan RS, Benjamin EJ, Levy D. Prevalence, clinical features and prognosis of diastolic heart failure: an epidemiologic perspective. J Am Coll Cardiol 1995;26(7):1565–74.

36. Cohn JN, Johnson G. Heart failure with normal ejection fraction. The V-HeFT Study. Veterans Administration Cooperative Study Group. Circulation 1990;81(Suppl 2):III48–53.

37. The effect of digoxin on mortality and morbidity in patients with heart failure. The Digitalis Investigation Group. N Engl J Med 1997;336(8):525–33.

38. Vasan RS, Larson MG, Benjamin EJ, et al. Congestive heart failure in subjects with normal versus reduced left ventricular ejection fraction: prevalence and mortality in a population-based cohort. J Am Coll Cardiol 1999;33(7):1948–55.

39. Yip GW, Wang M, Wang T, et al. The Hong Kong diastolic heart failure study: a randomised controlled trial of diuretics, irbesartan and ramipril on quality of life, exercise capacity, left ventricular global and regional function in heart failure with a normal ejection fraction. Heart 2008;94(5):573–80.

40. Cleland JG, Tendera M, Adamus J, et al. The perindopril in elderly people with chronic heart failure (PEP-CHF) study. Eur Heart J 2006; 27(19):2338–45.

41. Komajda M, Carson PE, Hetzel S, et al. Factors associated with outcome in heart failure with preserved ejection fraction: findings from the Irbesartan in Heart Failure with Preserved Ejection Fraction Study (I-PRESERVE). Circ Heart Fail 2011;4(1):27–35.

42. Yusuf S, Pfeffer MA, Swedberg K, et al. Effects of candesartan in patients with chronic heart failure and preserved left-ventricular ejection fraction: the CHARM-Preserved Trial. Lancet 2003;362(9386): 777–81.

43. Bergstrom A, Andersson B, Edner M, et al. Effect of carvedilol on diastolic function in patients with diastolic heart failure and preserved systolic function. Results of the Swedish Doppler-echocardiographic study (SWEDIC). Eur J Heart Fail 2004;6(4):453–61.

44. Klingbeil AU, Schneider M, Martus P, et al. A meta-analysis of the effects of treatment on left

ventricular mass in essential hypertension. Am J Med 2003;115(1):41–6.

45. van Veldhuisen DJ, Cohen-Solal A, Bohm M, et al. Beta-blockade with nebivolol in elderly heart failure patients with impaired and preserved left ventricular ejection fraction: data from SENIORS (Study of Effects of Nebivolol Intervention on Outcomes and Rehospitalization in Seniors with heart failure). J Am Coll Cardiol 2009;53(23): 2150–8.

46. Hernandez AF, Hammill BG, O'Connor CM, et al. Clinical effectiveness of beta-blockers in heart failure: findings from the OPTIMIZE-HF (Organized Program to Initiate Lifesaving Treatment in Hospitalized Patients with Heart Failure) Registry. J Am Coll Cardiol 2009;53(2):184–92.

47. Setaro JF, Zaret BL, Schulman DS, et al. Usefulness of verapamil for congestive heart failure associated with abnormal left ventricular diastolic filling and normal left ventricular systolic performance. Am J Cardiol 1990;66(12):981–6.

48. Hung MJ, Cherng WJ, Kuo LT, et al. Effect of verapamil in elderly patients with left ventricular diastolic dysfunction as a cause of congestive heart failure. Int J Clin Pract 2002;56(1):57–62.

49. Deswal A, Richardson P, Bozkurt B, et al. Results of the randomized aldosterone antagonism in heart failure with preserved ejection fraction trial (RAAM-PEF). J Card Fail 2011;17(8):634–42.

50. Edelmann F, Wachter R, Schmidt AG, et al. Effect of spironolactone on diastolic function and exercise capacity in patients with heart failure with preserved ejection fraction: the Aldo-DHF randomized controlled trial. JAMA 2013;309(8):781–91.

51. Patel K, Fonarow GC, Kitzman DW, et al. Aldosterone antagonists and outcomes in real-world older patients with heart failure and preserved ejection fraction. JACC Heart Fail 2013;1(1):40–7.

52. Shah SJ, Heitner JF, Sweitzer NK, et al. Baseline characteristics of patients in the treatment of preserved cardiac function heart failure with an aldosterone antagonist trial. Circ Heart Fail 2013;6(2): 184–92.

53. Ahmed A, Rich MW, Fleg JL, et al. Effects of digoxin on morbidity and mortality in diastolic heart failure: the ancillary Digitalis Investigation Group trial. Circulation 2006;114(5):397–403.

54. Guazzi M, Vicenzi M, Arena R, et al. Pulmonary hypertension in heart failure with preserved ejection fraction: a target of phosphodiesterase-5 inhibition in a 1-year study. Circulation 2011;124(2): 164–74.

55. Redfield MM, Chen HH, Borlaug BA, et al. Effect of phosphodiesterase-5 inhibition on exercise capacity and clinical status in heart failure with preserved ejection fraction: a randomized clinical trial. JAMA 2013;309(12):1268–77.

56. Gissi-HF Investigators, Tavazzi L, Maggioni AP, et al. Effect of n-3 polyunsaturated fatty acids in patients with chronic heart failure (the GISSI-HF trial): a randomised, double-blind, placebo-controlled trial. Lancet 2008;372(9645):1223–30.

57. Freedman RA, Hopper DL, Mah J, et al. Assessment of pacemaker chronotropic response: implementation of the Wilkoff mathematical model. Pacing Clin Electrophysiol 2001;24(12):1748–54.

58. Kass DA, Kitzman DW, Alvarez GE. The restoration of chronotropic competence in heart failure patients with normal ejection fraction (RESET) study: rationale and design. J Card Fail 2010;16(1):17–24.

59. O'Connor CM, Whellan DJ, Lee KL, et al. Efficacy and safety of exercise training in patients with chronic heart failure: HF-ACTION randomized controlled trial. JAMA 2009;301(14):1439–50.

60. Kitzman DW, Brubaker PH, Morgan TM, et al. Exercise training in older patients with heart failure and preserved ejection fraction: a randomized, controlled, single-blind trial. Circ Heart Fail 2010; 3(6):659–67.

61. Haykowsky MJ, Brubaker PH, Stewart KP, et al. Effect of endurance training on the determinants of peak exercise oxygen consumption in elderly patients with stable compensated heart failure and preserved ejection fraction. J Am Coll Cardiol 2012;60(2):120–8.

62. Edelmann F, Gelbrich G, Dungen HD, et al. Exercise training improves exercise capacity and diastolic function in patients with heart failure with preserved ejection fraction: results of the Ex-DHF (Exercise training in Diastolic Heart Failure) pilot study. J Am Coll Cardiol 2011;58(17):1780–91.

63. Zieman S, Kass D. Advanced glycation end product cross-linking: pathophysiologic role and therapeutic target in cardiovascular disease. Congest Heart Fail 2004;10(3):144–9 [quiz: 150–1].

64. Little WC, Zile MR, Kitzman DW, et al. The effect of alagebrium chloride (ALT-711), a novel glucose cross-link breaker, in the treatment of elderly patients with diastolic heart failure. J Card Fail 2005; 11(3):191–5.

65. Solomon SD, Zile M, Pieske B, et al. The angiotensin receptor neprilysin inhibitor LCZ696 in heart failure with preserved ejection fraction: a phase 2 double-blind randomised controlled trial. Lancet 2012;380(9851):1387–95.

66. McMurray JJ, Packer M, Desai AS, et al. Dual angiotensin receptor and neprilysin inhibition as an alternative to angiotensin-converting enzyme inhibition in patients with chronic systolic heart failure: rationale for and design of the Prospective comparison of ARNI with ACEI to Determine Impact on Global Mortality and morbidity in Heart Failure trial (PARADIGM-HF). Eur J Heart Fail 2013;15(9):1062–73.

67. Omori Y, Ohtani T, Sakata Y, et al. L-Carnitine prevents the development of ventricular fibrosis and heart failure with preserved ejection fraction in hypertensive heart disease. J Hypertens 2012;30(9):1834–44.

68. Reil JC, Hohl M, Reil GH, et al. Heart rate reduction by If-inhibition improves vascular stiffness and left ventricular systolic and diastolic function in a mouse model of heart failure with preserved ejection fraction. Eur Heart J 2013;34(36):2839–49.

69. Zouein FA, de Castro Bras LE, da Costa DV, et al. Heart failure with preserved ejection fraction: emerging drug strategies. J Cardiovasc Pharmacol 2013;62(1):13–21.

70. Dahlof B, Devereux RB, Kjeldsen SE, et al. Cardiovascular morbidity and mortality in the Losartan Intervention for Endpoint reduction in hypertension study (LIFE): a randomised trial against atenolol. Lancet 2002;359(9311):995–1003.

71. ALLHAT Officers and Coordinators for the ALLHAT Collaborative Research Group. The antihypertensive and lipid-lowering treatment to prevent heart attack trial. Major outcomes in high-risk hypertensive patients randomized to angiotensin-converting enzyme inhibitor or calcium channel blocker vs diuretic: the Antihypertensive and Lipid-Lowering Treatment to Prevent Heart Attack Trial (ALLHAT). JAMA 2002;288(23):2981–97.

72. Little WC, Zile MR, Klein A, et al. Effect of losartan and hydrochlorothiazide on exercise tolerance in exertional hypertension and left ventricular diastolic dysfunction. Am J Cardiol 2006; 98(3):383–5.

Adjunctive Therapy and Management of the Transition of Care in Patients with Heart Failure

Scott Feitell, DO, Shelley R. Hankins, MD,
Howard J. Eisen, MD, FACC, FAHA, FACP*

KEYWORDS

- Transition of care • Management • Adjunctive therapy • Heart failure

KEY POINTS

- Managing patients with heart failure in the outpatient setting is difficult, time consuming, and costly.
- A careful and well-orchestrated team of cardiologists, general practitioners, nurses, and ancillary support staff can make an important difference to patient care, improve quality of life, and improve mortality.
- A strong body of literature supports the appropriate use of pharmacologic therapy, and the careful implementation of evidence-based therapies can improve mortality and quality of life, and reduce hospital admissions.
- Adjunctive therapies such as exercise, diet, and quitting smoking can be important.
- Recognizing patients with refractory heart failure early on, investing extra time and resources in education and compliance, and taking a team approach can all help patients in the long term.
- Further research into pharmacologic therapies, new mechanical assist devices, and standardizations of care based on evidence-based approaches will continue to help these complicated patients and the clinicians responsible for their care.

INTRODUCTION: NATURE OF THE PROBLEM

More than 5.7 million people in the United States carry a diagnosis of heart failure, the incidence of which approaches 1 in 100 people more than 65 years of age.[1] The cost to society is estimated at $29 billion annually and more than 1.1 million hospital admissions.[1] Once hospitalized with heart failure, the 30-day readmission rate approaches 25%.[2] The cost to both the patient and society for these admissions is enormous and, as the population ages, these numbers are expected to grow.

To emphasize the importance of this cost, the US Centers for Medicare and Medicaid Services (CMS) began publishing outcome data for all patients with heart failure in 2007, with an emphasis on 30-day readmission and mortality for individual hospitals. To further reduce costs, effective October 1, 2012, 30-day readmission rates for heart failure play an active role in determining hospital reimbursements for care by CMS.[3]

These factors place further emphasis on the need for an integrated and seamless transition from inpatient care to the outpatient setting. This article reviews the current data and outlines various strategies entailed in discharging a patient with heart failure from the hospital. It also reviews current guidelines and recommendations regarding

The authors have no disclosures.
Division of Cardiology, Drexel University College of Medicine, 245 North 15th Street, Philadelphia, PA 19102, USA
* Corresponding author.
E-mail address: heisen@drexelmed.edu

Cardiol Clin 32 (2014) 163–174
http://dx.doi.org/10.1016/j.ccl.2013.09.007

patient monitoring in the outpatient setting and discusses how to prevent future readmissions.

MANAGEMENT GOALS

As noted earlier, the task at hand is daunting. Thus it is important to focus on several key factors that will facilitate a smooth transition from inpatient to outpatient care while preventing readmission and not exposing the patient to an increased risk of mortality (**Box 1**). It is important to emphasize that disposition planning should begin almost immediately from the time of admission, which allows the maximal amount of time to educate the patient, arrange for follow-up care, and ensure that both the resources and support will be available to keep the patient out of the hospital.

The first step in transitioning care to the outpatient setting is identifying patients with de novo heart failure, as distinct from those who already carry the diagnosis. De novo patients require significantly more education on their disease state, and most importantly an introduction to the multidisciplinary heart failure team approach to heart failure. A great deal of time must be spent on dietary education, the importance of fluid balance and the meaning of congestion, and its effects on the body. The importance of pharmacologic therapy must be stressed, and access to what will likely be many new medications must be facilitated. Limitations in access, including a lack of insurance, a lack of social support, and a lack of understanding of the disease state, should immediately raise a red flag, and serve as a warning sign for future readmission.

Managing heart failure as an outpatient requires a multidisciplinary team approach and should take advantage of all resources available for the patient.

Several trials have evaluated approaches such as immediate follow-up at time of discharge, frequent nursing assessments, nurse-driven education on a rotating basis, and home-based approaches to care.[4] Although most of these approaches are both labor and cost intensive, to varying degrees most of these studies have shown either a reduction in cost or a reduction in readmission rates over a short span of time. It remains hard to make broad generalizations and definitive recommendations based on current literature. Readying a patient for discharge home after a heart failure admission should be individualized, and must make use of easy-to-use and inexpensive metrics that can guide therapy and progress.

We emphasize a symptoms-driven approach that allows patients to approximate their functional status and alert our clinicians to any red flags that warrant immediate evaluation. Although patients do not necessarily need to correlate their own symptoms with a New York Heart Association (NYHA) functional class, having patients assess their ability to walk up and down a flight of stairs or a trip to the mailbox each day can serve as a good measure of their functional class. Assessing a 6-minute walk test and a careful assessment by a physical and occupational therapy team at time of discharge can help patients identify their performance status. Thus, on arriving home, any decrease in exercise tolerance should warrant an immediate call to the clinician and heart failure team so that medications may be adjusted or a more urgent outpatient appointment be made to assess a potentially deteriorating patient. Being mindful of other symptoms, including the need for additional pillows to sleep at night (orthopnea), waking up short of breath (paroxysmal nocturnal dyspnea), and the development of dizziness or lightheadedness, can be helpful as well. Assessing ankle/leg edema can be another useful tool for patients to assess volume status. Noting the height up the leg and the severity of pitting can be useful and easy enough for patients to understand.

In the outpatient setting, the use of a home scale for weight checks is essential. Checking a daily weight and recording it in a journal can allow patients to have an easy-to-use monitoring system of their heart failure. A steady increase in weight over a short period of time can immediately alert both the patient and clinician that the current regimen is failing, or that perhaps compliance with salt and fluid intake are not ideal. It is important to establish a dry weight for the patient either at time of discharge from the hospital or when medically optimized in the clinic. It is essential for patients to check their weight at home to allow for any discrepancies in calibration between a

---

Box 1
Factors that facilitate the transition from inpatient to outpatient care

- Identify patients with de novo heart failure
  - Educate patients on the disease state
  - Introduce patients to the multidisciplinary heart failure team
- Teach patients to approximate their functional status and alert clinician to any red flags that warrant immediate evaluation
- Use a home scale for weight checks
- Address comorbid conditions
- Frequent and thorough reconciliation of medications at each office visit

hospital or clinic scale and the home scale. Weight gains of as little as 0.9 kg (2 pounds) more than a 1-week period have predicted hospitalization.[5] We routinely send all patients with heart failure home from the hospital with a scale that is provided free of charge to the patient. Thus a weight can be documented at time of discharge, and monitored easily and with little effort by the patient. Instructions are provided to immediately call the heart failure clinic once a weight gain is noted. A heart failure nurse coordinator can then instruct the patient to increase diuretic dosing for a period of time, reinforce dietary restrictions, and then follow up in a short period of time (often over the phone), to ensure that an effective volume status has been obtained.

In addition to treating heart failure and its symptoms, it is important to address the multitude of comorbid conditions in this patient population. Uncontrolled hypertension, diabetes, obstructive sleep apnea, obesity, and the associated metabolic syndrome can all play a role in deteriorating health, and can complicate care of heart failure. Renal disease is another severe comorbidity common in this population and can further complicate medical management and fluid balance. Close teamwork with the primary care physician, and, if needed, an endocrinologist or nephrologist, is essential in successfully managing these patients.

Medical reconciliation is also a key part of successful heart failure management. Frequent and thorough reconciliation of medications at each office visit can ensure proper dosing, frequency, and adherence. We encourage patients to bring any and all pill bottles to every clinic appointment to ensure that every list is updated and accurate. It is crucial that any over-the-counter medications, particularly nonsteroidal antiinflammatory drugs, herbal supplements, and vitamins, be accounted for.

The Hospital to Home (H2H) initiative, established by the American College of Cardiology (ACC) and the Institute for Healthcare Improvement, provides specific tools and strategies for clinicians to facilitate the transition from hospital to home to reduce readmissions. These tools can be accessed through the H2H Web site (http://www.h2hquality.org).

PHARMACOLOGIC STRATEGIES

Pharmacologic therapy remains the mainstay of therapy for heart failure. Pharmacologic therapy plays a key role not only in improving symptoms but also in improving mortality and decreasing hospitalizations. Numerous studies have evaluated several classes of drugs, showing various degrees of success in the treatment of heart failure. A stepwise approach to therapy is important, because rapid additions and titrations of medications may not be well tolerated in patients with heart failure. The current recommended therapies for heart failure management (**Box 2**), and how to approach each therapy in the outpatient setting, are reviewed later. Most therapies approved for heart failure are in the setting of a reduced ejection fraction. Although it has become clear that heart failure with preserved ejection fraction makes up a sizable percentage of patients with heart failure, few data support specific therapy tailored to this disease.

Diuretics

Diuretics remain the mainstay of therapy in most patients with heart failure. Volume overload remains the driving force in symptoms and hospitalization of patients with heart failure. Thus it is essential to manage volume status aggressively. Loop diuretics remain a mainstay of therapy for heart failure, providing both symptomatic relief and clinical improvement of vascular congestion. Few data suggest an advantage of one loop diuretic rather than another, and so furosemide, bumetanide, or torsemide may be used interchangeably at equivalent doses. Furosemide remains the most commonly used loop diuretic; however, if an appropriate response to therapy is not achieved with appropriate dose titration, it is reasonable to switch to either bumetanide or torsemide. Dosing of diuretics as an outpatient can represent a major challenge to the clinician caring for the patient with heart failure. Although hospitalized, complete control of intake, accurate measurements of output, and, if needed, nearly hourly assessment of the patient can achieve an ideal regimen. With outpatients, the clinician

---

Box 2
Current recommended therapies for heart failure management

- Diuretics
- Angiotensin-converting enzyme inhibitors/angiotensin receptor blockers
- β-Blockers
- Aldosterone antagonists
- Digoxin
- Hydralazine and nitrates
- Antiarrhythmics
- Inotropic support

must contend with dietary indiscretions, a lack of measurement of outputs, and less than weekly clinical assessments. We advocate a patient-centered approach, with an attempt to correlate weight gain and symptoms with titration of diuretic dosing. Loop diuretics function on a dose-responsive curve, so it is better to increase individual doses of a loop diuretic than to increase the frequency of dosing. Failure of escalating diuretic therapy should be an automatic red flag of worsening heart failure, or more commonly noncompliance with diet or medical therapy, and should be addressed with additional education and assessment. When titrating diuretic therapy, it is advisable to monitor serum chemistry values of potassium, blood urea nitrogen, and creatinine. A routine basic metabolic profile should be obtained within a week after increasing diuretic dosing. Hypokalemia should be treated aggressively with either supplements or a potassium-sparing diuretic to lower the risk of arrhythmias.

Angiotensin-converting Enzyme Inhibitors/ Angiotensin Receptor Blockers

Angiotensin-converting enzyme (ACE) inhibitors are essential for all patients with heart failure. A multitude of groundbreaking clinical trials have shown survival benefit in patients with heart failure with reduced ejection fraction.[6–8] Although most trials have evaluated individual drugs, there is enough evidence to suggest that the benefit of ACE/angiotensin receptor blocker (ARB) is a class effect. Although most early trials studied the use of enalapril and captopril, lisinopril and quinapril provide ease of use with once-daily dosing, which makes it easy to use in the outpatient setting. ACE therapy should always be initiated before hospital discharge. Starting a low-dose ACE before discharge ensures that the patient tolerates the dose, and allows screening for hypotension and azotemia in a monitored clinical setting. Titration of an ACE can occur at regular intervals as an outpatient at each outpatient visit until an optimal dose is achieved. Although most patients tolerate a reasonable dose of ACE, limitations such as hypotension may limit titration. Spacing medical therapy apart, or timing medications at different times of the day, can be a helpful way to maximize dose titration. ACE inhibitors have side effects, and require careful monitoring. The most frequent side effect is cough, occurring in some studies in up to 10% of patients.[9] Switching these patients to an ARB can often alleviate symptoms. Challenging patients with a different ACE is not advised, because the recurrence rate has been well documented in up to two-thirds of patients. Angioedema is a rarer and life-threatening event and warrants lifelong discontinuation of these drugs.

All patients on an ACE/ARB should have frequent monitoring of renal function and serum potassium levels. Initiation of an ACE may lead to a significant increase in serum creatinine (up to 30%).[10] This increase should not warrant a discontinuation of therapy, and should be monitored. We routinely screen our patients 1 week after initiation of therapy, again at 6 weeks, and then as clinically warranted.

β-Blockers

Another mainstay of heart failure management to reduce morbidity and mortality is the use of β-blockers.[11] Unlike ACE inhibitors, β-blockers do not show a class effect. The only β-blockers approved for heart failure therapy are carvedilol, metoprolol succinate (long-acting metoprolol), and bisoprolol. The initiation of β-blocker therapy can present many concerns to the clinician caring for a patient with heart failure. Concerns including hypotension, bradycardia, evidence of heart block, underlying lung disease, and evidence of volume overload can all make the use of β-blockers difficult and dangerous. Side effects notwithstanding, the initiation of this therapy is crucial to obtain survival benefit in heart failure. Therapy should ideally be administered when a patient has been maximally diuresed and has begun ACE therapy. Initial β-blocker therapy should be started at a low dose to ensure that the patient tolerates it. As care is transitioned to the outpatient setting, it is important to continue titrating the β-blocker as the patient tolerates it. Careful monitoring of heart rate, blood pressure, and orthostatic monitoring can ensure safe titration. We routinely increase doses of β-blockers incrementally at 2-week intervals in the outpatient setting until a reasonable dose is obtained. Patients are advised to take ACE inhibitors and β-blockers, especially carvedilol, at least 1 hour apart.

Although the 3 β-blockers mentioned earlier have shown survival benefit, we routinely choose carvedilol as the β-blocker of choice in patients with concomitant hypertension, because of its nonselective activity and vasodilatory effect. For patients intolerant of carvedilol because of hypotension, we try to transition to metoprolol succinate because the lack of vasodilatation may allow better tolerance of this agent.

Aldosterone Antagonists

The aldosterone antagonists, namely spironolactone and eplerenone, play a key role in heart failure therapy in specific subsets of patients.[12,13] Subsets of patients who have shown a survival benefit from these agents include patients with NYHA class 3 or 4 symptoms and an ejection fraction less than 35%, patients with NYHA class 2 symptoms and an ejection fraction less than 30%, patients after ST elevation myocardial infarction with an ejection fraction less than 40% and on ACE inhibitor therapy.[12–14] Although a clear survival benefit has been shown in each of these subsets of patients, risk factors for complications such as hyperkalemia must be assessed. We cautiously start these agents in patients with any degree of renal dysfunction, but we generally avoid use of these agents in patients with glomerular filtration rate less than 30 mL/min per 1.73 m^2.[12] We also do not initiate therapy if the serum potassium concentration is greater than 5.0 meq/L.[12] Initiation of therapy should occur before discharge from the hospital, with a serum potassium measured at 1 week and again at 1 month from discharge. Although spironolactone and eplerenone both confer survival benefit, the significant cost difference between the two agents favors initiating therapy with spironolactone. However, side effects such as gynecomastia and impotence in men and menstrual irregularities in women can make it difficult to tolerate. If these side effects develop, switching to eplerenone may be beneficial. There are no data to support the aggressive titration of aldosterone antagonists, and higher doses may lead to higher risk of hyperkalemia.

Digoxin

Although not indicated as a first-line agent, digoxin can still serve as a particularly useful agent in certain subsets of patients who are already on appropriate medical therapy for heart failure. It should be considered an adjunctive therapy in patients with reduced ventricular function who remain symptomatic despite appropriate volume removal and drug therapy with ACE and β-blocker.[15] Although there are limited data that digoxin maintained in a narrow therapeutic range of between 0.5 ng/mL and 1.0 ng/mL may confer some survival benefit, its use to reduce annual hospitalization rates has been well documented.[16,17] In patients with systolic heart failure and concomitant atrial fibrillation, digoxins added suppression of atrioventricular (AV) nodal conduction can provide added rate control, which is beneficial. Despite these benefits, digoxin has a narrow therapeutic window and should be used with extreme caution or avoided altogether in patients with underlying renal disease. Furthermore, patients with known sinus or AV nodal disease

should not be given digoxin. Patients with stable renal function on a low dose of digoxin do not require routine measurement of their serum digoxin levels.

Hydralazine and Nitrates

The combination of hydralazine and isosorbide dinitrate can be used in select subsets of patients, but should not be routinely used as a primary heart failure regimen. Several studies of this combination have found that select populations may benefit from its use. We routinely implement hydralazine and isosorbide dinitrate in African American patients with NYHA class 3 or 4 symptoms despite maximal medical therapy on an ACE and β-blocker.[18] This combination is also useful in patients who are intolerant of ACE/ARB because of the drug's side effect profile.[19] The addition of this regimen to non–African American patients with NYHA class 3 or 4 symptoms despite maximal medical therapy is also reasonable. The side effect profile of this combination is generally well tolerated and is generally limited to hypotension. The greatest limitation to this regimen involves its frequent dosing regimen, which requires dosing 3 times a day for maximum efficacy. Hydralazine and nitrate should only be initiated after maximal titration of first-line therapy has been achieved. Thus therapy is often initiated in the outpatient setting. Low doses of each agent should be started and monitored closely for hypotension. If tolerated, doses should be titrated at subsequent office visits as blood pressure tolerates.

Other Pharmacologic Agents

There are numerous other drugs that may play a role in heart failure management. The robust data behind aspirin use in atherosclerotic disease support routine use in any patient with ischemic cardiomyopathy.[20] There is little support for aspirin use in patients with nonischemic heart failure unless another indication exists.[21] Data supporting statin use in patients with heart failure are less clear. Several trials have shown no benefit in patients with heart failure with reduced ejection fractions, regardless of cause.[22,23] Unless there are strong indications to start a statin, current data suggest withholding statin therapy in heart failure populations with reduced ejection fractions.

Antiarrhythmics are another class of drugs that can play a crucial role in patients with heart failure. Many of these patients show the deleterious effects of both atrial and ventricular arrhythmias that may require suppression. The use of antiarrhythmics is reviewed elsewhere in this issue.

Inotropic support with agents such as home dobutamine or milrinone infusion can be an option in NYHA class 4 patients who have failed all other therapies and show an improvement in hemodynamic measurements during hospitalization, or for patients waiting for cardiac transplants. Although these agents may improve quality of life and time spent out of the hospital, they have never been documented to improve mortality and, in most studies, have led to an increase in mortality.[24–27] Transitioning patients to home inotropic support as palliation is an important undertaking, because it signifies that all other pharmacologic therapies have failed. These agents can be proarrhythmogenic, and require permanent intravenous access, and the ability to properly care for and maintain such access at home. We favor milrinone rather than dobutamine for home infusion in patients who can tolerate the potential hypotensive side effects of its vasodilatory action. Using milrinone allows the effective and continued use of a β-blocker when tolerated, thus potentially lowering its arrhythmogenic properties and allowing the continuation of appropriate heart failure therapy.

NONPHARMACOLOGIC STRATEGIES

Nonpharmacologic strategies for the management of heart failure in the outpatient setting should complement pharmacologic therapy (**Box 3**). A multifaceted approach focusing on diet and exercise can improve symptoms. Management of comorbid conditions such as renal disease, diabetes, and hypertension is essential. Evaluating patients for a defibrillator or cardiac resynchronization therapy is crucial to successfully treating the patient with heart failure in the clinic setting.

Diet in Heart Failure

Although little evidence exists that a cardiac-prudent diet with 2 g sodium restriction improves

---

Box 3
Nonpharmacologic strategies for managing heart failure in the outpatient setting

- Diet
- Cardiac rehabilitation and exercise
- Evaluation for implantable cardioverter-defibrillator
- Cardiac resynchronization therapy
- Smoking, alcohol, and substance abuse cessation
- Self-management strategies

---

survival, it remains part of the American Heart Association guidelines for the management of heart failure.[19] A routine part of transitioning care from the hospital to the outpatient setting should include a consultative visit with a nutritionist or dietician. Involving family members in these meetings can help reinforce healthy eating habits and ensure compliance. The ability to read food labels and calculate daily sodium intake can be reviewed during these meetings. Further complicating dietary compliance for heart failure involves other comorbid conditions such as diabetes, renal disease, coronary artery disease, or hypertension that have other dietary restrictions. Poor understanding of these disease states, and understanding the correlation between compliance and symptoms, can create severe limitations in care.[28] Frequent education and an outpatient dietician can help implement and maintain an appropriate diet.

Cardiac Rehabilitation and Exercise

Although it remains unclear whether an aggressive exercise or rehabilitation program can improve survival in patients with heart failure, multiple studies have examined quality of life, symptomatic relief, hospitalization rates, and improved oxygen capacity (Vo_2) and 6-minute walk tests.[29–32] The American Heart Association recommends cardiac rehabilitation and routine exercising for all NYHA class 2 and 3 patients.[33] No recommendations are made for class 4 patients. Careful considerations to evaluate before recommending a patient to rehabilitation include a history of arrhythmias and other comorbidities that may limit exercise. Only severe arrhythmias that may portend instability and are resistant to therapy should limit routine exercise.[31] Patients with de novo ischemic cardiomyopathy (ie, those immediately after myocardial infarction with a depressed ejection fraction) have been shown to have a survival benefit from cardiac rehabilitation, and thus should routinely be referred for it immediately at time of discharge.[34]

Evaluation for Implantable Cardioverter-Defibrillator

All patients with a reduced ejection fraction, less than 35%, and at least NYHA class 2 heart failure symptoms, should be evaluated for a defibrillator, unless expected life expectancy is less than 1 year caused by other comorbidities such as cancer. This evaluation is particularly important in the transition to outpatient care, because any patient with de novo heart failure does not meet initial criteria for an implantable cardioverter-defibrillator (ICD). Current guidelines recommend that an ICD not be implanted after myocardial infarction in patients with reduced ejection fraction until at least 40 days from the event and on maximal medical therapy.[19] In patients with nonischemic de novo heart failure, current guidelines recommend a period of at least 3 months on maximal medical therapy before implanting a defibrillator. This waiting period allows for possible recovery of function. Thus all patients discharged with de novo heart failure, particularly those with reduced ejection fraction, should be monitored closely and assessed regularly for symptoms of worsening heart failure because the risk of sudden cardiac death remains high in these populations.

Because many patients discharged from the hospital do not meet initial criteria for an ICD, evaluation for a wearable cardiac defibrillator should be performed before discharge from the hospital.[35] A wearable cardiac defibrillator provides the protection necessary from a ventricular tachycardia or fibrillation arrest, but still provides a window of time in which to assess for myocardial recoverability. Assessing patients for a wearable defibrillator requires compliance (because the defibrillator only works if the patient is wearing it) and a basic ability to push buttons as instructed to avoid inappropriate shocks. The greatest limitation of the wearable defibrillator is that it does not provide any pacing function; thus patients who meet indications for a pacemaker still require implantation of a device. A seamless transition of care between the inpatient and outpatient setting is crucial, because sudden cardiac death is a real and preventable form of death in this cohort of patients. We routinely seek a consult with an electrophysiologist for all patients being discharged with a wearable cardiac defibrillator. This consult ensures close monitoring of any potential life-threatening arrhythmias and ensures timely placement of an implantable device when the patient is ready for it. Regular assessment of ejection fraction after discharge from the hospital via two-dimensional echocardiography allows an assessment of recovery. In patients who have started with markedly reduced ejection fractions and who show moderate improvement over a short period of time (eg, 40 days from infarct), we may continue the wearable cardiac defibrillator for an additional period of time, especially in patients without evidence of an arrhythmic event; however, few data support this approach. We routinely use additional imaging modalities in patients who have ill-defined echocardiographic windows, or those patients whose echocardiograms are interpreted precisely at the 35% mark (or those whose echocardiograms are read in a range encompassing the 35% mark). Often an echocardiogram is repeated with an intravenous contrast agent if poor windows have limited interpretation. For those with borderline ejection fractions, we routinely refer the patient for a multigated acquisition scan for definitive assessment of ejection fraction.

Cardiac Resynchronization Therapy

For some patients, despite maximal medical therapy, close adherence to diet and exercise, and full compliance, a continued deterioration in NYHA functional class occurs. In patients who continue to be symptomatic despite maximal medical therapy, have an ejection fraction less than 35%, and have evidence of a bundle branch block on electrocardiogram (ECG) with a QRS complex wider than 120 milliseconds, evaluation for biventricular pacing should be done.[36] By placing leads in the right ventricle and the coronary sinus (the left ventricle lead), improved synchronization of ventricular contraction can occur. Several trials have evaluated biventricular function and shown a significant survival benefit in patients with NYHA class 2, 3, or 4 heart failure who have an ejection fraction less than 35% and a wide QRS complex (>120 milliseconds).[36–38] There has been no survival benefit seen in patients with NYHA class 1 symptoms. Subgroup analysis of some trial data suggests that patients with even wider QRS complexes (>150 milliseconds) may benefit more from cardiac resynchronization therapy than those with narrower bundle branch blocks.[39] We routinely refer all our patients with heart failure with NYHA class 2 or greater symptoms and evidence of a bundle branch block on ECG to electrophysiologists for evaluation for resynchronization therapy.

Smoking, Alcohol, and Substance Abuse Cessation

The immediate cessation of all harmful substances should be addressed in any patient diagnosed with heart failure. Smoking, alcohol, and many illicit substances such as cocaine and stimulants are directly cardiotoxic.[19] Reviewing the harmful effects of these agents with patients with heart failure should occur at every possible opportunity. We routinely offer smoking cessation aids to patients interested in smoking. There is evidence to suggest that simple counseling at each physician encounter can have a positive effect on quitting smoking.[40] Patients with substance abuse and/or alcohol abuse problems should be provided with resources that can provide psychological and social support and assistance in quitting.

Self-management Strategies

The ability to transition the patient with heart failure from inpatient care to outpatient management and, more importantly, to keep from readmission requires patients to take ownership of the disease and empower themselves to make careful decisions regarding their health. Maximizing educational opportunities, reinforcing key points, and involving family in care while the patient remains hospitalized can all be valuable tools to empower individual patients to take charge of their disease.

As noted previously, numerous studies have evaluated successful programs to prevent heart failure readmission rates.[4] Although most of these studies involve small patient populations at a single medical center, often with carefully screened patient populations, some important concepts can be extrapolated from these studies.

Eliminating the physician-driven top-down approach to care is essential. A fully integrated heart failure team is needed, comprising physicians, nurse practitioner/physician assistants, nurse educators, social workers, and dieticians, all of whom must play an active role in preparing the patient for discharge. The message delivered to the patient must be simple to understand, and should be reinforced at all times. We routinely focus on medication compliance, diet compliance, and symptom awareness. To be successful, it is important to first appreciate the patient's ability to grasp the information that is being provided. A brief assessment of reading comprehension skills, educational background, and language barriers is essential. Despite all this, assessing a patient's ability to manage the disease remains difficult. To create a patient-managed care approach, we routinely start with a broad overview of heart failure, including a rudimentary explanation of what heart failure is, and how it affects the patient's body. Most of this education is provided by nurse coordinators who specialize in heart failure. All patients in our hospital are given a standardized heart failure booklet that outlines everything that is reviewed with the nurse.

Having patients take ownership of their medication regimens remains the cornerstone of heart failure therapy, and self-management of medications at home remains a challenge. Compliance rates vary widely in even the best clinical trials, implying that, in real world clinical settings with unscreened patients, compliance rates are likely even lower.[41,42] To maximize patient compliance, we routinely use some simple techniques to maximize compliance. We simplify medicine regimens to include essential medications only. We eliminate as many as-needed medications as possible, and try to eliminate any vitamins and supplements with little proven benefit. We involve case managers and social workers in our medical reconciliation process to ensure that all medications prescribed are either covered by the patient's insurance or are available as easily affordable generic medications. We simplify all medication regimens to daily or twice-daily dosing whenever possible, and try to create an easy-to-use schedule that allows patients to take the same medication at the same time every day.

The most important aspect of self-management of heart failure often involves the dosing of a diuretic. Although most patients remain on a single stable dose of diuretic, the ability to adjust diuretic doses in the setting of weight gain or symptoms can be important in keeping patients out of the hospital. Allowing the patient to manage the diuretic dosing independently can also eliminate a sizable burden to the clinicians and office staff, because patients who can titrate their diuretic doses successfully do not have to call the clinic and speak to a clinician. We ask patients to weigh themselves daily, and monitor for symptoms. A gain of 1.4 kg (3 pounds) or a change in NYHA functional class triggers the patient to reflexively take an additional dose of diuretic until a return to baseline is noted. If the change in diuretic dosing does not make a difference in weight or symptoms within 3 to 5 days, we encourage a call to the clinic for further instructions. Thus the patient can be appropriately triaged over the phone, and a clinic appointment can be made sooner, and thus a possible hospital admission is avoided.

EVALUATION, ADJUSTMENT, RECURRENCE

Transitioning patients with heart failure from the hospital back to their homes remains the most difficult task for clinicians caring for these patients. The hospital represents a closely monitored, carefully regulated environment, accounting for every gram of sodium consumed, every liter of fluid removed, and every pill administered. As soon as the patient steps through the hospital's doors, clinicians must rely solely on that patient's discipline and prudence. There remains a lack of definitive research and guidelines to help improve the transition of health care from the inpatient to outpatient environment. However, some observational studies and small trials, as well as some commonsense approaches, can help guide clinicians and patients through this difficult time.

When to evaluate patients as they leave the hospital remains an unanswered question. Perhaps the best data come from a large observational study of 30-day readmission rates in patients with heart failure more than 65 years of age. Hospitals that had the highest 30-day readmission rates had the lowest rates of follow-up from initial discharge within 7 days.[43] Thus, although the additional resources and burdens this can place on a health care system can be challenging, and there remains a lack of randomized controlled trials proving that a 7-day follow-up can improve morbidity or mortality, it provides one of the few suggestions on when first to evaluate the patient from time of discharge.

However, it must be left for the individual clinician to assess each patient's needs and determine what resources may be worthwhile to each individual patient in each setting. Patients who continue to present with recurrent symptoms and/or compliance issues require more careful evaluation and a more aggressive, and perhaps more frequent, evaluation approach to prevent recurrent decompensation.

Once the initial evaluation has been made in the outpatient setting, the question then becomes how often should a patient be seen, and how often should contact be made between the patient and a care provider. Again, the data are lacking. A multitude of small, single-center trials have implemented various models including frequent phone calls, various degrees of clinic assessments, home nursing visits, and even telemedicine approaches.[44,45] Although many of these studies have proven small benefits in readmission rates and even mortality outcomes, the limitations of broad acceptance and applicability are numerous because of cost and access to such services. Several studies have noted improved outcomes in patients with heart failure cared for by both an internist/general practitioner and a cardiologist.[46,47] Thus, it is reasonable to suggest that all patients with heart failure discharged from the hospital have appropriate cardiology follow-up.

Adjustments

There is a well-established correlation between hospitalization and 1-year mortality.[48] Any patient admitted with heart failure, particularly one who has remained a stable outpatient for some time, should automatically be placed in a high-risk cohort of patients who are monitored closely and carefully. Adhering to guideline-based therapy and adjusting medications and treatment strategies is crucial to help lower mortality. Medications should be adjusted frequently and aggressively in all patients with heart failure to maximize the proven benefits of pharmacologic therapy in heart

failure. Frequent monitoring of side effects and clinical responses can allow doses of medications to be titrated often to ensure that maximal doses of medications such as ACE inhibitors and β-blockers are achieved. Current guidelines recommend titrating doses approximately every 2 weeks, thus allowing a pharmacologic steady-state to be achieved, and screening for the development of any potential side effects or intolerability (such as orthostatic hypotension or symptomatic bradycardia). Patients who are intolerable to dose titrations or the addition of other mortality-lowering drugs should alert the clinician that perhaps the patient's heart failure is more advanced or progressing more rapidly than anticipated and that consideration of more advanced therapies should be made. The need for further escalation of diuretic dosing should also serve as a warning sign of impending decompensation. Patients who have been maintained on a steady regimen for some time and suddenly become intolerant to a drug or a certain dose of drug should further warn the clinician that something is amiss. Careful screening for compliance with medications, diet, and activity should be performed immediately and care/therapy should be escalated quickly to prevent further decompensation.

Recurrence

As discussed earlier, despite the best efforts of clinicians and their patients to manage heart failure, effective treatment strategies can still remain ineffective or fail over time. Even in the most carefully screened heart failure populations receiving the best standards of care, more than 1 in 5 patients who are initially admitted for heart failure return to the hospital within 30 days.[2] Patients who present with recurrent heart failure decompensation require a thorough evaluation to pinpoint a cause. Although compliance, or lack thereof, may provide the answer for most patients, a careful evaluation of comorbid conditions and other factors is essential. Any reversible cause should be identified. Certain subsets of patients also may benefit from further testing and work-up. Patients with ischemic cardiomyopathies who present with recurrent symptoms should have a careful evaluation of their ischemic burden of disease. Any pertinent cardiac catheterization or stress tests should be reviewed carefully to ensure that further revascularization is not necessary. Patients with valvular disease should have a careful evaluation of echocardiograms, and if necessary further imaging involving a transesophageal echocardiogram to better evaluate valvular disorders, particularly if symptoms are disproportionate to what is seen on a transthoracic echocardiogram. Further evaluation of comorbid conditions that may be contributing to recurrent symptoms is also important, in particular worsening renal function, which may impair responsiveness to diuretics and cause significant metabolic derangements.

However, because of the natural progression of heart failure over time, recurrence of symptoms and decompensation may happen despite optimal medical therapy and close follow-up. In this subset of patients with refractory heart failure, more aggressive therapies may be warranted. As discussed earlier, cardiac resynchronization therapy should be considered in any patient who meets the aforementioned criteria for biventricular pacing. In addition, these patients should be evaluated for inotropic support with agents such as dobutamine or milrinone. As already mentioned, inotropes may improve symptoms and allow a patient to leave the hospital, but they do not improve mortality. Thus, to improve survival, further evaluation for mechanical circulatory support, such as a left ventricular assist device or heart transplantation, may also be warranted. Patients with refractory heart failure should be referred to a cardiologist with advanced heart failure training to evaluate these options.

PALLIATIVE CARE IN HEART FAILURE

Sadly, despite our best medical therapies and treatment options, heart failure remains a progressive disease with progressively worsening symptoms for some patients. While it is difficult to determine which patients will fail therapy and decline over time, several predictive models and trials have looked at factors to identify such patients.[49,50] Perhaps the best validated model is the Seattle Heart Failure Model which takes into account multiple clinical parameters and can be easily calculated via a free website.[50,51] For patients with a poor prognosis an open and honest discussion with the patient and his family is crucial. Discussions should include what to expect as symptoms worsen and what can be done about them. It is also important to discuss the possible termination of defibrillation therapy from an implantable defibrillator.[52] We will routinely consult a palliative care team to aid with symptom management and aid in these difficult discussions with the patient and family. A coordinated effort that manages symptoms of pain, dyspnea and anorexia is crucial. Maintaining heart failure therapies such as ACE Inhibitors, Beta blockers, loop diuretics and even intravenous inotropes can all help with symptoms.[53] Opioids can be crucial to minimizing symptoms of shortness of breath.[54] Ultimately, as in so many other facets of heart

failure management, a multidisciplinary team including the patient's cardiologist, internist, a palliative care team, as well as psychosocial supports such as family, clergy and social workers can all help make the transition to palliation and even hospice care seamless and provide the patient with optimal care.

SUMMARY

Heart failure remains, and likely will remain, a costly and difficult disease to treat for the foreseeable future. The ability to manage these patients in the outpatient setting is difficult, time consuming, and costly. However, new quality metrics such as 30-day readmission tracking with penalties for high readmission rates make it an imperative to keep these patients out of the hospital. Although successful therapies do exist, implementing and maintaining patients on successful treatment plans is difficult. A multitude of factors make transitioning care to the outpatient setting difficult. Patient compliance, the cost of resources needed to help patients, and the time needed to educate and follow these patients are all factors that limit success.

A careful and well-orchestrated team of cardiologists, general practitioners, nurses, and ancillary support staff can make an important difference to patient care, improve quality of life, and improve mortality. Although a lack of clear evidence-based approaches may not provide guidance, a commonsense approach and taking advantage of all the resources available to the patient can help. The tools and information available at the ACC-sponsored H2H Web site may provide considerable guidance.

Despite these limitations, a strong body of literature supports the appropriate use of pharmacologic therapy, and the careful implementation of evidence-based therapies can improve mortality and quality of life, and reduce hospital admissions. Adjunctive therapies such as exercise, diet, and quitting smoking can be equally important. Recognizing patients with refractory heart failure early on, investing extra time and resources into education and compliance, and taking a team approach can all help patients in the long term. Further research into pharmacologic therapies, new mechanical assist devices, and standardizations of care based on evidence-based approaches will continue to help these complicated patients and the clinicians responsible for their care.

REFERENCES

1. Russo CA, Andrews RM. The national hospital bill: the most expensive conditions, by payer, 2004.

HCUP statistical brief no. 13. Rockville (MD): Agency for Healthcare Research and Quality; 2006.

2. Elixhauser A, Steiner C. Readmissions to U.S. hospitals by diagnosis, 2010. HCUP statistical brief #153. Rockville (MD): Agency for Healthcare Research and Quality; 2013.

3. Available at: http://www.cms.gov/Medicare/Quality-Initiatives-Patient-Assessment-Instruments/Hospital QualityInits/OutcomeMeasures.html. Accessed July 30, 2013.

4. McAlister FA, Stewart S, Ferrua S, et al. Multidisciplinary strategies for the management of heart failure patients at high risk for admission: a systematic review of randomized trials. J Am Coll Cardiol 2004;44:810.

5. Chaudhry SI, Wang Y, Concato J, et al. Patterns of weight change preceding hospitalization for heart failure. Circulation 2007;116:1549.

6. Effects of enalapril on mortality in severe congestive heart failure. Results of the Cooperative North Scandinavian Enalapril Survival Study. N Engl J Med 1987;316:1429.

7. Effect of enalapril on survival in patients with reduced left ventricular ejection fractions and congestive heart failure. N Engl J Med 1991;325:293.

8. Pfeffer MA, Braunwald E, Moyé LA, et al. Effect of captopril on mortality and morbidity in patients with left ventricular dysfunction after myocardial infarction. Results of the survival and ventricular enlargement trial. N Engl J Med 1992;327:669.

9. Matchar DB, McCrory DC, Orlando LA, et al. Systematic review: comparative effectiveness of angiotensin-converting enzyme inhibitors and angiotensin II receptor blockers for treating essential hypertension. Ann Intern Med 2008;148:16.

10. Bakris GL, Weir MR. Angiotensin-converting enzyme inhibitor-associated elevations in serum creatinine: is this a cause for concern? Arch Intern Med 2000;160:685.

11. Foody JM, Farrell MH, Krumholz HM. Beta-blocker therapy in heart failure: scientific review. JAMA 2002;287:883.

12. Pitt B, Zannad F, Remme WJ, et al. The effect of spironolactone on morbidity and mortality in patients with severe heart failure. Randomized Aldactone Evaluation Study Investigators. N Engl J Med 1999;341:709.

13. Zannad F, McMurray JJ, Krum H, et al. Eplerenone in patients with systolic heart failure and mild symptoms. N Engl J Med 2011;364:11.

14. Pitt B, White H, Nicolau J, et al. Eplerenone reduces mortality 30 days after randomization following acute myocardial infarction in patients with left ventricular systolic dysfunction and heart failure. J Am Coll Cardiol 2005;46:425.

15. Gheorghiade M, van Veldhuisen DJ, Colucci WS. Contemporary use of digoxin in the management of cardiovascular disorders. Circulation 2006;113:2556.

16. Ahmed A, Rich MW, Love TE, et al. Digoxin and reduction in mortality and hospitalization in heart failure: a comprehensive post hoc analysis of the DIG trial. Eur Heart J 2006;27:178.

17. The effect of digoxin on mortality and morbidity in patients with heart failure. N Engl J Med 1997;336:525.

18. Taylor AL, Ziesche S, Yancy CW, et al. Early and sustained benefit on event-free survival and heart failure hospitalization from fixed-dose combination of isosorbide dinitrate/hydralazine: consistency across subgroups in the African-American Heart Failure Trial. Circulation 2007;115:1747.

19. Hunt SA, Abraham WT, Chin MH, et al. 2009 Focused update incorporated into the ACC/AHA 2005 Guidelines for the Diagnosis and Management of Heart Failure in Adults: a report of the American College of Cardiology Foundation/American Heart Association Task Force on Practice Guidelines: developed in collaboration with the International Society for Heart and Lung Transplantation. Circulation 2009;119:e391–479.

20. Antithrombotic Trialists' Collaboration. Collaborative meta-analysis of randomized trials of antiplatelet therapy for prevention of death, myocardial infarction, and stroke in high risk patients. BMJ 2002;324:71.

21. Seshasai SR, Wijesuriya S, Sivakumaran R, et al. Effect of aspirin on vascular and nonvascular outcomes: meta-analysis of randomized controlled trials. Arch Intern Med 2012;172:209.

22. Kjekshus J, Apetrei E, Barrios V, et al. Rosuvastatin in older patients with systolic heart failure. N Engl J Med 2007;357:2248.

23. Tavazzi L, Maggioni AP, Marchioli R, et al. Effect of rosuvastatin in patients with chronic heart failure: a randomized, double-blind, placebo-controlled trial. Lancet 2008;372:1231.

24. Cuffe MS, Califf RM, Adams KF Jr, et al. Short-term intravenous milrinone for acute exacerbation of chronic heart failure: a randomized controlled trial. JAMA 2002;287:1541.

25. Yamani MH, Haji SA, Starling RC, et al. Comparison of dobutamine-based and milrinone-based therapy for advanced decompensated congestive heart failure: hemodynamic efficacy, clinical outcome, and economic impact. Am Heart J 2001;142:998.

26. Sindone AP, Keogh AM, Macdonald PS, et al. Continuous home ambulatory intravenous inotropic drug therapy in severe heart failure: safety and cost efficacy. Am Heart J 1997;134:889.

27. Oliva F, Latini R, Politi A, et al. Intermittent 6-month low-dose dobutamine infusion in severe heart failure. Am Heart J 1999;138:247.

28. Peterson PN, Shetterly SM, Clarke CL, et al. Health literacy and outcomes among patients with heart failure. JAMA 2011;305:1695.

29. Belardinelli R, Georgiou D, Cianci G, et al. Effects of exercise training on left ventricular filling at rest and during exercise in patients with ischemic cardiomyopathy and severe left ventricular systolic dysfunction. Am Heart J 1996;132:61.

30. Belardinelli R, Georgiou D, Cianci G, et al. Randomized, controlled trial of long-term moderate exercise training in chronic heart failure: effects on functional capacity, quality of life, and clinical outcome. Circulation 1999;99:1173.

31. Hambrecht R, Fiehn E, Weigl C, et al. Regular physical exercise corrects endothelial dysfunction and improves exercise capacity in patients with chronic heart failure. Circulation 1998;98:2709.

32. Haykowsky MJ, Liang Y, Pechter D, et al. A meta-analysis of the effect of exercise training on left ventricular remodeling in heart failure patients: the benefit depends on the type of training performed. J Am Coll Cardiol 2007;49:2329.

33. Piña IL, Apstein CS, Balady GJ, et al. Exercise and heart failure: a statement from the American Heart Association Committee on Exercise, Rehabilitation, and Prevention. Circulation 2003;107:1210.

34. Taylor RS, Brown A, Ebrahim S, et al. Exercise-based rehabilitation for patients with coronary heart disease: systematic review and meta-analysis of randomized controlled trials. Am J Med 2004; 116:682.

35. Feldman AM, Klein H, Tchou P, et al. Use of a wearable defibrillator in terminating tachyarrhythmias in patients at high risk for sudden death. Pacing Clin Electrophysiol 2004;27:4.

36. Bristow MR, Saxon LA, Boehmer J, et al. Cardiac-resynchronization therapy with or without an implantable defibrillator in advanced chronic heart failure. N Engl J Med 2004;350:2140.

37. Cleland JG, Daubert JC, Erdmann E, et al. The effect of cardiac resynchronization on morbidity and mortality in heart failure. N Engl J Med 2005;352: 1539.

38. Abraham WT, Fisher WG, Smith AL, et al. Cardiac resynchronization in chronic heart failure. N Engl J Med 2002;346:1845.

39. Sipahi I, Carrigan TP, Rowland DY, et al. Impact of QRS duration on clinical event reduction with cardiac resynchronization therapy: meta-analysis of randomized controlled trials. Arch Intern Med 2011;171:1454.

40. Ockene JK. Physician-delivered interventions for smoking cessation: strategies for increasing effectiveness. Prev Med 1987;16:723.

41. Roe CM, Motheral BR, Teitelbaum F, et al. Compliance with and dosing of angiotensin-converting-enzyme inhibitors before and after hospitalization. Am J Health Syst Pharm 2000;57:139.

42. Lamb DA, Eurich DT, McAlister FA, et al. Changes in adherence to evidence-based medications in the first year after initial hospitalization for heart failure: observational cohort study from 1994 to 2003. Circ Cardiovasc Qual Outcomes 2009;2:228.

43. Hernandez AF, Greiner MA, Fonarow GC, et al. Relationship between early physician follow-up and 30-day readmission among Medicare beneficiaries hospitalized for heart failure. JAMA 2010; 303:1716.

44. Leff B, Burton L, Mader SL, et al. Hospital at home: feasibility and outcomes of a program to provide hospital-level care at home for acutely ill older patients. Ann Intern Med 2005;143:798.

45. Inglis SC, Clark RA, McAlister FA, et al. Structured telephone support or telemonitoring programmes for patients with chronic heart failure. Cochrane Database Syst Rev 2010;(8):CD007228.

46. Ansari M, Alexander M, Tutar A, et al. Cardiology participation improves outcomes in patients with new-onset heart failure in the outpatient setting. J Am Coll Cardiol 2003;41:62.

47. Go AS, Rao RK, Dauterman KW, et al. A systematic review of the effects of physician specialty on the treatment of coronary disease and heart failure in the United States. Am J Med 2000;108:216.

48. Curtis LH, Greiner MA, Hammill BG, et al. Early and long-term outcomes of heart failure in elderly persons, 2001-2005. Arch Intern Med 2008;168:2481.

49. Lee DS, Austin PC, Rouleau JL, et al. Predicting mortality among patients hospitalized for heart failure: derivation and validation of a clinical model. JAMA 2003;290(19):2581.

50. Levy WC, Mozaffarian D, Linker DT, et al. The Seattle Heart Failure Model: prediction of survival in heart failure. Circulation 2006;113(11):1424.

51. Available at: http://depts.washington.edu/shfm.

52. Lampert R, Hayes DL, Annas GJ, et al. HRS Expert Consensus Statement on the Management of Cardiovascular Implantable Electronic Devices in patients nearing end of life or requesting withdrawal of therapy. Heart Rhythm 2010;7(7):1008.

53. Hershberger RE, Nauman D, Walker TL, et al. Care processes and clinical outcomes of continuous outpatient support with inotropes in patients with refractory end-stage heart failure. J Card Fail 2003;9(3):180.

54. Johnson MJ, McDonagh TA, Harkness A, et al. Morphine for the relief of breathlessness in patients with chronic heart failure–a pilot study. Eur J Heart Fail 2002;4(6):753.

Index

Cardiol Clin 32 (2014) 175–180
http://dx.doi.org/10.1016/S0733-8651(13)00119-7
0733-8651/14/$ – see front matter © 2014 Elsevier Inc. All rights reserved.

Moving?

Make sure your subscription moves with you!

To notify us of your new address, find your **Clinics Account Number** (located on your mailing label above your name), and contact customer service at:

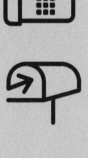

Email: journalscustomerservice-usa@elsevier.com

800-654-2452 (subscribers in the U.S. & Canada)
314-447-8871 (subscribers outside of the U.S. & Canada)

Fax number: 314-447-8029

Elsevier Health Sciences Division
Subscription Customer Service
3251 Riverport Lane
Maryland Heights, MO 63043

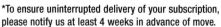